Pathophysiology of the Enteric Nervous System

A basis for understanding functional diseases

Pathophysiology of the Enteric Nervous System

A basis for understanding functional diseases

EDITED BY

Robin Spiller MD FRCP

Professor of Gastroenterology, Wolfson Digestive Diseases Centre, University Hospital Nottingham, UK

AND

David Grundy PhD

Professor of Biomedical Science, The University of Sheffield, UK

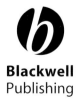

Blackwell
Publishing

© 2004 by Blackwell Publishing Ltd

Blackwell Publishing, Inc., 350 Main Street, Malden, Massachusetts 02148–5020, USA
Blackwell Publishing Ltd, 9600 Garsington Road, Oxford OX4 2DQ, UK
Blackwell Publishing Asia Pty Ltd, 550 Swanston Street, Carlton, Victoria 3053, Australia

First published 2004

ISBN 1-4051-2361-3

Library of Congress Cataloging-in-Publication Data

Pathophysiology of the enteric nervous system : a basis for understanding functional diseases / edited by Robin
Spiller and David Grundy.-- 1st ed.
      p.   ;   cm.
   Includes bibliographical references and index.
   ISBN 1-4051-2361-3
1. Gastrointestinal system--Diseases. 2. Gastrointestinal system--Innervation.
   [DNLM: 1. Enteric Nervous System--physiopathology. 2. Gastrointestinal Diseases--etiology. 3. Gastrointestinal
Diseases--physiopathology. WI 140 P2975 2004] I. Spiller, Robin C. II. Grundy, David.
   RC817.P385 2004
   616.3'3--dc22

                                                                                                              2004013802

A catalogue record for this title is available from the British Library

Set in Minion 9.5/12pt by Sparks – www.sparks.co.uk
Printed and bound in Slovenia by Mladinska Knjiga Tiskarna dd, Ljubljana
Commissioning Editor: Alison Brown
Development Editor: Claire Bonnett
Production Controller: Kate Charman

For further information on Blackwell Publishing, visit our website:
http://www.blackwellpublishing.com

Contents

Contributors

Fernando Azpiroz MD PhD
Chief of the Section of GI Research, Digestive System Research Unit, Hospital General Vall d'Hebron, Spain

Qasim Aziz PhD, MRCP
Senior Lecturer and Honorary Consultant Gastroenterologist, Section of Gastrointestinal Sciences, Hope Hospital, UK

Giovanni Barbara MD
Assistant Professor of Medicine, Department of Internal Medicine and Gastroenterology, University of Bologna, Italy

Adil E Bharucha MD
Associate Professor of Medicine, Mayo Clinic College of Medicine, Mayo Clinic, USA

Klaus Bielefeldt MD PhD
Associate Professor, Division of Gastroenterology, Department of Internal Medicine, University of Pittsburgh, Pittsburgh, USA

L Ashley Blackshaw PhD
Associate Professor, Nerve-Gut Research Laboratory, Hanson Institute, Australia

Simon Brooks PhD
Associate Professor, Senior Research Fellow, Department of Human Physiology and Centre for Neuroscience, Flinders University, Australia

Lionel Bueno MD
Head of the Department of Neurogastroenterology, Neurogastroenterology Unit INRA Toulouse, France

Lin Chang MD
Centre for Neurovisceral Sciences and Women's Health, Division of Digestive Diseases, David Geffen School of Medicine at UCLA, USA

Marcello Costa MD FAA MS&D
Professor of Neurophysiology, Department of Human Physiology and Centre for Neuroscience, Flinders University, Australia

Roberto De Giorgio MD PhD
Assistant Professor of Medicine, Department of Internal Medicine and Gastroenterology, University of Bologna, Italy

Fabrizio De Ponti MD PhD
Professor of Pharmacology, University of Bologna, Italy

Anton Emmanuel BSc MD MRCP
Senior Lecturer in Gastrointestinal Physiology and Honorary Consultant, St Marks Hospital, Harrow, UK

GF Gebhart PhD
Professor and Head, Department of Pharmacology, University of Iowa, USA

Shaheen Hamdy MRCP PhD
MRC Clinician Scientist/Honorary Consultant Gastroenterologist, Department of Gastrointestinal Sciences, Hope Hospital, UK

Ikuo Hirano MD
Assistant Professor of Medicine, Division of Gastroenterology, Feinberg School of Medicine, USA

Anthony R Hobson PhD
Research Fellow, Section of GI Sciences, Hope Hospital UK

Peter Holzer PhD
University Professor, Department of Experimental and Clinical Pharmacology, Medical University of Graz, Austria

Peter J Kahrilas MD
Gilbert H Marquardt Professor of Medicine, Chief, Division of Gastroenterology, Northwestern University, Feinberg School of Medicine, USA

John Kellow
Associate Professor of Medicine, University of Sydney, Director, Gastrointestinal Investigation Unit, Royal North Shore Hospital, Sydney, Australia

David R Linden PhD
Department of Anatomy and Neurobiology, University of Vermont, USA

Gary M Mawe PhD
Professor, Department of Anatomy and Neurobiology, University of Vermont, USA

Peter J Milla PhD
Professor of Paediatric Gastroenterology and Nutrition, Department of Surgery and Gastroenterology, Institute of Child Health, and Honorary Consultant Paediatric Gastroenterologist, Great Ormond Street Hospital, UK

Mulugeta Million DVM PhD
Associate Adjunct Professor, CURE: Digestive Diseases Research Center, USA

Charles Murray MA MB MRCP
Research Fellow, Physiology Unit, St Marks Hospital, Harrow, UK

Virpi V Smith MD
Department of Histopathology, Great Ormond Street Hospital, UK

Robin Spiller MD FRCP
Professor of Gastroenterology, Wolfson Digestive Diseases Centre, University Hospital Nottingham, UK

Yvette Taché PhD
Co-Director Center for Neurovisceral Sciences, CURE: Digestive Diseases Research Center, USA

Jan Tack MD PhD
Professor of Medicine, University of Leuven, Head of Clinic, Department of Gastroenterology, University Hospitals Leuven, Belgium

Heng Y Wong BM BCh MRCP (UK)
Centre for Neurovisceral Sciences and Women's Health, Division of Digestive Diseases, David Geffen School of Medicine at UCLA, USA

Preface

These are exciting times for neurogastroenterology. Over the last ten years, substantial advances have been made in describing the anatomy, physiology and pathophysiology of the enteric nervous system and its relation to the clinically important functional gastrointestinal diseases. We felt it was important to bring together these ideas, which are often published in very different journals, to help workers in the field see the whole picture. The book has been conceived in four parts.

The first four chapters deal with neuroanatomy, neurophysiology, how the gut signals to the brain and how these signals are centrally processed to generate symptoms. The next four chapters then cover the pathophysiology of the enteric nervous system, considering the general processes that may cause disease, including disordered development, inflammation and stress. There then follow sections on functional disorders of the esophagus, stomach, small and large bowel, and the anorectal region. Finally, we have four chapters on pharmacotherapy, with separate chapters for tachykinin and serotonin receptor modulators. The last chapter deals with emerging transmitters that may form the basis of future treatments.

As you can see from the author list, we have been lucky in attracting some of the most knowledgeable people in the field. Thanks to very rapid processing of the manuscripts, these authors are up to date with the latest developments in this fast-moving field. We hope that you will enjoy reading them and that you will find it useful both in your current and future clinical practice.

Robin Spiller
David Grundy

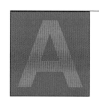

SECTION A
Basic Principles

CHAPTER 1

Functional Neuroanatomy

Simon Brookes and Marcello Costa

Introduction

In this chapter we review how enteric neuronal structure may be related to function, based on the large number of studies carried out by many groups over the last three decades. We believe that it is useful to consider a hierarchy of structural features of enteric neurons which vary in importance. Some are crucial to neuronal function (e.g. their targets and primary transmitters), while others are of less functional significance (such as dendritic morphology and the modulatory substances that nerve cells contain). Despite extensive studies in gut tissue from mice, rats, pigs and humans over the last decade, the benchmark for detailed understanding of the enteric nervous system is still the guinea-pig small intestine. Many of the findings originally made in guinea-pigs have later turned out to apply to other mammals, including humans, although there are some notable exceptions. In this review we will refer to the guinea-pig small intestine, but where appropriate will point out important species differences.

The enteric nervous system comprises the third major division of the autonomic nervous system[1] and consists of ganglionated plexuses which extend from the esophagus to the internal anal sphincter (Fig. 1.1). The myenteric plexus is located between the longitudinal and the circular smooth muscle layers. Closer to the mucosa lies the submucous plexus (or plexuses), located between the muscularis mucosa and the circular muscle layer. There are marked differences in the functional types of cells located in the different plexuses. The myenteric plexus is largely associated with the control of motility. In larger species (pig, dog, man), the submucous plexus is divided into two or three layers.[2] The outer submucous plexus layer contains nerve cells which are also associated with motor control, while the

inner submucous plexus (closer to the mucosa) mainly contains neurons that are associated with control of blood flow and secretion.

There are complete reflex circuits present within the enteric nervous system that allow adaptive behavior to occur when the gut is isolated from the central nervous system.[3] Ordinarily, however, the enteric nervous system is subject to powerful modulation by sympathetic and parasympathetic neurons. A third major source of extrinsic input to the enteric nervous system arises from extrinsic sensory neurons. A brief discussion of the functional anatomy of these pathways will be included in this review.

The myenteric plexus contains about two-thirds of all enteric neurons, including cell bodies of enteric

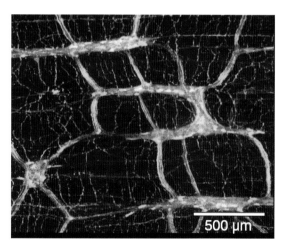

Fig. 1.1 Low-power micrograph of a wholemount of myenteric plexus of the guinea-pig ileum stained immunohistochemically. Cell bodies (red) are concentrated in ganglia: there is extensive labeling of axons (green) in internodal strands (joining ganglia) and in the fine tertiary plexus innervating the longitudinal muscle.

primary afferent neurons, interneurons, excitatory and inhibitory motor neurons, viscerofugal neurons (which project out of the gut) and some secretomotor and vasomotor neurons that project to epithelia and blood vessels in the mucosa. Different types of enteric neurons have been classified in several ways, including soma-dendritic morphology (numbers of axons, types of dendrites)[4] or on the basis of their electrophysiological features (action potential shape, afterhyperpolarizations, types of synaptic input, patterns of firing).[5] Enteric nerve cells have also been distinguished by the immunohistochemical markers, or rather the combinations of such markers ('chemical coding'; Fig. 1.2) that they contain.[6] Using lesions or neuroanatomical tracing techniques, the projections of enteric neurons have been used to distinguish the major functional classes. All of these different types of information have now been combined to provide one of the more comprehensive descriptions of any part of the mammalian nervous system.[7] To aid understanding of the functional anatomy of the enteric nervous sys-

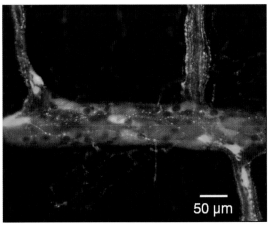

Fig. 1.2 Chemical coding of nerve cell bodies in the myenteric plexus. Primary afferent neurons were labeled immunohistochemically for the calcium-binding protein calbindin (red); longitudinal muscle motor neurons contain calretinin (green) and inhibitory motor neurons to the circular muscle are immunoreactive for nitric oxide synthase (blue). With this particular combination of antisera, no single neuron contained more than one marker.

Tools of the trade

Visualizing nerve cells in the brain, spinal cord or enteric nervous system under the microscope is relatively easy as many histochemical stains reveal a dense mass of cell bodies and processes in nervous tissue. However, visualizing nerve cells in a way that aids understanding how they are organized is considerably more challenging. It requires the ability to stain selectively just a few cells, which can then be characterized in detail without being obscured by the surrounding neurons, dendrites and axons. Several approaches have been used to achieve this, including the capricious ability of certain silver stains or histochemical stains to reveal a small proportion of nerve cell bodies and their soma-dendritic organization. This has allowed some types of cells to be distinguished morphologically,[4] although the targets of their axons have not usually been revealed. Multiple-labeling immunohistochemistry has been used to reveal combinations of peptides and proteins, which can be used to distinguish different classes of neurons (Fig. 1.2). This method can be used systematically to give a comprehensive account of the dif-

ferent classes. The likely projections of some classes can be deduced by observing the disappearance of axons with particular chemical coding, after lesions to the enteric plexuses.

A more direct and quantitative approach to the identification of classes of nerve cells, their projections, functions, chemical coding and morphology has been developed by the application of neuroanatomical tracing techniques. Briefly, a dye is applied selectively to a small region of gut tissue (usually *in vitro*), where it is taken up by axons innervating that particular target (Fig. 1.3). Sufficient time is allowed for the dye to be transported back to the cell bodies of origin (usually in organotypic culture), thus identifying the cell bodies that project to that one target tissue. After fixation, multiple-labeling immunohistochemistry can be carried out to determine the chemical coding of the retrogradely labeled cell bodies. This provides a systematic and quantitative means of analyzing nerve cell morphology, coding, projections and, by deduction, the function of all classes of enteric neurons.

tem, we will briefly summarize important features of the different classes of enteric neurons and then discuss their functional significance.

Circular muscle motor neurons

The motor neurons that innervate circular muscle are either excitatory cholinergic cells or inhibitory nitrergic cells. Motor neurons located 0.5 to 25 mm oral to the site where a retrograde label was applied are consistently immunoreactive for inhibitory neurotransmitters [nitric oxide synthase or peptides such as vasoactive intestinal polypeptide (VIP)], but not for the cholinergic enzyme choline acetyltransferase (ChAT).[8] Nerve cell bodies under the application site, or aboral to it, are consistently immunoreactive for ChAT and usually tachykinins, but not for VIP (Fig. 1.3). Since nitric oxide and VIP have inhibitory effects on the circular muscle, and acetylcholine and tachykinins both cause contraction, it can be deduced that motor neurons with descending projections are inhibitory while those that project locally or orally are excitatory. Excitatory motor neurons make up about 70–75% of the full comple-

ment of motor neurons and have shorter projections and smaller cell bodies than inhibitory motor neurons. In most regions of the gut, excitatory motor neurons outnumber inhibitory, except in sphincteric regions such as the lower esophageal sphincter.[9]

The projections of inhibitory and excitatory motor neurons are likely to contribute to the polarized responses of the 'law of the intestine' described by Bayliss and Starling in 1899.[3] If sensory neurons excite motor neurons in one region of gut, this will cause contraction of the circular muscle orally and relaxation aborally. When excitation and inhibition overlap, inhibition usually dominates, leading to local accommodation of the contents. In fact, in many regions of gut, there is considerable evidence for a net inhibitory tone that is driven by spontaneous activity of inhibitory motor neurons. This is well illustrated by the obstructive constriction that occurs in aganglionic regions of gut in Hirschsprung's disease, where all enteric neurons are absent (including both excitatory and inhibitory motor neurons).

Another consistent finding from retrograde labeling studies is that, no matter where the dye is applied, filled

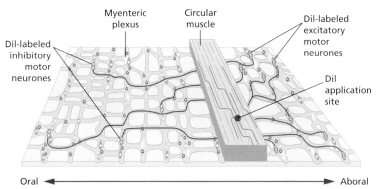

Fig. 1.3 Neuroanatomical tracing of enteric neurons. A water-insoluble dye, DiI, is applied on a bead to the surface of an intact strip of circular muscle in a dissected specimen of gut, which is then kept alive in organotypic culture. Over several days, the DiI is taken up by axons of motor neurons that contact the bead and is transported back to their cell bodies in the myenteric plexus (DiI-labeled cell bodies and axons are outlined in red). Every myenteric ganglion contains a random selection of different classes of enteric neurons (blue, yellow, green, purple, gray). However, DiI labeling of nerve cell bodies (red outlines) reveals a high degree of organization, based on the projections of the different classes. DiI-containing nerve cell bodies oral to the DiI application site consist exclusively of inhibitory motor neurons (with yellow cell bodies), whereas the labeled cells aborally are always excitatory motor neurons (green cell bodies). Other classes of cells (blue, gray and purple) do not project to the circular muscle and hence never contain DiI. Note that many inhibitory and excitatory motor neuron cell bodies in every ganglion are not labeled with DiI – these particular motor neurons project to regions of circular muscle that were not contacted by the DiI-coated bead. This approach allows different classifications of enteric neurons to be brought together, and has also been extended to targeted electrophysiological studies of live, retrogradely labeled cells.

What does chemical coding imply about neuronal function?

Chemical coding is a useful tool to identify enteric neurons. However, the significance of the molecules used to distinguish classes of cells is not always obvious, and the variability in chemical coding between apparently similar cells in different regions of gut and between species can appear confusing.

Synthetic enzymes for nitric oxide (nitric oxide synthase, NOS) and acetylcholine (ChAT) can be considered the defining markers for motor neurons in all regions of gut that have been tested to date. Essentially, every motor neuron contains one or other of these markers. This is not surprising, since nitric oxide and acetylcholine are the primary inhibitory and excitatory transmitters to gut smooth muscle. It appears that evolution has come up with few alternatives to these vital molecules and they are thus highly conserved in motor neurons between species and regions.

Gastrointestinal motor neurons often contain neuropeptides. Among these, VIP and tachykinins can be considered as secondary transmitters to gut smooth muscle.[10] Their role is typically less prominent than those of nitric oxide and acetylcholine and is usually revealed only after blockade of nitrergic and cholinergic transmission. VIP expression in inhibitory motor neurons is considerably more variable than NOS expression; many inhibitory motor neurons lack detectable VIP immunoreactivity, for example, in the human colon. There are a few alternative secondary transmitters. Thus, PACAP (pituitary adenylate cyclase-activating peptide), ATP and PHI (peptide histidine isoleucine) can substitute for (or complement) VIP in some cells, and both substance P and neurokinin A can act as excitatory secondary transmitters.[10]

Other neuropeptides present in gut motor neurons can be considered as tertiary transmitters or modulators, and usually have even fewer obvious functions. Typically, they modulate the release of primary and secondary transmitters. Thus, opioid peptides are present in many enteric neurons, but only when the gut is forced to work hard (for example, to empty against a resistance) are effects of endogenous opioids detectable. Immunoreactivity for enkephalin is highly variable among motor neurons, being present only in excitatory motor neurons in the human colon but in many inhibitory motor neurons in other species. Significantly, many other neurochemicals have similar modulatory effects, including dynorphin, GABA (γ-aminobutyric acid), neuropeptide Y, galanin, adenosine and ATP, and these often appear to substitute for enkephalin.

A fourth level of neurochemical used for chemical coding studies includes molecules such as calcium-binding proteins, receptors, ion channels and second messengers. Usually, many alternatives to these molecules exist and the exact ones present in particular neurons vary greatly between cell types, species and regions.

From this very brief consideration, it is clear that specific chemical coding can be a useful tool to identify unequivocally the functional class to which a particular neuron belongs. However, the functional significance of each marker may vary widely and great care has to be taken in extrapolating between species or regions of the gut, particularly as one moves down the hierarchy of markers from primary transmitters to modulators.

---

motor neuron cell bodies are spread across the width of the preparation. This shows that both excitatory and inhibitory motor neurons have long circumferential projections within the circular muscle. One obvious consequence of this arrangement is that stimulation at any localized point in the intestine will tend to lead to annular contractions of the circular muscle layer, rather than just contractions in line with the stimulus.

Longitudinal muscle motor neurons

Longitudinal muscle motor neurons are smaller, have less complex dendritic morphology and a single axon, and have very short projections (less than 3 mm in any direction). In the guinea-pig ileum the great majority (>97%) are cholinergic,[11] but this paucity of inhibitory motor neurons is not typical of the whole gut; in the guinea-pig colon there is significantly more inhibitory input, and inhibitory motor neurons with polarized projections are present in the guinea-pig proximal colon.[12] One of the most surprising findings about longitudinal muscle motor neurons in the ileum is that they constitute more than one-quarter of all myenteric neurons, despite the thinness of this muscle layer.[13] This might reflect the innervation of each region of longitudinal muscle by many converging inputs, making finely graded control possible. However, the most important point is that longitudinal muscle motor neurons form a population separate from the circular muscle motor neurons. Thus, the two layers can potentially be activated independently under neuronal control.

Enteric primary afferent neurons

Distension or mucosal chemicals evoke reflexes in segments of ileum that have previously been extrinsically denervated,[14] indicating that there must be enteric primary afferent (sensory) neurons in the gut wall. Direct identification of enteric primary afferents was made by making intracellular recordings from neurons close to nearby intact mucosa and showing that they responded to a variety of chemical stimuli applied to villi. These cells had large, smooth cell bodies and several axons with either no dendrites or short filamentous dendrites (Dogiel type II morphology). Some primary afferent neurons can also be activated by stretch stimuli applied to the gut, and this is probably mediated by specific mechanosensitive sites located in myenteric ganglia.[15] Similar enteric primary afferent neurons are also found in the submucous plexus. The proportions of these neurons activated by mucosal stimuli and by stretch stimuli add up to more than 100%, indicating that some Dogiel type II cells are likely to respond to both types of stimulus.

Enteric primary afferent neurons have extensive projections in the circumferential axis of the gut, and give rise to varicose endings in many myenteric ganglia. This projection pattern must help ensure the spread of responses to local stimuli around the circumference of the gut wall. All Dogiel type II neurons have projections to the mucosa and this may allow them to transduce signals at multiple points and then give outputs to other neurons over a wide area of the circumference. Their long circumferential projections probably contact most other

types of enteric neurons, making excitatory cholinergic or tachykinin-mediated synapses. Thus, they probably provide the major excitatory drive to all enteric neuronal circuits controlling gut functions.

Enteric interneurons

To date, four classes of interneurons have been distinguished in the small intestine.[13] Three classes have descending projections and are cholinergic, but also contain somatostatin, 5-hydroxytryptamine (5-HT, or serotonin) or NOS. The NOS-containing interneurons may also use other transmitters, particularly ATP, as a fast transmitter. All three classes of descending interneurons have very long descending projections (much longer than motor neurons) and innervate both myenteric and submucous ganglia. In addition, all three classes make dense baskets of varicosities around other interneurons of the same type, while also contacting other classes of enteric neurons. The functional consequences of this arrangement are worth considering. The NOS-containing descending interneurons probably spread the descending inhibitory reflex further down the gut than would be the case if only inhibitory motor neurons and enteric primary afferent neurons were involved. If somatostatin- and 5-HT-containing interneurons make strong excitatory synaptic connections with their own kind, it is possible that activation at one point in the gut would lead to firing of the whole chain of interneurons further down the gut. By releasing modulatory transmitters, such interneurons could then alter the state of enteric circuitry over long distances, perhaps switching from one pattern to another. It is not hard to imagine that such switching could occur ahead of a migrating myoelectric complex, or during the transition from fasting to fed motor behavior after a meal. Some of these classes of descending interneurons may also be involved in other pathways, such as the descending excitation that has been shown to occur under some circumstances.

In the guinea-pig small intestine, there is just one class of ascending interneuron. This is a small cholinergic neuron with a single orally directed axon that makes synaptic contact with a few other classes of myenteric neurons. In comparison with descending interneurons, these cells have much shorter projections (up to 14 mm long), but they also make functional chains, one ascending interneuron synapsing onto another further up the gut. Evidence suggests that at least three ascending interneurons in a chain can contribute to the spread of the ascending excitatory reflex up the gut, via fast cholinergic (nicotinic) synapses. Because of their relatively short length, ascending interneurons appear to be suited to a role in rapid reflex responses rather than to pattern switching behavior.

Viscerofugal neurons

This special type of interneuron, with cell bodies in enteric ganglia and axons that project out of the gut, have short lamellar or filamentous dendrites and a single axon. They do not make synaptic outputs within the gut, but are driven by prominent nicotinic fast excitatory synaptic inputs[16] from other enteric neurons. Thus, viscerofugal neurons act simply as interneurons, relaying integrated information from enteric circuitry to the sympathetic ganglia. In guinea-pigs and rats, viscerofugal neurons are restricted to the myenteric plexus, but in the pig they are also found in the outer submucous plexus layer, which shares much of the motor circuitry of the gut. Another class of viscerofugal neurons in rats, the rectospinal neurons, have cell bodies in the wall of the rectum and project directly into the sacral spinal cord. There may be similar viscerofugal neurons in the stomach and duodenum which project to the brainstem.[17] It is possible that these last two types of viscerofugal neurons contact central parasympathetic nuclei and thus play a part in vagal and sacral parasympathetic reflexes to the gut, while other viscerofugal neurons project to prevertebral ganglia and influence inhibitory sympathetic reflex pathways.

Secretomotor and vasomotor neurons

Two classes of secretomotor neurons have been identified, largely confined to the submucous plexus. One class is cholinergic and the other releases non-cholinergic peptidergic transmitters, particularly VIP. Non-cholinergic secretomotor neurons project both to the subepithelial plexus of the mucosa and to submucous arterioles, where they may mediate non-cholinergic vasodilation. Thus, these cells stimulate secretion and simultaneously increase mucosal blood flow. In

the guinea-pig small intestine, none of the secretomotor neurons show polarized projections along the gut, but elegant studies in the colon have shown that non-cholinergic secretomotor neurons project down the gut, whereas cholinergic secretomotor neurons project orally.[18] The functional significance of this arrangement is not yet clear. Another class of submucous neurons provides cholinergic vasodilator input to blood vessels in the submucosa that is potentially independent of increases in secretion.

Sympathetic innervation of the gut

Sympathetic and parasympathetic inputs to the gut contribute to the control of motility, secretion and blood flow. Sympathetic postganglionic neurons, located in the prevertebral ganglia, provide a substantial input to both myenteric and submucous ganglia, with some innervation of the muscle and mucosa and a dense plexus of fibers on submucous blood vessels. There is also an innervation of blood vessels by paravertebral sympathetic chain neurons (Fig. 1.4). In enteric ganglia, sympathetic axons typically form dense networks of varicosities coursing through all parts of the ganglion and closely approaching most, if not all, enteric nerve cell bodies (Fig. 1.5). Several different classes of sympathetic axons can be distinguished by their chemical coding and targets.[19] Those supplying blood vessels contain tyrosine hydroxylase (TH)/neuropeptide Y, those that innervate the submucous plexus contain TH/somatostatin, and those innervating myenteric ganglia contain TH alone. This anatomical arrangement potentially allows independent control of motility, secretion and blood flow according to the body's requirements. In enteric ganglia, sympathetic neurons directly inhibit non-cholinergic secretomotor neurons and possibly some descending interneurons. Generally, however, sympathetic neurons release norepinephrine throughout the enteric ganglia, causing presynaptic inhibition of synaptic activity and thus a reduction in nerve-mediated reflexes.[10]

Parasympathetic innervation of the gut

Parasympathetic input to the gut follows either the vagus nerve or the pelvic nerves (Fig. 1.4). Vagal parasympathetic axons form branching varicose endings

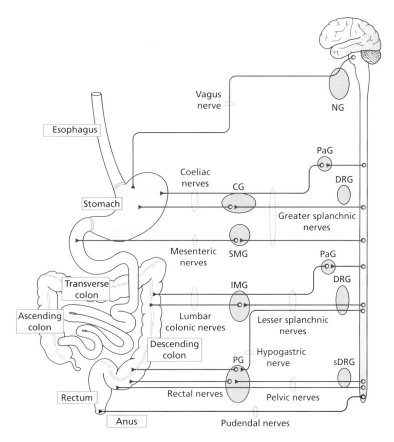

Fig. 1.4 Major extrinsic efferent pathways to the gut. Sympathetic pathways (red) have preganglionic cell bodies in the spinal cord which synapse onto postganglionic sympathetic neurons mostly located in the prevertebral ganglia (CG, SMG, IMG, PG), but with a few located in paravertebral chain ganglia (PaG). Parasympathetic pathways (purple) have cell bodies in the brainstem that project to the upper gut or cell bodies in the sacral spinal cord, which either project directly to the lower bowel or synapse onto another neuron in the pelvic ganglia (PG). CG, coeliac ganglion; DRG, dorsal root ganglia; IMG, inferior mesenteric ganglia; NG, nodose ganglion; PaG, paravertebral chain ganglia; PG, pelvic ganglia; sDRG, sacral dorsal root ganglia; SMG, superior mesenteric ganglion.

that course through myenteric and, to a lesser extent, submucous ganglia, with a physical appearance similar to sympathetic axons,[17] although transmission from vagal efferents is mediated by fast synaptic transmission. Vagal inputs are mostly concentrated in the upper gut (esophagus, stomach and duodenum). Unlike sympathetic axons, which directly innervate blood vessels and mucosal cells, all effects of vagal efferent activity are mediated via excitation of enteric neurons. Early studies suggested that relatively few enteric 'command neurons' received inputs from vagal efferents, but it is now clear that most gastric enteric neurons are contacted by parasympathetic axons.[17] To date, there are relatively few data regarding the chemical coding of different functional classes of vagal efferent, although it is known that different populations can activate excitatory or inhibitory motor pathways selectively.

The pelvic viscera receive parasympathetic input from cells in the sacral parasympathetic nucleus of the caudal spinal cord, which either project directly to enteric ganglia or synapse onto other autonomic nerve cells in the pelvic ganglia, which then project to the gut. It should be noted, however, that the pelvic ganglia also contain some sympathetic neurons, which receive preganglionic input from the thoraco-lumbar spinal cord. Again, sacral parasympathetic efferents form branching varicose axons that appear to contact many enteric neurons as they run through the ganglia. Like vagal efferents, they make fast synaptic contacts onto enteric neurons,[20] but they also use slow excitatory synaptic transmission, unlike their vagal counterparts.

Extrinsic afferent input to the enteric nervous system

Extrinsic afferent pathways (Fig. 1.6) are responsible for sensations arising from the gut and for activating many of the sympathetic and parasympathetic reflex

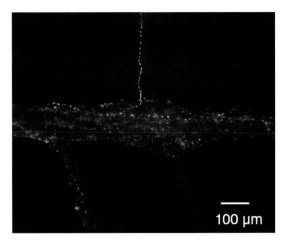

100 µm

Fig. 1.5 Varicose nerve fibers in a myenteric ganglion. Sympathetic nerve fibers, labeled for tyrosine hydroxylase immunoreactivity (blue), branch extensively throughout the ganglion and approach most, if not all, myenteric nerve cell bodies. In contrast, a subset of extrinsic sensory axons (labeled for CGRP, in green) are much sparser and probably contact just a few cells in the ganglion. In red are shown axons of one class of intrinsic (enteric) descending interneuron (labeled for 5-HT immunoreactivity). Note how all varicose axons have a similar appearance despite having very different targets and modes of action.

pathways. Vagal afferent neurons form three types of endings in the gut. Endings in the mucosa of the stomach and duodenum correspond to the electrophysiologically recorded afferent fibers that respond to chemical or mechanical stimuli applied to the mucosa. The second major functional type of vagal afferent unit[21] is sensitive to stretch, or more precisely, to intramural tension, and is responsible for sensations arising from esophageal, gastric or duodenal distension and for the vago-vagal reflexes that these stimuli evoke (such as gastric accommodation). The anatomical identity of these endings has been the subject of much speculation. Intramuscular arrays of densely branching axons, which run parallel to circular or longitudinal smooth muscle fibers, were one candidate. Another possibility was the intraganglionic laminar endings (IGLEs), which consist of flattened branching processes concentrated on the surfaces of myenteric ganglia. By recording and dye-filling vagal trunks close to the gut, vagal tension receptors were shown to be mechanically sensitive at a few tiny hotspots, which correspond exactly to IGLEs.[22,23] Thus, IGLEs are the

transduction sites of the tension-sensitive receptors. The function of intramuscular arrays is currently uncertain. They appear well situated to function as stretch (length)-sensitive endings,[24] but clear evidence that any vagal afferents actually detect length (rather than tension) is lacking.

Because IGLEs lie close to many myenteric nerve cell bodies, it has been speculated that they might also directly activate enteric circuits. They contain proteins associated with synaptic release and vesicular glutamate transporters, and have some ultrastructural specializations of transmitter release sites. However, to date there is no clear evidence that they excite enteric neurons; rather, they work primarily by activating vago-vagal reflex pathways via synaptic connections in the brainstem.

Spinal afferent neurons, which carry nociceptive information from the gut, have long been believed to make unspecialized endings in the gut wall.[21,25,26] Calcitonin gene-related peptide (CGRP) immunoreactivity in many of these neurons revealed unspecialized varicose axons in enteric ganglia, in the muscle layers and mucosa, and on submucosal and mesenteric blood vessels.[27] CGRP-immunoreactive endings in enteric ganglia release excitatory transmitters onto enteric neurons and their endings on blood vessels cause vasodilation, increasing blood flow during damage or inflammation of the gut wall. However, studies have repeatedly shown that many spinal afferents to the gut do not contain CGRP. Some may contain vesicular glutamate transporters, but we currently cannot visualize these non-peptidergic spinal afferents in a way that distinguishes them from enteric neurons. Thus, we know little about the neuroanatomy of a major group of spinal afferents.

A recent study has shown the presence of specialized mechanosensitive afferents in the guinea-pig rectum which are not present in the colon. These are similar in many ways to vagal tension receptors, having low thresholds, wide dynamic ranges and transduction sites comprising flattened branching endings in myenteric ganglia ('rectal IGLEs'). These afferents probably have nerve cell bodies in sacral dorsal root ganglia and are immunoreactive for vesicular glutamate transporters, but not for CGRP.[28,29] It seems likely that these and other sacral sensory neurons may form a specialized subgroup of spinal afferents, similar to vagal afferents, and are involved in rectal reflex control and sensation, rather than nociception, like the thoraco-lumbar spinal afferents.

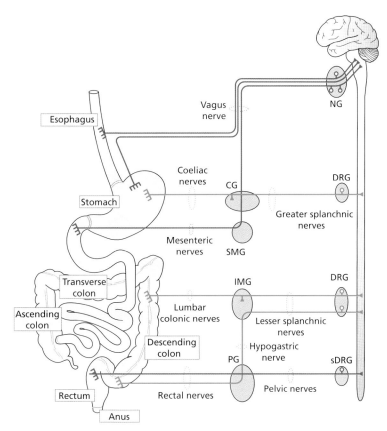

Fig. 1.6 Extrinsic afferent innervation of the gut. Spinal afferent pathways are shown in green and have cell bodies in thoraco-lumbar dorsal root ganglia and axons that project to the gut in parallel with sympathetic efferents. Note that these neurons make synaptic contacts in prevertebral ganglia, en route to the spinal cord. Vagal afferents (blue) have cell bodies in the nodose ganglion and travel with vagal parasympathetic efferent pathways, mostly to the esophagus, stomach and duodenum. Sacral spinal afferent pathways are also shown in blue as they appear to share many features with vagal afferents, traveling with parasympathetic axons and giving rise to graded sensations rather than just nociception. CG, coeliac ganglion, DRG, dorsal root ganglia; IMG, inferior mesenteric ganglia, NG, nodose ganglion; PG, pelvic ganglia; sDRG, sacral dorsal root ganglia; SMG, superior mesenteric ganglion.

Conclusions

This account has given a short summary of the major types of nerve cells in the ganglionated enteric plexuses, linking their anatomical features with their functions where possible. It is clear, even from such a brief account, that the enteric nervous system is highly organized. The different plexuses show some specialization in the functional types of nerve cells that they contain. Apart from this constraint, ganglia contain random assortments of many types of nerve cells. However, each nerve cell within a ganglion has predictable polarity and length of projection, characteristic soma-dendritic morphology, and electrophysiological and synaptic features. The chemical coding of enteric neurons is a powerful means to distinguish the different functional classes of neurons, but the functional implications of immunohistochemical markers are often far from clear. Markers for primary transmitters (choline acet-yltransferase and nitric oxide synthase) appear to be well conserved between equivalent cells in different regions and species, but secondary transmitters and modulators show much more variability. Enteric neuronal circuits appear relatively simple, but nevertheless have a highly organized structure that allows them to fulfill their vital roles in controlling the gut functions of motility, blood flow and secretion.

References

1 Langley JN. *The Autonomic Nervous System.* Cambridge: Heffer, 1921.
2 Hens J, Schrodl F, Brehmer A *et al.* Mucosal projections of enteric neurons in the porcine small intestine. *J Comp Neurol* 2004; **21**: 429–36.
3 Bayliss WM, Starling EH. The movements and innervation of the small intestine. *J Physiol* 1899; **24**: 99–143.
4 Dogiel AS. Über den Bau der Ganglien in den Geflechten

des Darmes und der Gallenblase des Menschen und der Säugethiere. *Arch Anat Physiol Leipzig, Anat Abt* 1899; 130–58.

5   Hirst GDS, Holman ME, Spence I. Two types of neurones in the myenteric plexus of duodenum in the guinea-pig. *J Physiol (Lond)* 1974; **236**: 303–26.

6   Costa M, Furness JB, Gibbins IL. Chemical coding of enteric neurons. *Progr Brain Res* 1986; **68**: 217–39.

7   Brookes SJH, Costa M. Cellular organisation of the mammalian enteric nervous system. In: Brookes SJH, Costa M, eds. *Innervation of the Gastrointestinal Tract*. London: Taylor and Francis, 2002: 393–467.

8   Brookes SJH, Steele PA, Costa M. Identification and immunohistochemistry of cholinergic and non-cholinergic circular muscle motor neurons in the guinea-pig small intestine. *Neuroscience* 1991; **42**: 863–78.

9   Brookes SJH, Chen BN, Hodgson WM, Costa M. Characterization of excitatory and inhibitory motor neurons to the guinea pig lower esophageal sphincter. *Gastroenterology* 1996; **111**: 108–17.

10 Tonini M, De Ponti F, Frigo G, Crema F. Pharmacology of the enteric nervous system. In: Brookes SJH, Costa M, eds. *Innervation of the Gastrointestinal Tract*. London: Taylor and Francis, 2002: 213–94.

11 Brookes SJH, Song ZM, Steele PA, Costa M. Identification of motor neurons to the longitudinal muscle of the guinea pig ileum. *Gastroenterology* 1992; **103**: 961–73.

12 Neunlist M, Michel K, Aube AC, Galmiche JP, Schemann M. Projections of excitatory and inhibitory motor neurones to the circular and longitudinal muscle of the guinea pig colon. *Cell Tissue Res* 2001; **305**: 325–30.

13 Costa M, Brookes SJH, Steele PA, Gibbins I, Burcher E, Kandiah CJ. Neurochemical classification of myenteric neurons in the guinea-pig ileum. *Neuroscience* 1996; **75**: 949–67.

14 Furness JB, Johnson PJ, Pompolo S, Bornstein JC. Evidence that enteric motility reflexes can be initiated through entirely intrinsic mechanisms in the guinea-pig small intestine. *Neurogastroenterol Motil* 1995; **7**: 89–96.

15 Kunze WA, Clerc N, Furness JB, Gola M. The soma and neurites of primary afferent neurons in the guinea-pig intestine respond differentially to deformation. *J Physiol* 2000; **526**: 375–85.

16 Sharkey KA, Lomax AE, Bertrand PP, Furness JB. Electrophysiology, shape, and chemistry of neurons that project from guinea pig colon to inferior mesenteric ganglia. *Gastroenterology* 1998; **115**: 909–18.

17 Holst MC, Kelly JB, Powley TL. Vagal preganglionic projections to the enteric nervous system characterized with Phaseolus vulgaris-leucoagglutinin. *J Comp Neurol* 1997; **381**: 81–100.

18 Neunlist M, Frieling T, Rupprecht C, Schemann M. (1998). Polarized enteric submucosal circuits involved in secretory responses of the guinea-pig proximal colon. *J Physiol* 1998; **506**: 539–50.

19 Furness JB, Costa M. *The Enteric Nervous System*. Edinburgh: Churchill-Livingstone, 1987.

20 Tamura K. Synaptic inputs to morphologically identified myenteric neurons in guinea pig rectum from pelvic nerves. *Am J Physiol* 1997; **273**: G49–55.

21 Grundy D, Scratcherd T. Sensory afferents from the gastrointestinal tract. In: Wood J, ed. *Handbook of Physiology. Section 6. The Gastrointestinal System, Vol. 1.* Bethesda (MD): American Physiological Society, 1989: 593–620.

22 Zagorodnyuk VP, Brookes SJH. Transduction sites of vagal mechanoreceptors in the guinea pig esophagus. *J Neurosci* 2000; **20**: 6249–55.

23 Zagorodnyuk VP, Chen BN, Brookes SJH. Intraganglionic laminar endings are mechano-transduction sites of vagal tension receptors in the guinea-pig stomach. *J Physiol* 2001; **534**: 255–68.

24 Phillips RJ, Powley TL. Tension and stretch receptors in gastrointestinal smooth muscle: re-evaluating vagal mechanoreceptor electrophysiology. *Brain Res Rev* 2000; **34**: 1–26.

25 Cervero F. Sensory innervation of the viscera: peripheral basis of visceral pain. *Physiol Rev* 1994; **74**: 95–138.

26 Sengupta JN, Gebhart GF. Gastrointestinal afferent fibers and sensation. In: Johnson LR, ed. *Physiology of the Gastrointestinal Tract*. New York: Raven Press, 1994: 483–519.

27 Gibbins IL, Furness JB, Costa M, MacIntyre I, Hillyard CJ, Girgis S. Co-localization of calcitonin gene-related peptide-like immunoreactivity with substance P in cutaneous, vascular and visceral sensory neurons of guinea pigs. *Neurosci Lett* 1985; **57**: 125–30.

28 Lynn PA, Olsson C, Zagorodnyuk V, Costa M, Brookes SJH. Rectal intraganglionic laminar endings are transduction sites of extrinsic mechanoreceptors in the guinea pig rectum. *Gastroenterology* 2003; **125**: 786–94.

29 Olsson C, Costa M, Brookes SJH. Neurochemical characterisation of extrinsic innervation of the guinea pig rectum. *J Comp Neurol* 2004; **470**: 357–71.

CHAPTER 2

Neurophysiology

David R Linden and Gary M Mawe

Introduction

The enteric nervous system (ENS) is capable of providing precise control of gastrointestinal functions because it is composed of several classes of neurons that contribute to distinct motor and secretory activities of the bowel. For example, in the guinea-pig ileum, where these populations of neurons are best characterized, there are at least 14 functionally defined classes of enteric neurons.[1] Comprehensive understanding of the pathophysiology of enteric neurons in the malfunctioning bowel requires a thorough examination of changes in enteric neurons at several levels, including changes in ion channel function, how these changes contribute to altered excitability of individual neurons, and how these alterations contribute to disordered reflex physiology. This comprehensive characterization requires the combined use of several techniques to assess changes adequately. This chapter will provide insight into the tools used by enteric neurobiologists to study the neurophysiology of the gastrointestinal tract, describe what is currently known about the electrical and synaptic properties of individual enteric neurons, the intrinsic reflex circuitry of the intestines, and a brief description of recently identified pathological changes in enteric neurophysiology. We will begin with a description of the current techniques used by enteric neurobiologists, which can be divided into two categories, electrophysiological and imaging.

Neurophysiological techniques

Electrophysiology

The electrical behaviors of enteric neurons are studied using three electrophysiological recording techniques: extracellular electrophysiology, intracellular electrophysiology and patch-clamp electrophysiology. Each of these approaches is associated with advantages and disadvantages with regard to determining details about the integrated network properties, and molecular mechanisms of electrical and synaptic behavior.

Extracellular electrophysiology

Extracellular recording of enteric neurons is accomplished by using fine metal electrodes or suction electrodes. This technique provides information in the form of patterns of spontaneous and stimulus-evoked action potential discharges. This is accomplished by placing the electrode in close contact with the nerve fiber such that rapid changes in extracellular ion concentrations can be detected and amplified as rapid changes in voltage. Metal electrodes can be adjusted in size to record from multiple neurons simultaneously, down to a single active unit. Suction electrodes are typically used to record from all axons within a nerve fiber bundle. A comprehensive review of the information gathered from extracellular recordings of enteric nerves has been published.[2]

Extracellular electrophysiology is also the technique of choice for studying the discharge patterns of extrinsic afferent and efferent pathways. These are the nerves supplying sensory information to the central nervous system and those providing parasympathetic preganglionic or sympathetic postganglionic input to the gastrointestinal tract, respectively. For these studies, mesenteric, dorsal root or vagal nerve fibers are laid over a bipolar wire electrode.[3] Voltage differences between the two wires are detected with a differential amplifier, and action potentials passing along these axons are registered as both a rise and a fall in voltage. This technique has been instrumental in defining classes of afferent neurons that innervate the gastrointestinal tract and how they respond to chemical or mechanical stimuli. This technique has also been critical in demonstrating the sensitization of afferent fibers in conditions such as inflammation, which can account for peripheral mechanisms of allodynia and/or hyperalgesia.

Intracellular electrophysiology

Intracellular recording is an excellent technique for acquiring information about the electrical and synaptic properties of intact neurons in whole-mount preparations. This has the advantage of preserving much of the neural circuitry that exists *in vivo*. Intracellular recording involves the use of sharp glass microelectrodes (<0.5 μm tip diameter) filled with electrolyte solution,

typically KCl. The fine tip of the electrode is used to impale individual neurons in an intact whole-mount preparation, so that the voltage difference between the electrode tip and a reference (ground) electrode in the extracellular space is amplified (Fig. 2.1). Current can be injected through the recording electrode to control the membrane potential, thus allowing the investigator to activate action potentials or change the membrane potential of the cell. The types of information regarding electrical properties of the neurons include the passive membrane properties of a neuron, such as resting membrane potential and membrane input resistance, as well as active membrane properties such as action potentials and afterhyperpolarizations. In addition to

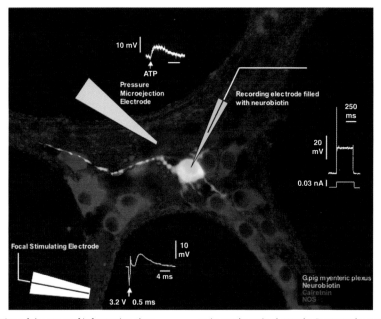

Fig. 2.1 Representation of the types of information that can be obtained from an intracellular electrophysiological recording. Impaling a neuron with a microelectrode allows the investigator to measure voltage changes across the cell's membrane. Voltage changes in response to current injected through the recording electrode (right trace) can be used to determine the membrane input resistance and the tonic versus phasic nature of the neuron. A separate stimulating electrode placed near the interganglionic fibers can activate synaptic inputs to the cell (bottom trace). Pharmacological manipulation of the neuron can occur by placing compounds directly in the bathing solution, by pressure-ejecting compounds near the recording site via a pressure microejection electrode (top trace), or by a more controlled local release via an iontophoretic electrode. Because the recording electrode can be filled with neurobiotin, which can be injected into the cell, the cell can be identified microscopically (green fluorescence). The cell's morphology (Dogiel type I) and projection pattern (orally projecting) can be determined. Combining this with immunohistochemistry allows the neurochemistry of the neuron to be identified. This particular cell is immunoreactive for calretinin (red) but not nitric oxide synthase (blue). By these combined techniques and comparison with our knowledge of projection patterns and neurochemical coding, we can establish that this neuron is a rapidly accommodating (phasic), ascending excitatory motor neuron that projects to the longitudinal smooth muscle, receives fast excitatory synaptic input and expresses purinergic receptors.

their use in the study of the electrical properties of a given neuron, intracellular recording techniques can be used to evaluate the types of synaptic input that a given neuron receives. In studies of synaptic potentials in the ENS, stimulating electrodes are placed on interganglionic fiber bundles leading to the ganglion containing an impaled neuron. Brief individual pulses of the stimulating electrode are used to activate fast synaptic responses, and trains of high-frequency pulses are used to elicit slow synaptic responses. When intracellular electrophysiological experiments are being performed, the microelectrode can be filled with an ionic substance, such as neurobiotin or biocytin, and iontophoretically injected into the cell. Once the recording session is complete, the impaled cell can be visualized and morphologically characterized. Furthermore, single- or dual-labeled immunohistochemistry can be performed on these preparations to determine the neurochemicals expressed by the neuron that has already been electrically and morphologically characterized. With these combinations of information, it has become possible to identify with certainty the neuronal elements of intrinsic reflex circuits.

Intracellular recording techniques can also be used to investigate the ionic currents that contribute to a given neuron's passive and active electrical properties. These investigations can involve ion substitution or the use of ion channel blockers while measuring membrane voltage. In addition, current recordings can be obtained using the single-electrode voltage clamp (SEVC) technique, which involves the use of a feedback amplifier that uses alternating membrane potential measurement and current injection.[4] Unfortunately, because of the small tip size and high resistance of intracellular microelectrodes it is difficult to pass current. Therefore, ionic conductances with fast kinetics, such as those contributing to the action potential, cannot be controlled. The use of SEVC is therefore limited to investigations of slower events, such as conductances associated with prolonged afterhyperpolarizations or slow synaptic responses.

Patch-clamp electrophysiology

In order to optimally obtain information related to the individual ionic conductances that contribute to the passive and active electrical properties of enteric neurons and to identify the ion channels that are involved, patch-clamp recording is the method of choice. Patch-clamp recording involves the use of large-bore, low-resistance micropipettes that are placed against a neuronal cell membrane. Different configurations of patch-clamp recording can provide different types of information. In the whole-cell configuration, in which the electrode is attached to the cell and the membrane within the electrode pore is removed, ensemble currents from the entire cell are integrated. Isolation of classes of ion channels is accomplished pharmacologically or by utilizing unique biophysical properties of the ion channel, such as its activation voltage. In cell-attached, inside-out or outside-out patches, only channels that are within the pore of the electrode provide currents that are amplified and measured. In this manner, currents from individual ion channels can be measured and the biophysical properties, such as single-channel conductance, can be characterized.

Enteric ganglia are surrounded by a basement membrane that prevents the formation of the high-resistance seal required between the neuron and the patch pipette. To overcome this obstacle, several approaches have been used. First, individual enteric neurons can be isolated by enzymatic and mechanical dissociation. These neurons can be studied with patch-clamp recording techniques in the acutely dissociated state, or after being maintained in primary culture conditions for up to several days. When maintained in culture, the isolated neurons form synaptic contacts with one another. Another approach has been the enzymatic dissociation of an intact ganglionated plexus from muscle layers and connective tissue. Recently, enteric neurobiologists have used intact longitudinal muscle–myenteric plexus preparations that have been lightly treated with proteases, followed by mechanical scraping of individual ganglia to remove the basement membrane.[5] This approach leaves neurons and their networks relatively intact and still allows the seal formation required for patch-clamp electrophysiology. Although treatments needed to prepare neurons for patch clamp likely alter the properties of the neurons, most electrical and synaptic properties of these neurons are maintained.

The electrical properties of individual neurons are determined by the integrated contribution of many ion channels, and changes in the neurophysiological properties of enteric neurons involve discrete changes

---

Applications of electrophysiological approaches

1 **Extracellular recording techniques** are used for investigations of electrical activity in extrinsic afferent and preganglionic nerve fibers innervating the gut in response to physiological and pharmacological stimuli.

2 **Intracellular recording techniques** are used for investigations of enteric neurons in preparations that include intact neural circuits. Electrical, synaptic and pharmacological properties can be readily investigated.

3 **Patch-clamp recording techniques** are well suited for investigations of ionic conductances in enteric neurons under controlled electrical and pharmacological conditions. Patch-clamp studies typically involve acutely dissociated or cultured neurons, but can be conducted in intact preparations.

---

in ionic conductances. Therefore, the design of effective therapeutics for the pathological ENS requires the identification of these molecular targets, and patch-clamp electrophysiological studies will play a central role in elucidating what ion channels are involved and how they are affected by certain pathophysiological and pharmacological conditions.

Imaging

Physiology is typically the study of when biological events occur, whereas anatomy is the study of where biological structures or molecules are. New imaging techniques have been useful for defining both the 'when' and 'where' of active neural networks. These techniques use fluorescent molecules that shift their spectral properties (the wavelengths of light that the molecule absorbs and emits) with altered cellular events. By measuring the ratio of one fluorescent state to the other over time within a given region, the kinetics of an event can be measured. By measuring those changes simultaneously in a multitude of defined regions, the biological events can be localized to groups of cells or to individual cells, or even at the subcellular level. The broad range of imaging techniques available will be discussed below according to the biological events they are used to study. For a general overview of neuronal imaging techniques, the reader is referred to recent reviews.[6–8]

Calcium

Calcium is the most highly regulated ion in biological systems. In neurons, increases in intracellular Ca^{2+} levels mediate neurotransmitter release, modulate ion channel activity, or stimulate gene expression. While Ca^{2+} entry into the cell through the plasma membrane causes a current that can be detected using electrophysiology, Ca^{2+} mobilization (the release of calcium from intracellular stores) is not detectable electrophysiologically. To study these events, fluorescent probes that change their spectral properties with bound Ca^{2+} were developed to measure concentrations of intracellular free Ca^{2+}. Initially, these dyes were used to study whole-cell calcium levels in individual neurons. In this configuration, simultaneous electrophysiological recording and dynamic Ca^{2+} imaging have been used to determine the role of calcium mobilization and mitochondrial reuptake in the excitability of enteric neurons. Importantly, these contributions to neuronal excitability cannot be directly examined by electrophysiology alone. More recently, Ca^{2+} indicator dyes have been used to record Ca^{2+} signals simultaneously in multiple neurons, and to record neurons together with other cells such as interstitial cells of Cajal and smooth muscle cells. This approach will be very valuable in future efforts to resolve issues concerning neural networks and communication between motor neurons and smooth muscle. This approach is limited, however, by the fact that not all changes in neuronal excitability involve intracellular Ca^{2+}. Some neurons exhibit little detectable change in Ca^{2+} even with ongoing electrical activity.

Voltage

Voltage-sensitive dyes can be used to measure changes in membrane voltage optically. This is an exciting advance because these voltage changes reflect the excitability of the neurons being investigated and, unlike intracellular neuronal recording, several neurons can be evaluated simultaneously. New generations of voltage-sensitive dyes have important characteristics, such as rapid kinetics and large signal-to-noise ratios, that allow them to provide accurate monitoring of rapid membrane potential changes, such as action potentials and fast synaptic inputs. The ability to track these electrical events in many neurons allows the accurate determination of the spread of excitability and basic understanding of network connections (Fig. 2.2).

Although the approach has not been used in the ENS, voltage changes in single neurons can be imaged optically by injecting the voltage-sensitive dye directly. This approach allows the precise measurement of voltage changes in processes that are too small or fragile for electrode recording, and has been used in cerebral and cerebellar neurons. In enteric neurons, it would be useful to resolve electrical integration of inputs in neural processes of individual neurons, especially the vast, branching processes of AH cells (see below).

Fluorescence resonance energy transfer

Fluorescence resonance energy transfer (FRET) is a technique that is based on the principle that signal transduction occurs by the reorganization of intracellular molecules, such that two molecules will be in close proximity only when signal transduction pathways are active. Using the properties of FRET, the fluorescent emission of one molecule is used to excite the second. This relatively new technique has yet to be used in enteric neurons but has been used successfully in other neural networks to identify network activation of signal transduction pathways, such as protein kinases A and C.[9] FRET depends on genetic manipulation, such as the incorporation of DNA encoding fluorescent proteins into the sequence encoding signaling molecules. For this reason, its use is often limited to mice, and as enteric neurobiologists shift to murine studies this is likely to become a valuable approach.

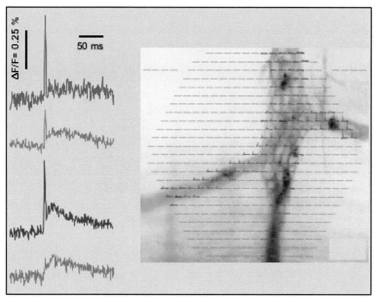

Fig. 2.2 Example of an experiment using optical imaging of the voltage-sensitive dye Di-8ANEPPS in the guinea-pig ileum myenteric plexus preparation. Multiple nerve cells within the ganglion, visualized in the image as black rings where the dye is incorporated into the membrane, can be simultaneously imaged over the same time course. Overlaid on the image is the 464 diode hexagonal array. Each trace is the condensed signal of one diode over time and reflects the response following a single-pulse electrical stimulation of the nerve fiber to the left of the ganglion. The four expanded traces on the left correspond to the like-colored traces in the array. From top to bottom, the traces are of a compound action potential from the stimulated fiber tract (in magenta), action potentials and fast EPSPs from cells at the bottom (in pink) and middle of the ganglion (in red), and a subthreshold fast EPSP from a cell at the top of the ganglion (in brown). The scale is for all expanded traces. Figure by courtesy of Drs Michael Schemann and Michal Ceregrzyn, Munich, Germany.

Applications of imaging approaches

1 **Calcium imaging techniques** are used to investigate signal transduction mechanisms in enteric neurons that involve changes in intracellular calcium concentrations. This is the only approach that can be used to evaluate calcium mobilization from intracellular stores. It allows the collection of data from several neurons simultaneously.

2 **Voltage imaging techniques** are used to investigate enteric neurons in intact preparations, such as human tissue samples, that are difficult to study with intracellular electrodes. This technique allows the collection of data related to synaptic and pharmacological responses from several neurons simultaneously.

Electrical and synaptic properties of enteric neurons

Most of our knowledge of the physiological properties of gut neurons comes from intracellular electrophysiological studies of the guinea-pig small intestine. Over the past decade and a half, a concentrated effort has been made to characterize enteric neurons in other gastrointestinal regions in the guinea-pig and enteric neurons in other species, including the human. Recent efforts have been made to characterize enteric neurons in mice because of the great potential for genetic manipulation in this species. The combination of all of these studies indicates that, with some exceptions, defining characteristics of enteric neurons are shared in different regions of the gut and between species. Two primary classes of neurons, AH and S, have been identified,[10,11] and the major features of myenteric AH and S neurons are described below (Fig. 2.3).

AH neurons

It has become clear that AH neurons act as multifunctional elements in the afferent limb of the intrinsic reflex circuitry. The AH neurons of the myenteric plexus and submucous plexus have been identified definitively as intrinsic primary afferent neurons in the guinea-pig ileum, as they respond to mucosal stimulation (mechanical, electrical and chemical) and are activated by stretching. In addition to acting as first-order afferent neurons, AH neurons can serve as interneurons since they form interconnected, self-reinforcing networks that act to synchronize motor events in the bowel.

AH neurons are multipolar (Dogiel type II morphology) and have many long processes extending to other ganglia and to the mucosa. The neurochemical characteristics of these neurons indicate that they are cholinergic, and most are immunoreactive for tachykinins and the calcium-binding protein calbindin. In the resting state, AH neurons have a more negative resting membrane potential and lower excitability than S cells. AH neurons are phasic, meaning that they typically do not fire repetitively, and their action potentials are followed by an afterhyperpolarization that lasts several seconds. This prolonged afterhyperpolarization is the defining characteristic (AH = afterhyperpolarization). In addition to the inward Na^+ and outward K^+ conductances that are typical of most neuronal action potentials, the action potential of AH neurons is also characterized by a shoulder on the repolarizing phase of the action potential that is due to an inward Ca^{2+} conductance. It is this influx of Ca^{2+}, and the subsequent release of Ca^{2+} from intracellular stores, that activates the long-lasting afterhyperpolarization. Conductances that contribute to the active properties of AH neurons are schematically represented in Fig. 2.4.

AH neurons provide tachykininergic slow excitatory synaptic input to one another, and these signals form the basis of the self-reinforcing network mentioned above. One of the puzzles concerning the synaptic properties of AH neurons is that evoked fast excitatory postsynaptic potentials (fEPSPs) are rarely detected despite the fact that AH neurons are cholinergic and express nicotinic acetylcholine receptors. The inability to detect fEPSPs may be due to the experimental limitations of intracellular electrophysiology, as the membrane potential is being monitored at the cell body and synaptic contacts are out on the processes. When fEPSPs are detected in these neurons they are almost always entirely cholinergic.

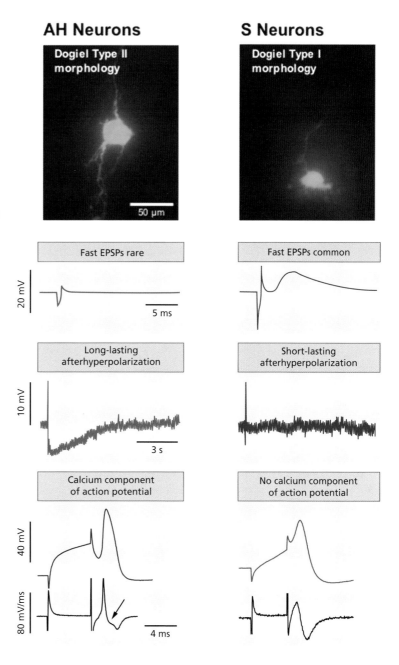

Fig. 2.3 Representative examples of the distinguishing characteristics of the two major classes of enteric neurons, AH neurons (left column) and S neurons (right column). AH neurons have a Dogiel type II morphology, with several long processes extending from a smooth cell soma, while S neurons have a Dogiel type I morphology, with one long axon and many short lamellar (pictured here) or filamentous dendrites. AH neurons rarely receive fast excitatory synaptic input, while most S neurons do. AH neurons exhibit a prolonged (3–10 s) afterhyperpolarization following a single action potential, while S neurons exhibit only a short afterhyperpolarization (20–60 ms). The action potential of AH neurons, shown here after a brief depolarizing current pulse, are composed of voltage-gated Na^+, K^+ and Ca^{2+} channels. The slower kinetics of the Ca^{2+} channels creates an observable shoulder on the repolarizing phase of the action potential. The change in the rate of repolarization is more easily recognized in a derivative of the time–voltage trace, where there is a prominent hump (arrow). The action potential of S neurons does not contain a Ca^{2+} component and therefore does not express a hump on the repolarizing phase of the action potential.

S cells

It is likely that S neurons serve as interneurons, excitatory motor neurons and inhibitory motor neurons, on the basis of their neurotransmitter phenotypes and projections. S cells are either unipolar with short processes emanating from the cell body (Dogiel type 1 morphology) or have a single axon and several filamentous dendritic processes (filamentous morphology). The various subpopulations of S cells in the guinea-pig enteric nervous system can be sorted on the

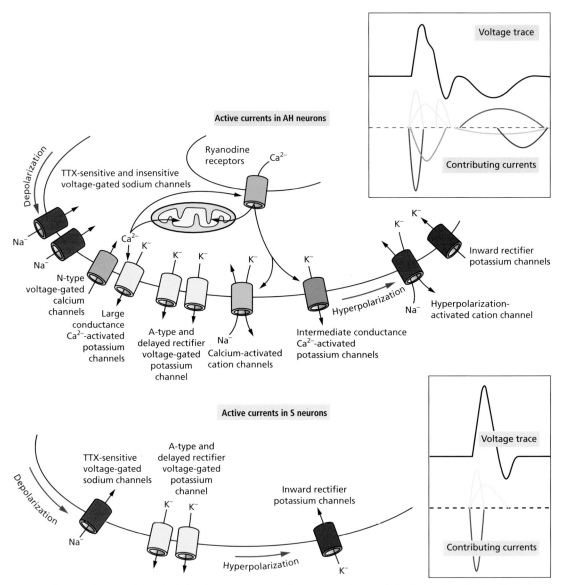

Fig. 2.4 Schematic diagram of the principal ionic currents that contribute to the active membrane properties of AH and S neurons. Cylinders represent classes of ion channels. In AH neurons, a depolarization causes the activation of voltage-gated Na+, Ca2+ and K+ ion channels. The calcium that enters through these ion channels activates a potassium current, which contributes to the repolarization and causes the release of calcium from intracellular stores. This calcium-induced calcium release, in turn, opens calcium-activated cation and potassium channels. The calcium-activated potassium current is responsible for the prolonged afterhyperpolarization, which, in turn, opens hyperpolarization-activated cation channels. This sequence of events is active upon initiation of each action potential. Modulation of each contributing current can alter the excitability of AH neurons, and the reflexes in which the AH neurons participate. In S neurons, the active currents presently identified include the voltage-gated Na+ and K+ channels that contribute to the action potential. Both AH and S neurons also express inward-rectifying K+ channels that are active during periods of hyperpolarization beyond the K+ equilibrium potential.

basis of unique projections and neurochemical coding patterns. These neurons can exist in several states of excitability: those that exhibit regular spontaneous action potentials in the absence of input whose firing rate can be modulated by increases or decreases in membrane potential; those that do not exhibit spontaneous action potentials but fire action potentials repetitively throughout a depolarizing current pulse (tonic neurons); those that exhibit action potentials only at the onset of a depolarizing current pulse (phasic neurons); and those that do not respond to any changes in membrane potential (silent neurons). In contrast to AH neurons, S cells have an action potential that is completely composed of inward Na^+ and outward K^+ conductances, and the action potential is not followed by a prolonged afterhyperpolarization. The conductances that are active in S neurons are represented in Fig. 2.4.

S neurons receive both fast and slow excitatory synaptic inputs. Almost all S neurons exhibit fast EPSPs, and this defining characteristic was used to name these cells (S = synaptic). These potentials are mediated mainly by acetylcholine acting at nicotinic acetylcholine receptors, but some cells also have a proportion of the EPSP mediated by ATP acting at purinergic P_2X receptors. A much smaller proportion of EPSPs in S neurons are also mediated by serotonin (5-HT) acting at $5\text{-}HT_3$ receptors. Only a proportion of S neurons (50–70%) receive slow excitatory synaptic inputs, and these are mediated by tachykinins or serotonin.

Enteric reflex circuitry

The normal physiology of the gastrointestinal tract relies on the precise coordination of the enteric neural reflexes that regulate motor activity, secretion and blood vessel diameter. Enteric neurobiologists have determined the individual neurons involved in reflex circuitry by using retrograde labeling techniques to determine the projection patterns of neurons that were then characterized further by intracellular recording and/or immunohistochemistry. Also, recording chambers that allow separation of the preparation into oral and aboral regions allow pharmacological manipulation of parts of the circuitry. In addition, evaluation of the responses of individual neurons to stimuli such as distension and mucosal stroking has been critical in the identification of intrinsic primary afferent neurons.

Despite their varied functions, enteric motor, secretory and vasodilatory reflexes share common elements.[1,12–15] All of these reflexes can be initiated by the release of paracrine substances from enteroendocrine cells in the mucosal epithelium that are activated by luminal mechanical and chemical stimuli. These paracrine compounds, which include serotonin and cholecystokinin, initiate activity in submucosal and myenteric AH neurons. In addition to mucosal stimuli, these reflexes can be initiated by stretching of the muscularis. AH neurons, as well as a small population of S neurons, are stretch-sensitive and respond to distending stimuli. At the efferent end of the reflexes are motor neurons that contract or relax smooth muscle, dilate blood vessels, and/or stimulate mucosal secretion. The submucous plexus is composed largely of primary afferent and motor neurons, whereas the myenteric ganglia house afferent neurons, motor neurons and a variety of interneurons, which can spread reflex signals along the gut in the oral and aboral directions. These reflex circuits are represented schematically in Fig. 2.5.

Pathological changes in neurophysiology

Collectively, the reflexes described above coordinate the effector functions of the gut, including the muscle contractions and relaxations that propel and mix the luminal contents, direct absorption and secretion and provide local control over blood supply to aid digestion throughout the gastrointestinal tract. Clearly, there are many stages in these precise reflex activities that can be modulated to alter gastrointestinal function. In addition to being influenced by paracrine compounds and neurotransmitters, enteric neuronal activity can be modulated by many substances that are present during intestinal inflammation, including histamine, prostaglandins, leukotrienes, interleukins, proteases and serotonin.

Changes in the electrical properties of enteric neurons have been demonstrated in a number of models of infectious and allergen-induced enteritis and in immune-mediated inflammation. AH neurons, which project to the mucosal layer, where the inflammatory response is typically centered, undergo the most dramatic changes. AH neurons are depolarized and are hyperexcitable in *Trichinella spiralis*-induced enteritis

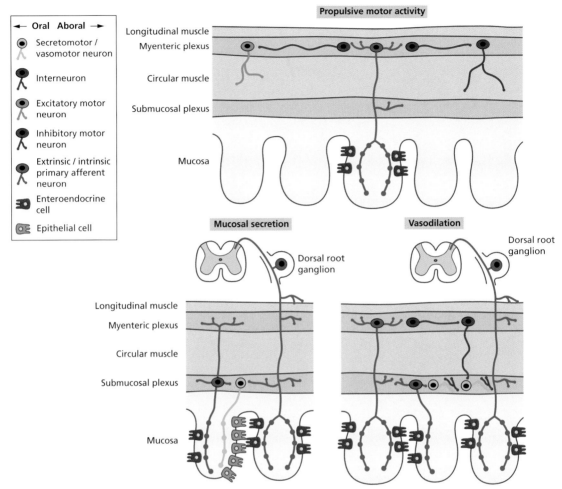

Fig. 2.5 Schematic illustrations of enteric reflex pathways that are involved in propulsive motor activity, mucosal secretion and vasodilation. Each of these reflexes can be initiated by mucosal activation of intrinsic primary afferent neurons via release of paracrine substances from enteroendocrine cells, or by circular muscle stretch. For propulsive motor activity, reflex initiation is followed by activation of ascending and descending interneurons. These stimulate excitatory motor neurons oral to the stimulus, causing contraction, and inhibitory motor neurons aboral to the stimulus, causing relaxation. The resulting pressure gradient causes the net propulsion of the luminal contents in an aboral direction. For secretory and vasodilatory reflexes, reflex initiation in the submucous plexus causes the local activation of secretomotor and vasomotor neurons. Recently, a long descending vasodilator reflex was discovered (by Vanner and colleagues), which is mediated by interneurons in the myenteric plexus. Extrinsic primary afferent neurons can contribute to secretion and vasodilation reflexes after noxious stimuli. During periods of intestinal distress, alteration in the physiology of the neurons involved in these reflexes can contribute to disordered motor, secretory and vasodilatory function.

and in allergen challenge following milk sensitization.[16–18] In these conditions, the neurons are able to fire repetitive action potentials and have a smaller afterhyperpolarization. In TNBS (trinitrobenzene-sulfonic acid) colitis, which is a model of an immune-mediated inflammatory response, the AH neurons are hyperexcitable but maintain a normal resting membrane potential.[19] The differences between these models in the changes in electrical properties of AH neurons suggest that the mechanisms leading to altered AH neuronal function differ in these types of inflammation.

Synaptic activity is also augmented in infectious and immune-mediated intestinal inflammation. As described above, fast excitatory synaptic input to AH neurons is relatively rare under normal conditions. However, in both TNBS colitis and *Trichinella spiralis* enteritis, fast EPSPs in AH neurons are frequently encountered and they are larger.[17,18] In TNBS colitis, both fast and slow excitatory potentials are enhanced in S neurons.[19] These findings suggest that inflammation leads to facilitation of synaptic transmission in enteric ganglia, possibly through a presynaptic mechanism.

Neurophysiological changes in enteric neural circuitry such as those described above are likely to contribute to the alterations in bowel function that are commonly associated with gastrointestinal inflammation. Similar alterations in gut function are also common symptoms of functional disorders such as irritable bowel syndrome. As animal models of functional disorders, such as those involving postinflammatory time points, are developed, enteric neurobiologists will be able to resolve sites of altered neuronal function in the enteric neural circuitry. As we gain a more comprehensive understanding of the sites and mechanisms of neuroplasticity in inflammatory and functional disorders, it is quite possible that novel therapeutic targets will be identified.

References

1 Furness J, Clerc N, Gola M, Kunze W, Fletcher E. Identification of component neurons and organisation of enteric nerve circuits. In: Krammer H, Singer M, eds. *Neurogastroenterology from the Basics to the Clinics*. Dordrecht: Kluwer Academic, 2000: 137–50.

2 Wood JD. Physiology of the enteric nervous system. In: Johnson LR, ed. *Physiology of the Gastrointestinal Tract*. New York: Raven Press, 1994: 423–82.

3 Grundy D. Neuroanatomy of visceral nociception: vagal and splanchnic afferent. *Gut* 2002; **51** Suppl 1: i2–5.

4 Galligan J. In vitro electrophysiological methods in gatrointestinal pharmacology. In: Gaginella T, ed. *Handbook of Methods in Gastrointestinal Pharmacology*. Boca Raton (FL): CRC Press, 1996: 247–72.

5 Rugiero F, Gola M, Kunze WA, Reynaud JC, Furness JB, Clerc N. Analysis of whole-cell currents by patch clamp of guinea-pig myenteric neurones in intact ganglia. *J Physiol* 2002; **538**: 447–63.

6 Yuste R, Lanni F, Konnerth A, eds. *Imaging Neurons. A Laboratory Manual*. Plainview (NY): Spring Harbor Laboratory Press, 2000.

7 Van den Berghe P, Bisschops R, Tack J. Imaging of neuronal activity in the gut. *Curr Opin Pharmacol* 2001; **1**: 563–7.

8 Schemann M, Michel K, Peters S, Bischoff SC, Neunlist M. Cutting-edge technology. III. Imaging and the gastrointestinal tract: mapping the human enteric nervous system. *Am J Physiol Gastrointest Liver Physiol* 2002; **282**: G919–25.

9 Sekar RB, Periasamy A. Fluorescence resonance energy transfer (FRET) microscopy imaging of live cell protein localizations. *J Cell Biol* 2003; **160**: 629–33.

10 Wood JD. Application of classification schemes to the enteric nervous system. *J Auton Nerv Syst* 1994; **48**: 17–29.

11 Bornstein JC, Furness JB, Kunze WA. Electrophysiological characterization of myenteric neurons: how do classification schemes relate? *J Auton Nerv Syst* 1994; **48**: 1–15.

12 Vanner S, MacNaughton WK. Submucosal secretomotor and vasodilator reflexes. *Neurogastroenterol Motil* 2004; **16** (Suppl. 1): 39–43.

13 Cooke HJ. Neurotransmitters in neuronal reflexes regulating intestinal secretion. *Ann N Y Acad Sci* 2000; **915**: 77–80.

14 Reed DE, Vanner SJ. Long vasodilator reflexes projecting through the myenteric plexus in guinea-pig ileum. *J Physiol* 2003; **553**: 911–24.

15 Bornstein J, Furness J, Kunze W, Bertrand P. Enteric reflexes that influence motility. In: Costa M, Brookes S, eds. *Innervation of the Gastrointestinal Tract*. London: Taylor & Francis, 2002: 1–56.

16 Liu S, Hu HZ, Gao N, Gao C, Wang G, Wang X *et al*. Neuroimmune interactions in guinea pig stomach and small intestine. *Am J Physiol Gastrointest Liver Physiol* 2003; **284**: G154–64.

17 Frieling T, Palmer JM, Cooke HJ, Wood JD. Neuroimmune communication in the submucous plexus of guinea pig colon after infection with *Trichinella spiralis*. *J Auton Nerv Syst* 1997; **66**: 131–7.

18 Palmer JM, Wong-Riley M, Sharkey KA. Functional alterations in jejunal myenteric neurons during inflammation in nematode-infected guinea pigs. *Am J Physiol* 1998; **275**: G922–35.

19 Linden DR, Sharkey KA, Mawe GM. Enhanced excitability of myenteric AH neurones in the inflamed guinea-pig distal colon. *J Physiol* 2003; **547**: 589–601.

CHAPTER 3

Gut-to-Brain Signaling: Sensory Mechanisms

Klaus Bielefeldt and GF Gebhart

Introduction

Intrinsic and extrinsic sensory neurons provide information about visceral distension, which generally corresponds to the volume of luminal contents, the chemical composition and temperature of ingested material and its movement along the mucosal surface of the gut. This input generates signals that regulate intestinal motility, blood flow, secretion and absorption and is thus critical for normal digestion. Most of these stimuli, however, are processed within the enteric nervous system and are thus not perceived. Similarly, much of the sensory information carried by extrinsic afferents serves homeostatic functions and does not reach the brain areas involved in conscious sensation. If we perceive changes within the gastrointestinal tract, either as innocuous or painful

stimuli, our ability to discriminate the location and type (modality) of a given stimulus is poor. This is due to the low density of visceral innervation and the polymodal character of visceral afferents, which typically can be activated by several stimulus modalities. Afferent pathways converge within spinal cord and supraspinal areas, resulting in referral of visceral stimuli, especially painful stimuli, to somatic sites, such as the right shoulder in a patient with acute cholecystitis. Finally, intense visceral stimulation often triggers strong autonomic and emotional responses. In the following sections, we will summarize current understanding and emerging concepts related to visceral sensation, principally discomfort and pain.

As already discussed in Chapter 1, the anatomical basis of gastrointestinal innervation is quite complex,

---

Gastrointestinal tract sensory pathways

Intrinsic primary afferent neurons (IPANs)
- Located within the submucosal and myenteric plexuses.
- Activate enteric reflexes that regulate motility, secretion and blood flow.

Extrinsic primary afferent neurons (EPANs)
Vagal afferents:
- Activated by mechanical (low-intensity), thermal and chemical stimuli.
- Cell bodies in nodose ganglion and central terminals in brainstem nucleus tractus solitarius.
- Input to brainstem and higher centers that regulate

autonomic function are generally not perceived.
- Contribute to chemonociception and autonomic and emotional responses to painful stimuli.

Spinal afferents:
- Activated by low- and high-intensity mechanical stimuli.
- Cell bodies in dorsal root ganglia and central terminals in superficial dorsal horn of spinal cord.
- Generally polymodal (i.e. respond also to chemical and thermal stimuli).
- Convey information about painful stimuli.

with intrinsic primary afferent neurons in the sub-mucosal and myenteric plexuses and a dual extrinsic primary afferent innervation. While we have gained significant insight into the structure and function of the sensory innervation of the gut, surprisingly little is known about interactions between extrinsic and intrinsic sensory pathways and the contributions of intrinsic afferents in conscious sensation.

Mechanosensation and the gastrointestinal tract

The volume of hollow viscera changes frequently due to the ingestion, propulsion and expulsion of the luminal contents. Filling of any compartment within the gastrointestinal tract may trigger conscious sensation and – if the intraluminal pressure exceeds a value of around 30 mm Hg – discomfort or even pain. Therefore, controlled distension of hollow viscera is an appropriate mechanical stimulus to study sensory mechanisms. Studies in human volunteers demonstrate that intra-luminal pressures below 10 mm Hg typically elicit no or only vague sensations. When the pressure exceeds 30 mm Hg, the stimulus becomes unpleasant or painful. The quality of the sensation depends in part on the length of the balloon or bag used to distend the organ. Because of the low density of innervation, spatial summation plays an important role in sensations from the gut, explaining why high, very localized pressures along the gut are not normally associated with conscious sensation. Animal experiments with a variety of experimental approaches have allowed us to better define pathways and mechanisms mediating mechanical sensation in the gastrointestinal tract.

High- and low-threshold mechanoreceptors

By isolating a nerve, teasing it into small filaments and placing it on a recording electrode, it is possible to study the action potential firing of a single nerve fiber (axon). Distension of the esophagus activates vagal afferents, located within the muscle layer, as mucosal application of local anesthetics does not abolish this response. Studies in the esophagus and stomach have demonstrated that these vagal afferents appear to fall into a similar functional category: they have a low activation threshold and stimulus response functions that

encode intensities into the noxious range. Activation in response to muscle contraction (tension) or small volume changes (stretch) is certainly consistent with the role of the vagus nerve in regulating the normal function of the proximal gastrointestinal tract. Interestingly, two distinct populations of mechanoreceptive afferents can be identified in the spinal visceral afferent innervation. One group is activated by low-intensity stimuli, analogous to vagal afferents, whereas the second group, which comprises about 20–30% of the spinal afferents, responds to distending pressures exceeding 30 mm Hg. High-threshold mechanosensitive fibers have been found in spinal afferents innervating the stomach (Fig. 3.1), esophagus, gallbladder, urinary bladder, colon and uterus. The parallel between human data showing a pain threshold above 30 mm Hg intra-luminal pressure and the functional characteristics of high-threshold fibers suggest that these high-threshold mechanoreceptors function as nociceptors and mediate acute pain in response to noxious mechanical distension.

To examine whether spinal or vagal pathways mediate information about noxious mechanical stimulation of the stomach, we studied behavioral changes in response to noxious gastric distension. As expected, noxious intensities of gastric distension led to cessation of the normal exploratory behavior, which persisted after vagotomy and was abolished by splanchnic nerve resection. Thus, consistent with the potential role of high-threshold mechanoreceptors as nociceptors, behavioral data demonstrate that spinal pathways primarily mediate painful mechanical stimuli.

Mucosal mechanoreceptors

The most common and subtle mechanical stimulus along the gut is due to movement of the luminal contents, which deforms the mucosa. While this information is not consciously perceived, recent studies provide important insight into sensory mechanisms within the gastrointestinal tract. Nerve activity can be recorded *in vitro* when a hollow viscus and its nerves are dissected and placed in an appropriately designed recording chamber. The lumen can be exposed and subjected to defined stimuli. Gentle stroking of the mucosa triggers a rapidly adapting barrage of action potentials in some fibers, whereas high-intensity probing or stretching activates other fibers. Mucosal mechanore-

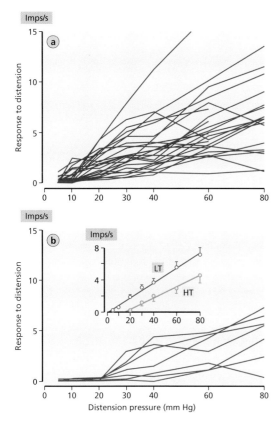

Fig. 3.1 Stimulus–response function of spinal afferents innervating the rat stomach. Whereas the majority of fibers are activated at distension pressures less than 10 mm Hg (a), a small population only responds to intragastric pressures exceeding 30 mm Hg (b). The insert summarizes the stimulus–response functions for low-threshold (LT) and high-threshold (HT) gastric splanchnic fibers. imps, impulses.

cells being the most abundant source. Intrinsic and extrinsic nerves within the gastrointestinal tract express 5-HT receptors, which in other experiments have been shown to be activated by 5-HT. Thus, 5-HT could function as one signal transmitting information about mucosal changes to afferent neurons. Consistent with this hypothesis, mechanical and chemical stimulation triggers 5-HT release from a cell line derived from human enteroendocrine cells. The most convincing evidence for a role of 5-HT in transducing mechanical stimulation comes from experiments demonstrating that mucosal stimulation does not elicit responses of submucosal neurons in the presence of 5-HT receptor blockers. The activation of these intrinsic primary afferent neurons by mucosally released 5-HT triggers enteric reflexes and alters secretion or muscle contraction. While a similar mechanism has not yet been directly shown for extrinsic afferents, 5-HT clearly affects vagal and spinal pathways and modulates gastric emptying, contributes to the gastrocolic reflex, and may be involved in triggering nausea. On the basis of these observations, several investigators have proposed a model according to which enteroendocrine cells and 5-HT play a pivotal role in the activation of intrinsic and possibly also extrinsic visceral afferents by mechanical and/or chemical stimulation of the gastrointestinal mucosa (Fig. 3.2). However, this concept needs to be extended to include other signaling molecules, as enteroendocrine and other epithelial cells release a variety of mediators that can affect nerve function.

Chemosensation and the gastrointestinal tract

The intestinal tract is continually exposed to changing luminal contents that contain different nutrients or even potentially noxious substances, such as high proton concentrations. While such alterations in luminal contents evoke neural responses and trigger changes in motility or secretion, we know relatively little about chemosensation within the gut. Duodenal infusion of nutrients or hypertonic saline relaxes the stomach and alters thresholds for discomfort and pain induced by gastric distension in healthy volunteers. When tested in animals, instillation of nutrients or hypertonic solutions into the duodenum activates vagal afferents. This may be due to direct activation of nerve endings located within

ceptors respond to very low-intensity, subtle mucosal stimuli and are potentially important in the regulation of blood flow, secretion or absorption. However, their physiological role is not fully understood.

Enteroendocrine cells, serotonin and mucosal mechanosensation

Stroking of the mucosa also triggers release of serotonin (5-HT) into the lamina propria of the epithelium and, to a lesser degree, the lumen of the gut. Serotonin is a monoamine neurotransmitter derived from the amino acid tryptophan. Most of the serotonin in the body is found within the gut, the specialized enteroendocrine

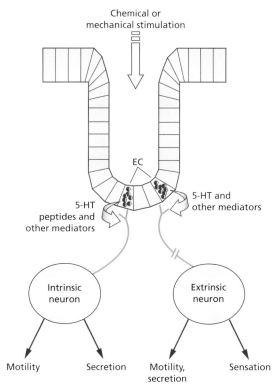

Fig. 3.2 Role of enteroendocrine cells and 5-HT in activating intrinsic and extrinsic sensory gastrointestinal neurons. Mucosal mechanical or chemical stimuli trigger release of 5-HT from enteroendocrine cells (EC) and other mediators from EC and other cells within the mucosa. The resulting increase in bioactive mediators in the lamina propria can activate intrinsic and extrinsic neurons, leading to changes in motility, secretion and sensation.

the mucosa or indirectly mediated by serotonin and/or other signaling molecules released by enteroendocrine or other cells. Using the single-fiber recording technique described above, acid-sensitive afferents have been identified in the esophagus, stomach and duodenum. In addition, by injecting a retrograde label into the intestinal wall, one can identify and selectively study the properties of the sensory neurons that innervate that area of the gastrointestinal tract. Using this approach, we recorded proton-gated currents in gastric neurons from nodose ganglia, the primary sensory ganglion of the vagus nerve, and T9–T10 dorsal root ganglia (Fig. 3.3), thus demonstrating that these neurons express ion channels that are directly activated by acid.

While vagal fibers are found within the mucosa, most spinal afferents terminate in the outer layers of the gut. The proximity of vagal endings to potentially noxious luminal stimuli raises the question of whether vagal fibers convey chemonociceptive information. Consistent with this hypothesis, instillation of high acid concentrations into the stomach activates only vagal and not spinal pathways (based on the expression of c-Fos, an immediate early gene that is transcribed after intense peripheral stimulation). The importance of the vagus is further supported by recent data showing that vagotomy, but not splanchnic nerve resection, abolishes the behavioral response to intragastric administration of acid. Thus, both spinal and vagal pathways are involved in gastric nociception. Accumulating evidence suggests that gastric spinal afferents convey mechanonociceptive information to the spinal cord, and that gastric vagal afferents convey chemonociceptive information to the brainstem and contribute to the autonomic and emotive response to noxious stimulation.

Specificity of gastrointestinal afferents

Appropriate discrimination of sensory information requires specific information about the location and modality of a given stimulus. Functional studies of gastrointestinal afferents have demonstrated that many fibers have more than one receptive field. Thus, peripheral visceral nerve terminals branch out and can collect information from different areas within a viscus, conveying the information along a single primary sensory neuron axon to the central nervous system. Importantly, the central terminations of visceral afferents typically diverge widely within the spinal cord, establishing synaptic contacts with several second-order neurons in different spinal segments. In addition, most visceral afferents are polymodal, i.e. respond to more than one stimulus modality, such as stretch and heat or chemical stimulation. This corresponds with clinical observations about the poor ability of patients to localize visceral pain and the unreliable discrimination of stimulus types, such as the sensation of heartburn during esophageal distension.

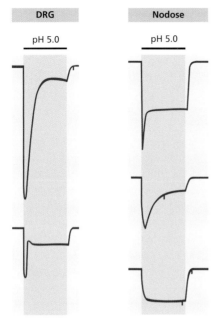

Fig. 3.3 Acid-sensitive ion currents recorded from gastric afferent neurons. Acid triggers transient inactivating inward currents in gastric dorsal root ganglion (DRG) sensory neurons (left). In contrast, only about half of the gastric nodose sensory neurons exhibit similar transient currents; the remaining half exhibit only a sustained current (right).

Visceral sensation and disease

Pain is a common symptom in patients with gastrointestinal diseases. Up to 25% of the adult population in the USA experiences abdominal discomfort or pain within a year and about 5–15% seek medical help. In about half of the cases, no structural or biochemical abnormality can be identified with appropriate clinical tests, leading to the diagnosis of functional diseases such as non-cardiac chest pain, non-ulcer dyspepsia or irritable bowel syndrome. Interestingly, patients with such functional disorders of the gastrointestinal tract experience pain or discomfort at lower distension pressures than healthy individuals, suggesting that changes in mechanosensation may contribute to their problem. Similarly, many patients with typical reflux symptoms do not have signs of esophageal injury (non-erosive reflux disease), raising the question of whether chemosensation is altered and is at least in part responsible for their symptoms.

Considering the pain associated with acute or chronic inflammation of the gastrointestinal tract, most experimental approaches investigating the possible contribution of changes in visceral afferents to pain syndromes study the effects of inflammation or inflammatory mediators and cytokines.

Sensitization of visceral afferent pathways

Acute or chronic visceral pain typically decreases exploratory behavior and triggers aversive reactions in experimental animals. However, observation of such behavioral changes is variable and subjective, and has limited sensitivity in detecting changes in visceral sensation. A component of the aversive response – the contraction of abdominal wall or other muscle groups

---

Sensitization

Sensitization of *peripheral* visceral sensory neurons is defined by:
- increase in the number of action potentials triggered by a stimulus
- decrease in stimulus intensity required for action potential generation
- lowering of the threshold for action potential generation

Sensitization of *peripheral* visceral sensory neurons may be associated with:

- increase in transmitter release at central synapses
- change in transmitters released at central synapses
- enhanced response (increased excitability) of postsynaptic neurons

Sensitization of *central* visceral sensory neurons is associated with:
- increase in response magnitude of central neurons
- increase in size of area of referred sensation
- increased excitability of spinal *and* supraspinal neurons

– can be monitored and quantified by recording electromyographic (EMG) activity in anesthetized or awake animals. This visceromotor response is a supraspinal reflex mediated within the brainstem and persists after decerebration. Visceral distension typically triggers a progressive increase in EMG activity when intraluminal pressure exceeds 20 mm Hg. Inflammation shifts this stimulus–response curve to the left, consistent with the development of hypersensitivity (Fig. 3.4).

Interestingly, the enhanced response to mechanical stimulation can persist for up to 6 weeks, long after repair of the initial injury, suggesting that inflammation can cause lasting changes in visceral sensation. Such

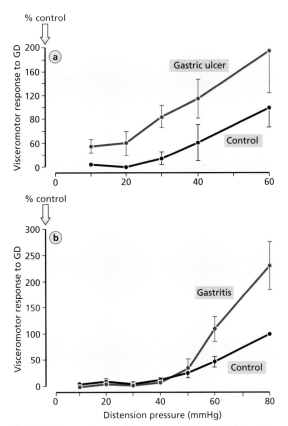

Fig. 3.4 Inflammation sensitizes responses to gastric distension (GD). The visceromotor response to gastric distension was quantified as EMG activity recorded from neck muscles in control animals and after induction of gastric ulcers (a) or mild gastritis (b). Inflammation shifted stimulus–response curves to the left, consistent with the development of gastric hypersensitivity.

changes may explain the persistence of symptoms after acute infections, such as postinfectious non-ulcer dyspepsia or irritable bowel syndrome. The hypersensitivity is not restricted to mechanical stimuli, as responses to acid are similarly enhanced.

Changes in the properties of extrinsic primary sensory neurons (*peripheral sensitization*) and processing centers at various levels within the spinal cord and/or brain (*central sensitization*) both play a role in the development of visceral hypersensitivity. Using different techniques, several investigators have studied the contribution of primary afferents. Recordings from single afferent fibers *in vivo* or *in vitro* demonstrate that sensory neurons can be acutely sensitized. Bradykinin, prostaglandin E_2, platelet-activating factor, histamine and other inflammatory mediators activate a subset of visceral afferents and in many cases enhance their response to subsequent mechanical stimulation (Fig. 3.5). Similarly, experimentally induced inflammation increases nerve responses to visceral distension or chemical stimulation.

Mechanisms of peripheral sensitization

On the cellular level, sensitization translates into increased excitability of a given afferent neuron; that is, lower stimulation intensity is needed to trigger an action potential, and/or a given stimulus triggers more action potentials. This is consistent with experimental results obtained in isolated neurons innervating the gastrointestinal tract. Stimulation of gastric sensory neurons with depolarizing current injections triggers action potentials. When cells obtained from animals with gastric ulcers are studied, the same stimulus elicits more action potentials (Fig. 3.6), reflecting an increase in neuron excitability.

Voltage-gated ion channels that are activated during depolarization form the basis of the action potential. The rapid upstroke is primarily due to the opening of sodium channels, with sodium influx into the cell and depolarization, while potassium channel opening causes potassium efflux and restoration of the negative membrane potential. Recent studies show that the expression of voltage-gated channels in visceral sensory neurons changes during inflammation. While sodium currents are increased and are more easily activated, potassium currents decrease, consistent with enhanced neuron excitability. Amitriptyline and κ-opioid ago-

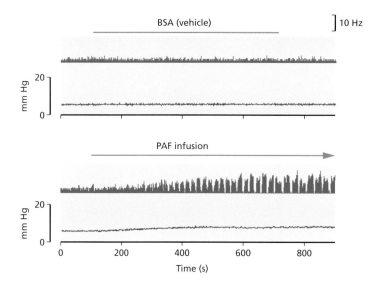

Fig. 3.5 Inflammatory mediators activate gastric vagal afferent fibers. While the vehicle did not affect the basal firing of mechanosensitive vagal afferent fibers, intra-arterial injection of platelet-activating factor (PAF) significantly increased firing.

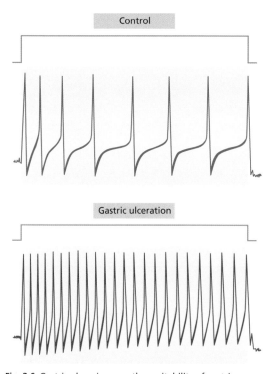

Fig. 3.6 Gastric ulcers increase the excitability of gastric sensory neurons. Depolarizing current injections trigger a short burst of action potentials in spinal gastric afferent neurons (control). When sensory neurons from animals with gastric ulcers were examined, the same stimulus intensity triggered significantly more action potentials (gastric ulceration).

nists have been used with some success in patients with functional bowel disorders. Interestingly, some κ-opioid agonists and tricyclic antidepressants use-dependently block voltage-gated sodium channels, which may contribute to their antinociceptive effects (Fig. 3.7). While these results suggest that these channels are interesting targets for pharmacological therapies, the lack of specific agents with low affinity for sodium channels in other areas, such as the central nervous system and the heart, currently limits its clinical application.

Multiple mechanisms probably lead to changes in neuron excitability during inflammation. Neurons express receptors for many inflammatory mediators, such as prostaglandins, histamine and serotonin, which can activate intracellular second-messenger cascades that in turn change the properties of ion channels (Fig. 3.8). In addition, some of these mediators and growth factors change the expression of ion channels and other proteins, thus leading to long-lasting alterations in neuron properties. One of these factors is nerve growth factor (NGF), which increases in gastrointestinal inflammation in humans and in animal models of inflammatory diseases. NGF regulates the expression of ion channels and causes functional changes that are similar to those seen during inflammation. Blocking the effects of NGF with neutralizing antibodies blunts the development of visceral hypersensitivity, further supporting the role of this mediator in the development of pain syndromes.

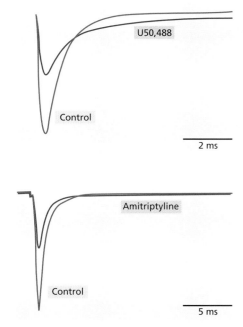

Fig. 3.7 Drugs used clinically affect inward, excitatory currents in visceral sensory neurons. Sample tracings show that the κ-opioid agonist U50,488 (10 μM) and the tricyclic antidepressant amitriptyline (10 μM) inhibit voltage-dependent sodium currents in visceral sensory neurons.

Serotonin and visceral hypersensitivity

As described above, 5-HT released from enteroendocrine cells plays an important role in activating sensory neurons. Mast cells are another potential source of 5-HT, as well as tryptase, histamine and other inflammatory mediators. Like enteroendocrine cells, mast cells are often found in close proximity to neurons. Enteroendocrine and mast cell numbers increase during inflammation and release more bioactive mediators. Interestingly, greater numbers of mast cells and enteroendocrine cells within the mucosa have also been reported in patients with functional bowel diseases. In experimental animals, inhibition of mast cell degranulation or administration of 5-HT receptor antagonists blunts responses to noxious visceral stimulation, supporting a possible role of this pathway in the sensitization of visceral afferents.

Despite these promising data, the contribution of 5-HT to human physiology and visceral pathophysiology is less clear. This is probably due to the multiple effects of 5-HT on different serotonin receptors at different sites within the body, including smooth muscle, intrinsic nerves, extrinsic afferents and various processing sites within the central nervous system. Moreover, few 5-HT agonists and antagonists are available that selectively act on one member of the seven distinct families of serotonin receptors, all of which contain several subtypes. The reuptake through specialized transport systems is important in terminating the effects of 5-HT. Many antidepressant drugs interfere with this process by blocking the specific transporter. However, serotonin reuptake inhibitors do not consistently affect visceral sensation in humans. Alosetron, a selective 5-HT_3 receptor antagonist, blunts the response to noxious colorectal distension in rats. While this agent showed some promise in women with diarrhea-predominant irritable bowel syndrome, concern about drug-induced ischemic colitis led to temporary removal of this agent from the US market. Tegaserod, a 5-HT_4 receptor agonist, has recently been approved for the treatment of patients with constipation-predominant irritable bowel syndrome. It enhances the peristaltic reflex and accelerates colonic transit. While it also blunts visceral sensation, this effect may be indirectly mediated by changes in muscle tone.

Central modulation of visceral sensation

Information flow through visceral afferent pathways is modulated by inhibitory and facilitating influences from higher centers within the brain. Stress affects these modulatory circuits and may alter responses to visceral stimulation. Acute and chronic stress or stressful life events during periods with high neuronal plasticity, such as early postnatal life, enhance reactions to visceral distension in experimental animals. The similarly enhanced startle response points to hypervigilance (increased responsiveness to a variety of stimuli independent of their nature or location), which may also contribute to symptoms in patients with functional bowel disease.

Conclusion

Visceral distension and other stimuli activate afferent pathways that are important in the regulation of

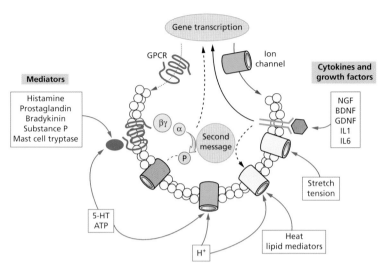

Fig. 3.8 Diagram of mechanisms of activation and sensitization of visceral sensory neurons. G protein-coupled receptors (GPCRs) and voltage/ligand-gated ion channels are synthesized in neurons and inserted into the cell membrane, where they are acted upon by extracellular and intracellular influences. Mediators such as bradykinin, substance P and serotonin (5-HT) act at bradykinin, neurokinin and 5-HT GPCRs (e.g. 5-HT4 receptors), respectively. In consequence, intracellular coupling of the heterotrimeric βγ and α G proteins activate second-messenger cascades that can lead to gene transcription and local activation of kinases and phosphorylation (P) of ion channels. For example, bradykinin phosphorylates the capsaicin receptor ion channel TRPV1. Ion channels that gate Na^+, K^+ and Ca^{2+} ions are activated by ATP (e.g. P2X receptors) protons (H^+), lipid mediators (e.g. HPETE), stretch/tension and 5-HT (e.g. 5-HT3 receptors). Finally, cytokines and growth factors acting at their receptors can influence gene transcription as well as modulate the activity of other receptors. When tissue is insulted, mediators, growth factors and cytokines in the extracellular environment increase in concentration, activate their respective receptors and contribute to processes of sensitization, typically associated with an increase in action potentials generated by a stimulus and a reduction in stimulus intensity to generate an action potential.

normal intestinal function and provide the basis for conscious sensation of visceral phenomena and pain. Convergence of different stimulus modalities from more than a single receptive field onto a second-order neuron in the central nervous system and divergence of that sensory information at the level of the spinal cord and higher centers contribute to the poor localization and discrimination of visceral stimuli. Both vagal and spinal pathways contribute to unpleasant visceral sensations, such as the pain, fullness and discomfort experienced by patients with organic and functional diseases of the gastrointestinal tract. Peripheral processes, such as inflammation, and central modulatory pathways can alter the function of visceral afferent inputs and contribute to the development of visceral hypersensitivity.

Selected references

1 Berthoud H-R, Lynn PA, Blackshaw LA. Vagal and spinal mechanosensors in the rat stomach and colon have multiple receptive fields. *Am J Physiol Regul Integr Comp Physiol* 2001; **280**: R1371–81.

2 Bielefeldt K, Ozaki N, Gebhart GF. Experimental ulcers alter voltage-sensitive sodium currents in rat gastric sensory neurons. *Gastroenterology* 2002; **122**: 394–405.

3 Gebhart GF, Kuner R, Jones RCW, Bielefeldt K. Visceral hypersensitivity. In: Handwerker HO, ed. *Hyperalgesia: Molecular Mechanisms and Clinical Implications*. Seattle (WA): IASP Press, 2004.

4 Grundy D. Speculations on the structure/function relationship for vagal and splanchnic afferent endings supplying the gastrointestinal tract. *J Autonom Nerv Syst* 1988; **22**: 175–80.

5 Hillsley K, Grundy D. Sensitivity to 5-hydroxytryptamine in different afferent subpopulations within mesenteric nerves supplying the rat jejunum. *J Physiol (Lond)* 1998; **509**: 717–27.

6 Holzer P. Sensory neurone responses to mucosal noxae in the upper gut: relevance to mucosal integrity and gastrointestinal pain. *Neurogastroenterol Mot* 2002; **14**: 459–75.

7 Kirkup AJ, Brunsden AM, Grundy D. Receptor and transmission in the brain–gut axis: potential for novel therapies. I. Receptors on visceral afferents. *Am J Physiol* 2001; **280**: G787–94.

8 Lamb K, Kang YM, Gebhart GF, Bielefeldt K. Gastric inflammation triggers hypersensitivity to acid in awake rats. *Gastroenterology* 2003; **126**: 1410–18.

9 Mayer EA, Collins SM. Evolving pathophysiologic models of functional gastrointestinal disorders. *Gastroenterology* 2002; **122**: 2032–48.

10 Ness TJ, Gebhart GF. Colorectal distension as a noxious visceral stimulus: physiologic and pharmacologic characterization of pseudaffective reflexes in the rat. *Brain Res* 1988; **450**: 153–69.

11 Ozaki N, Gebhart GF. Characterization of mechanosensitive splanchnic nerve afferent fibers innervating the rat stomach. *Am J Physiol* 2001; **281**: G1449–59.

12 Pan H, Gershon MD. Activation of intrinsic afferent pathways in submucosal ganglia of the guinea pig small intestine. *J Neurosci* 2000; **20**: 3295–309.

13 Sengupta JN, Gebhart GF. Mechanosensitive afferent fibers in the gastrointestinal and lower urinary tracts. In: Gebhart GF, ed. *Visceral Pain, Progress in Pain Research and Management*, Vol. 5. Seattle (WA): IASP Press, 1995: 75–98.

CHAPTER 4

Brain-to-Gut Signaling: Central Processing

Anthony R Hobson and Qasim Aziz

Introduction

The ability to dissociate the specific neurophysiological mechanisms of aberrant gastrointestinal sensory processing in patients with functional gastrointestinal disorders (FGID) has been the aspiration of an increasing number of gastrointestinal researchers. Improved access to state-of-the-art brain imaging techniques, previously the reserve of specialist neurology centers, has vastly increased our understanding of the central processing of gastrointestinal sensation and pain. In addition, the solid foundation based on this understanding of normal physiology has allowed us to investigate the effects that peripheral stimuli and psychological modulation have on central gastrointestinal sensory processing.

The predominant reason why FGID patients seek medical attention is chronic, episodic gastrointestinal pain. Heightened perception of gastrointestinal sensation (visceral hypersensitivity) is commonly observed in patients with FGID, and studies using mechanical and electrical stimulation have reproducibly demonstrated that these patients have lower gastrointestinal pain thresholds than healthy subjects.[1,2]

The pain experience is a multifaceted process that involves a complex interaction between sensory–discriminative, affective and cognitive dimensions.[3] Afferents capable of encoding a wide range of sensory events transmit information from the periphery to the brain. This input passes via the brainstem nuclei and midbrain structures to the cerebral cortex, where the activation of sensory–discriminative areas provides information about the site and intensity of sensation. Further processing occurs in limbic structures, allowing sensation to be judged in light of current physical and psychological context and the memories of similar past experiences. An emotional response is thus generated and cognitive judgments are made about coping with the sensation. Assessment of how this process becomes disturbed in FGID has led researchers to develop new techniques to investigate what has been called the visceral pain matrix.

Key points

1 While functional brain imaging studies have shown that there are many similarities between the cortical representation of somatic and visceral sensation/pain, the subtle differences demonstrated may help to explain some of the unique characteristics of visceral pain.

2 The visceral evoked potential allows an increase in the intensity of a reported sensation to be correlated with an objective, neurophysiological measure, thus reducing the inherent response bias commonly encountered in the clinical evaluation of visceral pain.

3 Understanding of the mechanisms of pain in functional gastrointestinal disorders will occur only if we use brain imaging as a complementary investigative tool in conjunction with psychological, physiological, pharmacological and biological profiling.

Positron emission tomography

Advantages
- PET has excellent spatial resolution (2–5 mm) and allows the operator to tag important biological molecules that bind to targeted receptor groups.

Disadvantages
- PET scanners are expensive and not readily available for most research groups.
- Subjects undergoing PET studies are exposed to a considerable dose of radiation, limiting serial studies.
- PET also has poor temporal resolution (1 minute) and requires group analysis from five or six subjects to obtain meaningful results.

Central representation of gastrointestinal sensory processing in health

There are important anatomical and physiological differences between the afferent innervations of the proximal and distal organs of the gastrointestinal tract. Proximal gut organs, such as the esophagus and duodenum, develop from the foregut and are innervated jointly by vagal and spinal afferents from the cervical and thoracic spinal cord segments.[4] In contrast, distal gut organs such as the rectum develop from the hindgut and are innervated solely by spinal afferents from the sacral spinal cord.[4] Despite these differences, electrophysiological studies in animals have shown convergence of afferent pathways from multiple visceral organs onto single cells in both the cortex and the thalamus.[5,6] Functional brain imaging has greatly enhanced our ability to evaluate gastrointestinal sensory-related cortical activity in

man. Techniques such as positron emission tomography (PET) and functional magnetic resonance imaging (fMRI) have allowed researchers to study the neuroanatomical representation of gastrointestinal sensory and pain processing, and the following section outlines our current understanding.

To date there have been approximately 30 studies of the processing by the brain of gastrointestinal sensation in health, and several studies have compared visceral and somatic stimuli. This was first demonstrated by stimulating the proximal (somatic) and distal (visceral) portions of the esophagus.[7] It suggested that, unlike somatic sensation, which has a strong homuncular representation in the primary somatosensory cortex (S1), visceral sensation is primarily represented in the secondary somatosensory cortex (S2), whereas representation in S1 is vague and potentially accounts for the poor localization of visceral sensation in comparison with somatic sensation.

Functional MRI

Advantages
- fMRI is totally non-invasive and is non-cumulative, allowing subjects to be studied many times.
- Single subjects may be studied with fMRI, although data are usually pooled.
- fMRI has comparable spatial resolution to PET, but fMRI has better temporal resolution, of approximately 1–3 seconds.

Disadvantages
- fMRI limits the use of ferromagnetic material inside the scanning environment.
- Limitations sometimes exist when imaging deeper brain structures, such as the brainstem and thalamus, due to pulsation artifacts.
- The fMRI environment is extremely noisy and claustrophobic in comparison with other techniques, which can have an effect when studying cognitive paradigms or when using a naive patient population.
- fMRI is limited to activation studies, giving no information regarding resting state, neurotransmitters or receptors.

However, in a manner similar to that of somatic sensation, visceral sensation is represented in the paralimbic and limbic structures, such as the insular, anterior cingulate and prefrontal cortices.[7] These areas are likely to mediate the affective and cognitive components of visceral sensation. A recent meta-analysis of these studies revealed that the esophagus is represented in all of the major cortical pain regions (S1, S2, insula and cingulate) in addition to the prefrontal cortex and motor cortex.[8]

In a further study, Strigo and colleagues compared cortical activity generated by distension of the esophagus and by thermal stimulation of the anterior chest wall.[9] Using psychophysical measures, the two stimuli were matched for intensity. However, esophageal stimulation was perceived to be more unpleasant than cutaneous stimulation. The major differences in cortical representation occurred in S1, the insula and the prefrontal cortex. Interestingly, both esophageal and chest wall stimulation activated S1 in the region associated with the homuncular representation of the trunk. However, esophageal stimulation alone activated the more lateral aspects of S1, often referred to as the gustatory cortex. The authors concluded that this diffuse representation of the esophagus in S1 was consistent with the fact that visceral pain can be referred to the skin but not vice versa.

An initially unexpected finding in this study revealed greater activation of the anterior portion of the insula (AI) to chest wall stimulation when compared to esophageal distension. Previous studies have shown bilateral activation of the AI to be the most consistent finding across all esophageal neuroimaging studies and this area plays an important role in the emotional modulation of esophageal sensory processing.[10] However, AI is also strongly activated by thermal stimulation and the differences seen here may merely reflect the fact that a higher number of somatic thermosensitive neurons are present in this region when compared with visceral specific neurons. Both visceral and somatic stimuli produced bilateral activation of the posterior insula, which is known to process somesthetic sensation, providing further evidence for the convergence of visceral and somatic pain processing. In summary, metabolic neuroimaging studies have revealed that esophageal sensation and pain are processed in a manner broadly similar to somatic pain processing, the main differences occurring in primary somatosensory and some limbic regions.

fMRI has also been used to study the cortical representation of anorectal stimulation. In a study by Hobday and colleagues,[11] rectal (visceral) stimulation resulted in bilateral activation of the inferior primary somatosensory, secondary somatosensory, sensory association, insular, peri-orbital, anterior cingulate and prefrontal cortices. Anal (somatic) canal stimulation resulted in activation of areas similar to those activated by rectal stimulation, but the primary somatosensory cortex was activated at a more superior level, and there was no anterior cingulate activation.[11]

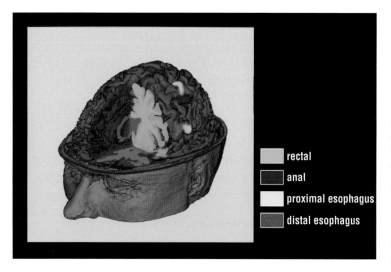

rectal
anal
proximal esophagus
distal esophagus

Fig. 4.1 A representation of somatic and visceral structures within the somatosensory cortex. While the visceral regions (distal esophagus and rectum) are represented in the lateral portion of S1, somatic regions (proximal esophagus and anal canal) are represented more medially. These images are taken from group functional MRI studies in eight healthy subjects after non-painful balloon distension.

This study concluded that anal and rectal sensation resulted in a similar pattern of cortical activation, including areas involved with spatial discrimination, attention and affect. The differences in sensory perception from these two regions could be explained by their different representations in the primary somatosensory cortex. The fact that the anterior cingulate cortex was activated only by rectal stimulation suggests that the viscera may have a greater representation on the limbic cortex than somatic structures. This may help to explain the greater autonomic responses evoked by visceral sensation than by somatic sensation.[11] Figure 4.1 shows a differential representation of somatic and visceral structures in S1.

Activation of subcortical regions such as the thalamus and periaqueductal gray in response to gastrointestinal stimulation has been demonstrated in approximately 50% of brain imaging studies,[8] predominantly in response to rectal distension. While the spatial resolution of these imaging techniques is insufficient for specific thalamic nuclei to be discerned, several authors have suggested that the ventroposterior lateral nucleus is the most commonly activated thalamic region.

Despite being few in number, these studies show relatively good concordance, giving us confidence that they are an accurate representation of gastrointestinal sensory processing. While there are many similarities between the cortical representation of somatic and visceral sensation/pain, the subtle differences demonstrated may help to explain some of the unique characteristics of visceral pain.

Temporal dynamics of gastrointestinal sensory processing in health

While PET and fMRI have revealed many salient features of pain processing, these techniques do not have sufficient temporal resolution to map cortical activity as it changes dynamically on a millisecond-by-millisecond basis. This is extremely important as different components of pain processing occur in different temporal time windows.[12] Therefore, identifying the sequence of activation of cortical structures within the visceral pain matrix would not only give us important information regarding the central conduction of the visceral pain pathways but also allow us to dissociate the functional relevance of specific cortical regions in the temporally distinct stages of pain processing.

Magnetoencephalography (MEG) is a non-invasive brain imaging tool that allows us to detect cortical neuromagnetic activity. The spatial resolution of MEG is comparable to those of PET and fMRI. However, it also has millisecond temporal resolution and can be used to study both group and individual data.[13] There have only been four MEG studies to date that have recorded cortical activity during experimental visceral sensation and pain.[23-27] These studies showed that activity in S1 and S2/posterior insula occurred approximately 70–190 ms after esophageal stimulation. Due to limitations in previous MEG analysis techniques, further information regarding other cortical structures was not reported.

Magnetoencephalography

Advantages
- Directly measures neuronal activity as opposed to metabolic changes, which are secondary to neural activity.
- Has a temporal resolution of milliseconds and is totally non-invasive.
- Studies take place in a quiet and pleasant environment.

Disadvantages
- MEG is not widely available, systems being present only in specialist centers.
- MEG is generally not sensitive to deep, subcortical sources.
- The exquisite sensitivity of the MEG sensors places some limitations on the equipment used to generate stimuli.
- An anatomical magnetic resonance scan is needed for each subject in order to co-register functional data, which adds to the expense of the procedure.

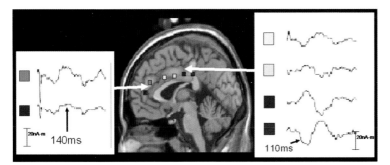

Fig. 4.2 Activation of the cingulate cortex in a healthy female subject after 50 painful electrical esophageal stimulations. The tomographic image in the center was generated using SPM99. In order to extract the temporal sequence of activation, virtual electrodes (represented by colored squares) were placed in the cingulate cortex and signal averaging was performed so that the evoked response was generated. This showed that activity occurred earlier (110 ms) in the mid-anterior cingulate than in the perigenual portion (140 ms). This may reflect the fact that these regions process different aspects of the pain experience.

We have recently used a new MEG analysis technique, synthetic aperture magnetometry (SAM), which allows us to record neural activity throughout the cortex. These data reveal that, following painful esophageal stimulation, activation first occurs in parallel within S1/S2/posterior insula approximately 80 ms after a stimulus. Activity is then seen in the mid-anterior cingulate (96 ms), followed by perigenual cingulate and anterior insula (115 ms). This temporal delay in processing esophageal pain in different cortical regions is consistent with the role of these areas in processing different aspects of the pain experience. Figure 4.2 shows the temporal sequence of activation within different regions of the cingulate cortex in one female subject.

Electrophysiological evaluation of visceral pain

While MEG is unlikely to become a widespread clinical tool (there is currently only one system in the UK), it has an additional advantage in that the recorded signal represents the magnetic component of the electromagnetic field generated by active cortical neurons. The electrical component can be recorded from the scalp using a simple electrophysiological technique known

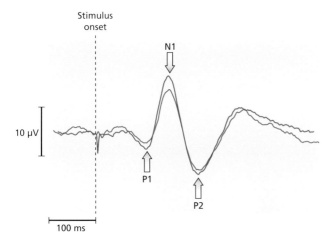

Fig. 4.3 A representative esophageal evoked response in a healthy male subject. The response was obtained after 200 non-painful esophageal electrical stimuli, acquired in four runs of 50 stimuli. After acquisition, signal averaging was performed to obtain the evoked response. A second trace is superimposed to demonstrate reproducibility.

as evoked potential (EP) recording. Therefore, extrapolation of the MEG data to the EP data would allow us to identify the cortical regions involved in the generation of each EP component. Development of EP for use in FGID has several advantages as the equipment required is cheap (less than £10 000), available in the majority of UK hospitals and can be used on individual patients, so there is no need to rely on group data.

The first EP responses to stimulation of the gastrointestinal tract were recorded by Frieling and colleagues 1989.[23] Since then, researchers have endeavored to establish the feasibility and reproducibility of visceral EP recordings. Subsequently, it has been shown that EP can be recorded in response to stimulation of virtually all regions of the gastrointestinal tract. Figure 4.3 shows a typical esophageal EP in response to electrical stimulation in one male subject. The response has been repeated on a second occasion to demonstrate reproducibility.

In addition, recent studies have shown that the characteristics of visceral EP correspond to known physiological differences in their innervation and function. For instance, despite the rectum lying distal to the esophagus, the latency of the rectal EP components is shorter and the response is elicited at significantly lower stimulation intensities. This is entirely in keeping with the role of the rectum as a sensory organ, with the rich afferent innervation that is essential for the maintenance of continence, while conscious sensations rarely arise from the esophagus.

One of the major reasons for developing visceral EP has been to develop an objective measure of visceral sensation. In order to address this question, several groups examined the effects of increasing the stimulation intensity on the amplitude and latency of the visceral EP components. These studies have shown that, as stimulation intensity and sensory perception increases, there is an associated reduction in the latency and an

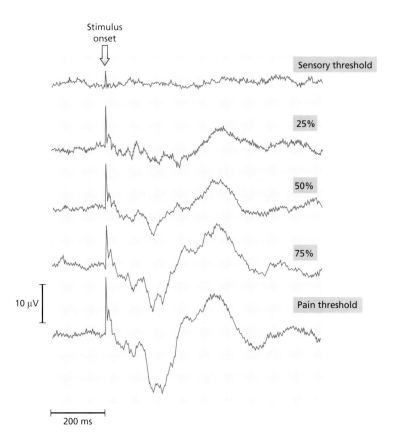

Fig. 4.4 Effect of increasing stimulation intensity on the rectal evoked response. Each trace represents the averaged response to 200 electrical stimuli at five intensities ranging from sensory threshold through to pain. It can be seen that at sensory threshold the response is not easily discernible from the background brain activity. However, as the stimulation intensity increases, the latency of the evoked potential components declines and their amplitude increases. This allows us to objectively correlate perceived sensations with neurophysiological measures. This trace was obtained from a single healthy female subject.

increase in amplitude of the EP components (Fig. 4.4). This phenomenon is common across all evoked potential modalities and reflects the recruitment of an increasing number of afferents. Visceral EP therefore allows an increase in the reported sensation to be correlated with an objective, neurophysiological measure, thus reducing the inherent response bias commonly encountered in the clinical evaluation of visceral pain. An example of these stimulus–response characteristics can be seen in Fig. 4.4, which shows EP recorded after electrical stimulation of the rectum.

MEG data reveal that the early component of the esophageal EP response (P1) relates to activation of brain regions involved in the sensory discriminatory aspect of pain processing. The later components (N1, P2) reflect an amalgamation of cortical activity in regions that process both the sensory–discriminatory and the cognitive/affective aspects of pain processing. It is this activity which is related to the secondary processing of esophageal sensation.

Proposed mechanisms of visceral hypersensitivity in FGID

Several hypotheses have been put forward about the mechanisms of visceral hypersensitivity in FGID. The first is that gut primary afferents become sensitized (peripheral sensitization) after an acute inflammatory or infectious episode. Evidence to support this comes from studies which have shown that, while treatment of these conditions can appear successful, many patients develop prolonged symptoms of pain after the original insult has passed.[14] New techniques are available to study these processes in biopsies taken from patients with chronic visceral hypersensitivity states without evidence of overt inflammation, and have shown demonstrable changes indicative of peripheral sensitization.[15] Therefore, peripheral sensitization may also contribute to visceral hypersensitivity in FGID.

A secondary consequence of peripheral sensitization is the development of an area of hypersensitivity in the surrounding uninjured tissue. This phenomenon is due to changes in the activity of spinal afferents and is called 'central sensitization'. Central sensitization is sustained by the phosphorylation of N-methyl-D-aspartate (NMDA) receptors expressed in dorsal horn neurons. This leads to an increase in the excitability and the receptive fields of the spinal neurons, and results in recruitment and amplification of both non-nociceptive and nociceptive inputs from the adjacent healthy tissue.[16]

We have recently developed an esophageal model of central sensitization, which has shown that infusion of hydrochloric acid (0.15 M for 30 minutes) into the distal esophagus can induce a prolonged reduction in pain threshold in the proximal, non-acid exposed esophagus. We have also shown that this response is exaggerated in patients with non-cardiac chest pain,[17] and that acid infusion into the duodenum can also lead to reproducible reductions in esophageal pain thresholds. Taken together, these findings provide compelling evidence that central sensitization plays an important role in the generation of visceral hypersensitivity.

The affective dimension of pain combines the degree of unpleasantness perceived with the emotions and cognitive appraisals associated with its present and future implications. It has long been recognized that the cognitive modulation of pain can have dramatic effects on its perception. In FGID, a high incidence (50–80%) of psychological disorders, such as heightened anxiety, depression, somatization, dysthymia and panic disorders, has been reported.[18]

The role that attentional state plays in modifying pain is the psychological variable that has been studied most commonly. Experiments have shown that pain is perceived as less intense when we are distracted from it and, in most cases, more intense when we focus our attention upon it. In FGID, it has been shown that patients often selectively attend to sensations that arise from the gut and it has been shown that this is an important factor in sustaining symptoms. Reasons why these patients selectively attend to gut sensations include factors such as exposure to family illness. The anxiety associated with disease attribution will in turn increase levels of arousal and attention, and this has been shown to result in a greater awareness and poorer tolerance of both experimental and endogenous gut sensations.[19]

Evidence from neuroimaging

Using the neuroscience tools described in earlier sections, several groups have embarked on studies aimed at modulating normal gastrointestinal sensory processing in health and comparing patterns of cortical activity in normal subjects and subjects with FGID. The following sections outline these findings.

The sensitization hypothesis

In our esophageal model of central sensitization, we demonstrated that pain thresholds declined for up to 5 hours after acid infusion. However, these data relied on subjective reporting of pain, and we were keen to demonstrate objective evidence for changes in the sensitivity of the central visceral afferent pathway. In order to achieve this, we recorded proximal esophageal EP before and after acid infusion of the distal esophagus. These studies revealed that, despite using the same intensity of stimulation throughout the study, the latency of the esophageal EP components reduced after acid, indicating potentiation of the response. This change in the sensitivity of the central afferent pathways provides further evidence that peripheral and central sensitization contributes to the development of visceral hypersensitivity and may be important mechanisms in FGID.

A recent study using fMRI in patients with irritable bowel syndrome lends further credence to this hypothesis. In this study, subjects received painful and non-painful stimulation of both the rectum (distension) and the foot (thermal). Comparison of group activation in FGID and control subjects revealed increased activity throughout the pain matrix in response to all stimuli in FGID. As increased activity was seen in regions that process both the sensory discriminatory aspects of pain processing (somatosensory cortex and thalamus) as well as in regions that process the cognitive and affective components (insula, anterior and posterior cingulate, prefrontal cortex), the authors proposed that this provided evidence that central afferent transmission was enhanced in FGID.[20] It was suggested that two major mechanisms may contribute to this enhanced nociceptive input from ascending spinal pathways. The first would be that tonic nociceptive input from the bowel may lead to sensitization of spinal dorsal horn neurons (central sensitization). The second would be that descending facilitation from 'on-cell' activity in the rostral ventromedial medulla region of the brainstem may also contribute.

Descending modulation of spinal afferent transmission via brainstem activity can be both facilitatory and inhibitory. Animal studies have shown that peripheral inflammatory events engage two concurrent but opposing descending modulatory systems.[21] This activity is mediated by the periaqueductal gray and rostral ventromedial medulla, with the excitatory component mediated via activation of NMDA receptors and the production of nitric oxide, while the inhibitory system is mediated via non-NMDA receptors.[21] It has been postulated that these systems interact with each other and that the difference in activity between the two determines the magnitude of hyperalgesia which develops. An imbalance in this descending modulatory system may well be a credible mechanism by which visceral hyperalgesia develops and is maintained. Further studies are required to investigate these possibilities with high-field fMRI techniques. In summary, there is now a growing body of evidence to suggest that the sensitization of gastrointestinal afferents is an important mechanism in the generation of visceral hypersensitivity.

The psychological hypothesis

Negative mood states, such as fear and sadness, are often associated with abnormal sensory perception, such as abdominal pain. In this study we examined the effects of negative emotional context on the perception of visceral sensations. It has been demonstrated that human facial expressions (considered to be the primary means of conveying emotional valence regarding a particular situation) depicting different emotions activate different brain neuronal networks. We therefore employed fearful and neutral facial expressions from a standardized series to provide negative and neutral emotional contexts, respectively, while healthy subjects experienced phasic, non-painful esophageal stimulation. We then compared the brain activation patterns using fMRI.[10]

These studies revealed that activation within the right insular and bilateral dorsal anterior cingulate cortex was significantly greater during esophageal stimulation with fearful rather than neutral facial expressions. These changes also correlated with behavioral ratings for increases in anxiety and discomfort, providing evidence for the modulation of neural responses and perceived discomfort during non-painful visceral stimulation by negative emotional context. These findings support the role of negative emotions as a mechanism of altered pain perception in functional gastrointestinal pain disorders.

Several studies in FGID have shown abnormal patterns of activation in limbic structures. This has shown increased activation in some studies, but decreased activation has also been demonstrated (for a review see Derbyshire, 2003).[8] This wide range of results probably reflects the heterogeneity of the FGID population and problems in the experimental design. For instance, the mid-anterior cingulate cortex is known to be important in sustained attention.[22] Therefore, in an anxious patient population it is feasible that this region may be activated in both control and stimulation conditions. Thus, subsequent subtraction of the images may indicate no activation in this region. This outlines one of the many pitfalls that researchers may encounter when using functional brain imaging in groups of FGID patients.

To date, functional imaging studies have shown only subtle differences in small groups of patients and controls, and these findings are yet to be of any pathophysiological significance. Current results are observations only and studies are largely hypothesis-generating rather than hypothesis-testing. Factors such as the variation in individual psychological circumstances have yet to be taken into account, and the normal variation in the brain activation patterns on repeated testing has not yet been identified in healthy subjects. In summary, we are still at a very early point in the development of functional brain imaging for FGID. It is clear that experimental paradigms targeted at investigating specific components of the cognitive and affective aspects of pain processing will yield results which provide more conclusive evidence of the importance of psychological factors in FGID.

Future directions

While great advances have been made over the last decade in our understanding of the central processing of gastrointestinal sensation, the time has arrived to develop pathophysiological models based on these findings in order to tease out the role of psychological factors and central sensitization. This will require a multidisciplinary approach combining information regarding the biological markers of peripheral sensitization, physiological/neurophysiological profiling and psychological/psychiatric assessment. Tests need to be developed that are sufficiently robust to study individual patients so that the novel visceral analgesic and anti-hyperalgesic compounds currently in development may be targeted to the specific mechanism of visceral hypersensitivity. This approach will have great benefits both for the well-being of patients and for health-care utilization in the future.

References

1   Chang L, Mayer EA, Johnson T, FitzGerald LZ, Naliboff B. Differences in somatic perception in female patients with irritable bowel syndrome with and without fibromyalgia. *Pain* 2000; **84**: 297–307.

2   Mayer EA, Collins SM. Evolving pathophysiologic models of functional gastrointestinal disorders. *Gastroenterology* 2002; **122**: 2032–48.

3   Price DD. Psychological and neural mechanisms of the affective dimension of pain. *Science* 2000; **288**: 1769–72.

4   Ness TJ, Gebhart GF. Visceral pain: a review of experimental studies. *Pain* 1990; **41**: 167–234.

5   Bruggemann J, Shi T, Apkarian AV. Viscero-somatic neurons in the primary somatosensory cortex (SI) of the squirrel monkey. *Brain Res* 1997; **756**: 297–300.

6   Bruggemann J, Shi T, Apkarian AV. Viscerosomatic interactions in the thalamic ventral posterolateral nucleus (VPL) of the squirrel monkey. *Brain Res* 1998; **787**: 269–76.

7   Aziz Q, Thompson DG, Ng VW *et al.* Cortical processing of human somatic and visceral sensation. *J Neurosci* 2000; **20**: 2657–63.

8   Derbyshire SW. A systematic review of neuroimaging data during visceral stimulation. *Am J Gastroenterol* 2003; **98**: 12–20.

9   Strigo I, Duncan G, Boivin M, Bushnell MC. Differentiation of visceral and cutaneous pain in the human brain. *J Neurophysiol* 2003; **89**: 3294–303.

10 Phillips ML, Gregory LJ, Cullen S *et al.* The effect of negative emotional context on neural and behavioural responses to oesophageal stimulation. *Brain* 2003; **126**: 669–84.

11 Hobday DI, Aziz Q, Thacker N, Hollander I, Jackson A, Thompson DG. A study of the cortical processing of anorectal sensation using functional MRI. *Brain* 2001; **124**: 361–8.

12 Bromm B, Lorenz J. Neurophysiological evaluation of pain. *Electroencephalogr Clin Neurophysiol* 1998; **107**: 227–53.

13 Vrba J, Robinson SE. Signal processing in magnetoencephalography. *Methods* 2001; **25**: 249–71.

14 Gwee KA, Leong YL, Graham C *et al.* The role of psychological and biological factors in postinfective gut dysfunction.

Gut 1999; **44**: 400–6.

15 Lowe EM, Anand P, Terenghi G, Williams-Chestnut RE, Sinicropi DV, Osborne JL. Increased nerve growth factor levels in the urinary bladder of women with idiopathic sensory urgency and interstitial cystitis. *Br J Urol* 1997; **79**: 572–7.

16 Woolf CJ, Salter MW. Neuronal plasticity: increasing the gain in pain. *Science* 2000; **288**: 1765–9.

17 Sarkar S, Aziz Q, Woolf CJ, Hobson AR, Thompson DG. Contribution of central sensitisation to the development of non-cardiac chest pain. *Lancet* 2000; **356**: 1154–9.

18 Creed F. Irritable bowel or irritable mind? Psychological treatment is essential for some. *BMJ* 1994; **309**: 1647–8.

19 Whitehead WE, Palsson OS. Is rectal pain sensitivity a biological marker for irritable bowel syndrome: psychological influences on pain perception. *Gastroenterology* 1998; **115**: 1263–71.

20 Verne GN, Himes NC, Robinson ME *et al.* Central representation of visceral and cutaneous hypersensitivity in the irritable bowel syndrome. *Pain* 2003; **103**: 99–110.

21 Coutinho S, Gebhart G. Descending modulation of visceral hyperalgesia. In: Holtmann G, Talley NJ, eds. *Gastrointestinal Inflammation and Disturbed Gut Function: The Challenge of New Concepts.* London: Kluwer Academic, 2003: 213–19.

22 Peyron R, Laurent B, Garcia-Larrea L. Functional imaging of brain responses to pain. A review and meta-analysis (2000). *Neurophysiol Clin* 2000; **30**: 263–88.

23 Frieling T, Enck P, Wienbeck M. Cerebral responses evoked by electrical stimulation of the esophagus in normal subjects. *Gastroenterology* 1989; **97**: 475–8.

24 Furlong PL, Aziz Q, Singh KD, Thompson DG, Hobson A, Harding GF. Cortical localisation of magnetic fields evoked by oesophageal distension. *Electroencephalogr Clin Neurophysiol* 1998; **108**: 234–43.

25 Hecht M, Kober H, Claus D, Hilz M, Vieth J, Neundorfer B. The electrical and magnetical cerebral responses evoked by electrical stimulation of the esophagus and the location of their cerebral sources. *Clin Neurophysiol* 1999; **110**: 1435–44.

26 Loose R, Schnitzler A, Sarkar S *et al.* Cortical activation during mechanical oesophagus stimulation: a neuromagnetic study. *Gastroenterology* 1997: A779.

27 Schnitzler A, Volkmann J, Enck P, Frieling T, Witte OW, Freund HJ. Different cortical organization of visceral and somatic sensation in humans. *Eur J Neurosci* 1999; **11**: 305–15.

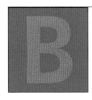

Mechanisms of Functional GI Disorders

CHAPTER 5

Developmental Disorders

Virpi V Smith and Peter J Milla

Introduction

Developmental disorders of the enteric nervous system (ENS) clinically present with signs of intestinal obstruction without mechanical occlusion of the gut usually in neonatal life or with constipation in infancy or later childhood.[1,2,3] The abnormalities may be confined to a variable length of the distal intestine or may affect the entire gastrointestinal tract. The child may also present with difficulty in swallowing and abnormalities in the esophagus without intestinal involvement.

The mature ENS is composed of neural plexuses situated in the submucosa (submucosal plexus) and between the layers of the muscularis propria (myenteric plexus of Auerbach). The submucosal plexus provides innervation to the mucosa and is involved in secretion and sensation, whereas the myenteric plexus is responsible for providing motor innervation to the muscle coats and the submucosal plexus.[4] These plexuses are referred to as the 'little brain' since they are capable of functioning independently from the 'big' brain, but they do communicate with each other and

the autonomic ganglia via the parasympathetic and sympathetic nerves, and ultimately with the brain.[5] The ganglia comprise neurons, glia and terminal bundles of nerve fibers and morphologically resemble the structure of the brain rather than the autonomic ganglia. There are more neurons in the ENS than in the spinal cord and the numbers of glial cells are greater than those of neurons.[4] Neuronal density varies from region to region of the gut.[6] The neurons in the ganglia consist of inhibitory and excitatory motor neurons and interneurons, which share a variety of neurotransmitters, all of which are found in the brain. Throughout the gastrointestinal tract there are also non-neural cells derived from the mesenchyme – the interstitial cells of Cajal, which generate and propagate slow waves.[7] The interstitial cells are important modulators of communication between nerves and muscle. The ENS is particularly concerned with the propulsion of the gut contents in an ordered, physiologically effective fashion and the control of secretion by the gut. In this chapter, the development of the ENS and known developmental defects will be discussed.

Key points

1 Development of the gut is controlled by homeobox (*Hox*) genes.

2 Expression of these genes is coordinated in time and space.

3 Knockouts of genes induce specific disorders of development.

4 Development of the enteric nervous system involves migration of neural crest cells into the developing gut.

5 Among the key genes are *Sox10* and *Hox B5*; expression of the tyrosine kinase receptor c-ret is also of critical importance.

6 Absence of c-ret or its ligand gdnf is associated with reduced numbers of enteric neurons.

7 Defects in chromosome 10q 11.2, which specifies the *RET* gene, are found in Hirschsprung's disease.

Normal development of the ENS

The gastrointestinal tract first appears at 4 weeks of gestation as a tube of stratified epithelium which extends from the mouth to the cloaca. Three major phases of development occur in the human gastrointestinal tract:[8]

- an early period of proliferation and morphogenesis
- an intermediate period of differentiation when many different and distinctive cell types appear
- a later period of maturation resulting in a bowel capable of transporting luminal contents and digesting and absorbing nutrients.

Three fundamental processes can be defined in the development of the gut from its primitive origins:

- regionalization of the gut tube along the anterior–posterior axis to form the foregut (esophagus, stomach, proximal duodenum, liver and pancreas), the prececal gut (small intestine) and postcecal gut (colon)
- radial patterning of the tube to achieve proper placement of the functional components of the gut, such as epithelium, nerve plexuses and muscle layers
- continuous self-renewal of the epithelium from stem cells or enteroblasts, which continues throughout life.

The structure and function of the gut result from a complex interplay between various cell types and components, which are regulated by growth factors and hormones together with immune and neural inputs. The gut develops from three germ layers: (i) the endoderm, which supplies the epithelial cells of the mucosa; (ii) the splanchnic mesoderm, which supplied the mesenchymal cell types, such as the muscle layers; and (iii) the ectoderm, the origin of the neural components.[8] In recent years, the importance of the formation of endodermal mesenchymal cell assemblages in generating form and in the cytodifferentiation of the mucosa has been appreciated,[9] as has the establishment of the intrinsic nervous system of the gut by neural crest cell migration and differentiation.[10] In the formation of the mucosa and the enteric neuromusculature, adhesive and other interactions between cells and the extracellular microenvironment are crucial. The extracellular microenvironment consists of a labile and developmentally regulated group of interacting molecules. Some of these will be located at the interface between endodermally and mesenchymally derived cells, where they are capable of directing specific cell behavior. Another group of interacting molecules are found associated with the extracellular matrix of the muscle coats of the gut, and are implicated in morphogenetic steps in the migration, homing and differentiation of both neural cells and smooth muscle cells. The development control mechanisms required for these processes are now beginning to be elucidated.

Developmental control regulatory genes

The above processes are controlled by a number of genes known as developmental control regulatory genes, which coordinate the control of many other genes at the transcriptional level. Genes which all contain the motif TAAT in their structure, known as homeobox genes, control these processes. *Hox* genes are particularly important in regionalization of the gut and Hedgehog signaling is important in endoderm–mesenchyme interaction.

Homeobox genes are a group of developmental control genes implicated in the positioning and patterning of organs in the embryo. These evolutionarily conserved genes encode transcription factors which self-regulate their own transcription or the transcription of other downstream effector genes in developing embryos ranging from *Drosophila* to humans. A group of genes which has been extensively studied is the antennapedia class of homeobox genes, the so-called *Hox* genes. *Hox* genes are evolutionarily highly conserved and derived from a common ancestral cluster, and are organized into four clusters, A, B, C and D, on four separate chromosomes in mammals. They comprise some 38 genes in total.[11] The genes are numbered 1 to 13 by virtue of their 3′ to 5′ position along each chromosome, the lowest number being at the 3′ prime end and the highest number at the 5′ end. A given gene may have up to three related genes in equivalent positions on the other three clusters, and the genes in such a group have sequence homology with each other and form a so-called paralogous group.[12] Such paralogues can display equivalent expression domains and may therefore have common functions during development, resulting in some functional redundancy. It is significant that *Hox* genes are expressed in precise patterns during early embryogenesis, particularly during critical periods of fate specification within a given morphogenetic field, such as a limb. The expression domains of the various groups overlap to differing extents within any particular field, leading to the concept that *Hox* genes have a combinatorial mode of action.[13] Along the body axis, these genes are generally expressed with discrete rostral cut-offs which coincide with either existing or emergent anatomical landmarks. It has therefore been suggested that they serve to specify component parts of the vertebrate body plan. This is particularly clear in segmented structures such as the branchial arches and the vertebral column.[14] Significantly, at least in these structures, the rostrocaudal sequence of the cut-offs map quite precisely with the 3′ to 5′ sequence of *Hox* genes within their respective cluster and with the order in which these genes are expressed. This phenomenon is known as spatial and temporal colinearity.[15] However, it is also clear that non-overtly segmented structures, such as limbs and internal organs, are also specified by *Hox* genes, and thus *Hox* genes could be upstream regulatory genes for the morphogenesis of the embryonal gut, and for the migration and maturation of neural crest cells and possibly splanchnic mesoderm.

Hox genes from the 5′ paralogous groups 12 and 13 are known to be involved in patterning of the hindgut.[16] *Hox* genes from paralogous groups 4 and 5 seem to be particularly good candidates for regulators of gut neuromusculature, for at least the foregut and midgut, since they are expressed in the developing hindbrain at the level of rhombomeres 6–8, from where a proportion of vagal neural crest cells migrate through the branchial arches into the intestine and differentiate into enteric ganglia.[17] In segmented structures such as the branchial arches, the branchial *Hox* code defined by the patterns of combinatorial *Hox* gene expression has been interpreted as a developmental strategy whereby positional specification made axially within the neural tube is transmitted to the periphery via the migrating neural crest, and is seen as an integral part of the mechanisms whereby the embryo develops an organ such as a head and face or a gut.[18]

Preliminary data on the expression of 3′ *Hox* genes in the gut of developing mouse embryos along the length of the gut primordium shows nested expression domains.[19]

Further studies delineated different spatial, temporal and combinatorial expression patterns in different morphological regions: foregut; prececal gut; cecum; and postcecal gut.[20] Two dynamic gradients, rostral and caudal, were coordinated with nested expression domains along the gut primordium. Region-specific domains were present in the stomach and cecum. The *Hox* gene transcripts in the mesoderm of the gut primordium were spatially colocalized to the same layer of outer mesoderm clearly preferred by migrating neural crest cells and the developing intestinal muscle coats. It was of particular interest that, in the postcecal gut, the appearance of enteric neuronal precursors was clearly preceded by the early presence of *Hox D4*, *C4* and *C5* transcripts in this region of the gut primordium between E9.75 and E12.5. This important study shows that specific spatial and temporal combinations of *Hox* genes are involved in the control of morphogenesis of the gut and that they are expressed in the form of an enteric *Hox* code.[20] The code provides correct positional information for migratory cells and for a permissive environment, the differentiation of developing tissues – particularly for the developing enteric neuromusculature. A few isolated observations of transgenic mouse models also suggest that *Hox* genes do indeed play an important role in gut morphogenesis. A transgenic knockout of *Enx*, *Hox 11L*[21] causes increased innervation of the hindgut and overexpression of *Hox A4* is associated with a megacolon.[22] Destruction of *Hox C4* severely affects the morphology of esophageal smooth muscle, while knockout of *Hox D13* affects anal sphincters.[23] It is clear that this family of genes is of importance within the genetic hierarchy of gut morphogenesis, and the delineation of the genes that constitute the human gut *Hox* code and of their spatiotemporal patterns of expression is an essential and integral part of understanding the molecular events underlying gut dysmorphogenesis in humans (Figs 5.1 and 5.2).

Although a number of critical molecules in the morphogenesis of the gut have been identified, it is still unclear how the embryonic gut tube is regionalized at the molecular level. It is very likely that it involves complex interactions between *Hox* genes and other transcription factors, such as *Parahox* genes (e.g. *Pdx1* and *Cdx*) and unclustered genes such as *Sox*, *Enx* and *Nkx*. A recent study has also involved the Hedgehog family

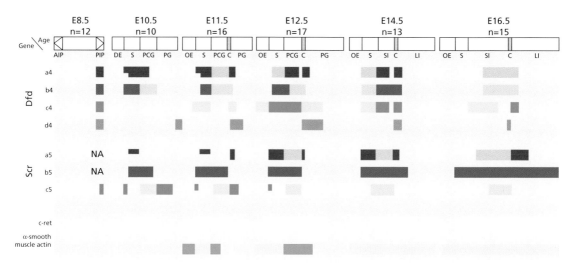

Fig. 5.1 Expression of *Hox* genes during the development of the gut from embryonal day 8.5–16.5. From *Gastroenterology* 1999;**117**:1341 (Pitera *et al.*). Redrawn with permission from *Gastroenterology*.

of cell signals, which are expressed in gut endoderm but have their target genes in the mesenchymal layers. Mice mutant for *Sonic Hedgehog* and *Indian Hedgehog* show abnormalities of muscle, nerve, epithelium and pancreas. Morphogenic abnormalities, including imperforate anus and malrotation, also occur.[24] How or whether these morphogen signaling molecules interact with *Hox* and other homeobox genes is at present not clear, but *Sonic Hedgehog* misexpression leads to ectopic *Hox d13* expression in the chick hindgut.[25]

Endodermal–mesenchymal interactions

Cell signaling events between the endodermal (epithelium) and mesenchymal layers are thought to play a major role in the coordination of the fundamental processes listed above.[26] Each of the intestinal endodermal and mesenchymal tissue components exerts an effect on the development of its associated counterparts and the contacts required to allow expression of the reciprocal permissive interaction.[27]

Cell interactions between embryonic endoderm and stromal cells (mesenchyme) are a prerequisite for intestinal morphogenesis and differentiation. Observations of the interactions between epithelial and mesenchymal cells may have important implications for the development of nerves and muscle layers of the gut, where similar interactions between neural crest cells and the mesenchyme have been observed in the developing enteric neuromusculature.

Development of the enteric nervous system

It has been known since the 1950s, following a series of *in ovo* microsurgical ablations of the dorsal neural primordium of chick embryos, that the ENS arises from the neural crest.[28] The neural crest arises on the dorsal midline as part of the neural tube, which later goes on to form the central nervous system. The neural crest gives rise to enteric neurons and their support cells, pigment cells and sympathetic nervous tissue, together with the adrenal medulla. More recently, much smaller-scale ablations have suggested that the neural crest between somites 3 and 5 is particularly important for ENS development.[29] The use of cell labeling techniques in chicken quail chimeric embryos by Le Douarin[10] confirmed that the enteric neurons arise from the vagal neural crest and that they colonize the gut in a rostrocaudal migration. However, some neural crest cells appeared to arrive in the hindgut from the lumbosacral level via a caudorostral wave of colonization. More recent studies in mice confirm these avian findings that the gut is colonized largely by vagal neural crest cells, but that some cells in the hindgut appear to have a lumbar–sacral origin.[30,31] The most recent of

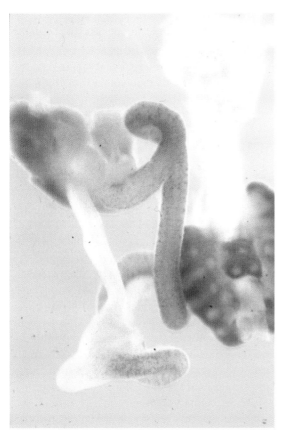

Fig. 5.2 Whole-mount immunostaining for Hox B5 protein expressed by neural crest cells in murine embryonal gut at embryonic day 12.5, showing the advancing migration front of neural crest cells. They have already colonized the stomach, small intestine and cecum, but have not reached the large intestine, which appears white.

these studies shows that in the mouse the enteric neuroblasts are derived from three distinct neural crest cell lines which express the control gene *Sox 10* and *Hox B5* and the transmembrane tyrosine kinase receptor c-ret. At the headfold stage embryo (E8.5) *Sox 10* and *c-ret* were expressed in neural crest cells, *c-ret* only being expressed in rhombomere 4 of the hindbrain and *Sox 10* in rhombomeres 2 and 4. In contrast, *Hox B5* first appeared later, at E9.5, and only occurred at the level of rhombomere 7. The cells from the vagal neural crest arrive at the gut by two pathways from the neural crest, one a dorsolateral route in a cell-free extracellular matrix between the epidermis and the somites, and a ventral route percolating through the sclerotomal

mesenchyme of the somites. In mice, the neural crest cells reach the foregut after passing through branchial arches 4 and 6. Cells expressing *Hox B5* only appear to arrive in the gut at the level of the stomach, most likely following the ventral route, whereas the *Sox 10/c-ret*-expressing cells appear to follow the dorsolateral route and enter via the primitive esophagus. Cells expressing these three genes coalesce together in the environment of the gut and by E12.5 many primitive neuroblasts are expressing all three genes (Fig. 5.3).

The foregut gives rise to the gut down to the duodenum and, given the compressed scale of the gut compared with the neural axis in these early developmental stages, the vagal neural crest cells require virtually no longitudinal movement to populate the gut down to the level of the second part of the duodenum. Caudal to this, the neural crest cells that have colonized the foregut migrate longitudinally within the gut mesenchyme in a caudal direction, favoring the region close to the serosal surface. The vanguard of cells colonizing the gut primordium advance at the rate of about 40 μm/hour[32] and the cells immediately behind the vanguard are found just outside the developing circular muscle layer; that is, they are already in position to form the myenteric plexus.[33] The cells that are going to form the submucous plexus are not seen until later, and it is not clear whether they are derived from a secondary migration from local myenteric cells or are a separate wave of immigrants. The sacral neural crest cells migrate ventrally through the adjacent somites before entering the hindgut at the cloaca near the stalk of the allantois. They then migrate rostrally in the gut mesenchyme layer. In the human, the vagal timetable appears to start at around 3–4 weeks and is complete by week 12. The presumed sacral input timetable is unknown. Those vagal neural crest cells that migrate and colonize the gut are committed to becoming neuroblasts or neuronal support cells (glioblasts). Differentiation into neurons and glial cells appears not to take place until they have reached their final resting places in the gut. The further movement through the gut mesenchyme, survival in the gut and differentiation into mature cells are strongly influenced by contacts with the microenvironment, which consists of other cells in the mesenchyme, neural crest and the extracellular matrix.[34] The extracellular matrix (ECM) components provide directional clues for migrating

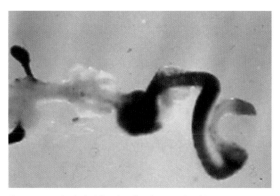

Fig. 5.3a *In situ* hybridization for the tyrosine kinase receptor *Ret* gene in a whole mount of murine embryonal gut at embryonal day E12.5, showing that vagal neural crest cells expressing the *Ret* gene have migrated as far as the cecum, but the sacral neural crest contribution is restricted to the extreme caudal region so that the colon appears pale.

neural crest cells and, together with neighboring cells, provide some of the signals for crest cell differentiation. In humans, for example, the appearance of neural crest cells in the gut is preceded by expression of ECM molecules, and these may play a role in migrational cues[35] or promote neuronal growth.[36] Other factors, such as glial-derived neurotrophic factor, ensure survival of committed neuroblasts.[37] Several transgenic knockout mouse models and naturally occurring strains of mice with particular genetic abnormalities have provided valuable evidence of some of the factors

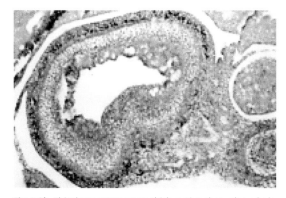

Fig. 5.3b This shows a transverse thick section through a whole mount of murine embryonal gut at embryonal day E13 in which *Ret* gene expressing cells staining dark brown are found just outside the developing circular muscle layer, that is, they are in position to form the myenteric plexus. The cells that are going to form the submucous plexus will appear later.

involved. Lethal spotted[38] and piebald spotting mice[39] have defects in the endothelin signaling pathway that result in an alteration of the microenvironment in which the neural crest cells find themselves. This curtails neural crest migration in the distal colon and is associated with localized overexpression of extracellular matrix molecules,[40] resulting in aganglionosis of the hindgut.

The intrinsic properties of the neural crest cells themselves are also important for migration survival and differentiation. Two knockout mouse models[37,41] and the human condition Hirschsprung's disease now have known genetic defects[42,43] and provide very powerful evidence for these intrinsic properties. The neural crest cells express a transmembrane tyrosine kinase receptor at the cell surface, the *RET* proto-oncogene. A transgenic knockout model of Ret in the mouse[37] shows total absence of the ENS, suggesting that normal ENS migration and/or the survival of migrating cells is dependent upon the functional integrity of this tyrosine kinase receptor and its ligand. We now know that the ligand for the Ret tyrosine kinase receptor is glial-derived neurotrophic factor and a knockout model of this gene shows a similar lack of expression of enteric neurons.[41] In Hirschsprung's disease, defects in chromosome 10q11.2[42,43] which specify the *RET* gene have been found and the defects extend all along the gene. It is of interest that other abnormalities of the *RET* gene result in multiple endocrine neoplasia type 2A and 2B, but these only occur at specific sites. In multiple endocrine neoplasia type 2B there is an association with hyperplasia of enteric neurons, resulting in enteric ganglioneuromatosis.[44] Abnormalities of *RET* are found in some 30% of patients with Hirschsprung's disease, and in families with Hirschsprung's disease there is incomplete penetrance of the genetic abnormality. While abnormalities of *RET* appear to account for a moderate proportion of patients with Hirschsprung's disease, other neural crest cell abnormalities, such as the provision of GDNF, only account for a very small proportion of patients with Hirschsprung's disease. A series of experiments[45] have suggested that glial-derived neurotrophic factor is required for the survival and differentiation of the vagal neural crest cells once they arrive in the gut, and some have suggested that the lumbar–sacral outflow into the gut is largely of cells which will become glial cells producing factors such as glial-derived neurotrophic factors, to ensure the survival of the migrating cells once they arrive in the hindgut.

The number of vagal neural crest cells colonizing the gut also seems to be important, since a gross reduction in the number leads to the development of the ENS in the rostral levels of the gut but its complete absence at caudal levels.[28] However, this information also suggests that perhaps there is some specification of different segment identity for potential enteric neurons before they leave the vagal neural crest, and this may be dependent upon the correct microenvironment in the gut primordium during the process of migration and ultimately differentiation. It has been suggested that spatially restricted differential expression of homeobox-containing regulatory genes along the hindbrain may be responsible for this.

Summary

For normal gut development, interactions of all three germ layers – the endoderm, the splanchnic mesoderm and the ectoderm – are crucial. After an early period of proliferation and morphogenesis, an intermediate period of differentiation is followed by a later period of maturation, resulting in a bowel capable of transporting luminal contents and digesting and absorbing nutrients. These different periods are controlled by a variety of developmental control genes. Developmental control genes encoding morphogens such as Hedgehog and BPM4 are particularly necessary for the initial phase and homeobox genes such as *Hox* and *Cdx* for the later periods.

It is important to note that ENS development does not arrest at birth. For a period of at least 2–5 years neural circuits and neurons themselves continue to mature.

Known developmental disorders of the enteric nervous system

Known defects of the development of the ENS may be familial, where a distinct pattern of inheritance is known, and there can also be sporadic cases, in which there are distinctive clinical and morphological findings.[46] A number of neuropathic motility disorders, including those that present with slow transit constipation in later childhood and adult life,[47] may be due to developmental defects, but at present this remains unclear. These conditions include familial visceral neuropathy without extra-intestinal manifestations,[48] familial visceral neuropathy with neuronal internuclear inclusions[49] and familial visceral neuropathy with neurological involvement.[50]

Hirschsprung's disease

First described by Harald Hirschsprung in 1887,[51] this is by far the commonest developmental disorder of the ENS. It occurs in about 1 in 4500 live births, and results in a distal aganglionic segment of bowel of variable length. There is a male predominance of 3.8:1. In about 75% of patients the abnormal segment is restricted to the rectosigmoid colon. In a small minority (about 5%) the condition may be more widespread, involving the whole colon (total colonic aganglionosis) or even the entire gastrointestinal tract.[52] In about 7% of those with the short-segment disease there is a familial tendency, increasing to about 21% in patients with total colonic aganglionosis. Most patients present in the first few days of life, 95% failing to pass meconium in the first 24 hours of life. Five percent may present later with constipation and 30% with symptoms of an

---

Hirschsprung's disease

1 Commonest developmental disorder of the ENS.
2 Male/female ratio is 3.8:1.
3 Incidence is 1 in 4500.
4 Caused by failure of migration of neural crest cells into gut.
5 Results in narrowed aganglionic distal segment.
6 Genetic basis involves defects in both *RET* and *SOX 10*.

7 Diagnosis by suction rectal biopsy, which shows hypertrophic nerve trunks and increased acetyl cholinesterase-positive fibers in the muscularis mucosae and lamina propria and absence of enteric neurons.
8 Treatment is resection of aganglionic segment and anastomosis of colon to the rectal stump.

enterocolitis. Fewer than 1% are not diagnosed until adult life.[53]

Pathogenesis

The loss of innervation of the distal segment of bowel is due to failure of colonization of the bowel by neural crest cells in early embryonic development. The resulting lack of neurons, with loss of inhibition of the enteric musculature, results in a contracted segment of gut and loss of the recto-anal sphincteric reflex. The normal ganglionic bowel is dilated, tapering to a narrowed aganglionic distal bowel.[54]

Genetic factors

The genetic mechanisms for Hirschsprung's disease appear to be multifactorial. A number of signaling systems, such as the *RET*/GDNF (glial-cell line derived neurotrophic factor)[37,41,42,43] and the endothelin systems[39,40] are implicated (see above) but mutations in other genes, such as *SOX 10*[38] and as-yet undefined genes, may be required for the Hirschsprung phenotype. In familial cases, in all families so far studied *RET* has always been involved, but mutations in at least two other genes are required for expression of the phenotype.[55] Hirschsprung's disease may also be associated with Waardenburg syndrome, Smith–Lemli–Opitz syndrome, Down syndrome and multiple endocrine neoplasia syndrome type 2A (MEN 2A).[56] The latter association ties up with the *RET* abnormalities encountered in Hirschsprung's disease as well as in MEN 2A. The former suggests that there may a relevant locus on the X chromosome resulting in the Hirschsprung phenotype.

Diagnosis

The most reliable diagnostic tool is a suction rectal biopsy, which must contain mucosa, muscularis mucosae and a sufficient amount of submucosa.[57] If even one submucosal neuron is present in an hematoxylin/eosin-stained section the diagnosis of Hirschsprung's disease can be excluded. The submucosa contains large hypertrophic nerve trunks instead of neurons in classical Hirschsprung's disease. Staining for acetyl cholinesterase activity reveals an increase in thick knotted fibers criss-crossing the muscularis mucosae even in a neonate. In an older baby there is also an increase in these fibers, which run not only vertically but also in a

horizontal direction in the lamina propria of the mucosa. These nerve trunks or acetyl cholinesterase-positive fibers, however, may not be evident in rare cases of total colonic aganglionosis. Thus, if total colonic aganglionosis is suspected, numerous serial sections must be examined to identify any possible neurons which may be present, particularly if the biopsy may have been taken from the physiologically hypoganglionic distal rectum (Fig. 5.4).

Treatment

Hirschsprung's disease is treated by surgical resection of the abnormal aganglionic segment followed by pulling through the normal ganglionic bowel, which is anastomosed to a rectal stump. Proximal to the aganglionic segment there is a variable length of a transitional zone before the bowel becomes fully ganglionic. This segment shows some hypertrophic nerve trunks but occasional neurons can also be identified. It is important that the hypoganglionic transitional zone is also removed. A variety of surgical procedures[58] (e.g. Duhamel, Swensson and Soave) exist for this, but the details of these procedures will not be discussed here. Until recently, the practice has been that, after the initial diagnosis has been made on a suction rectal biopsy, seromuscular biopsies are taken for frozen sections at laparotomy to establish the extent of aganglionosis. A stoma is then formed and the definitive surgery is per-

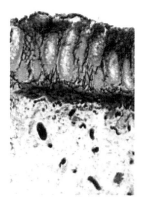

Fig. 5.4 Section of rectal mucosa showing acetyl cholinesterase positive thick nerve fibers criss-crossing in the muscularis mucosae. Acetyl cholinesterase positive fibers are also seen in the lamina propria and these fibers run horizontally as well as vertically. The submucosa shows the presence of nerve trunks with an absence of enteric neurons.

> ## Other disorders of ENS development
>
> ### Familial visceral neuropathy associated with multiple endocrine neoplasia
> - MEN 2A may be associated with aganglionosis.
> - MEN 2B may be associated with transmural intestinal ganglioneuromatosis.
> - *RET* gene abnormalities detected in both.
>
> ### Sporadic visceral neuropathies
> - Both hyper- and hypoganglionosis are reported.
>
> ### X-linked intestinal neuropathy
> - Linkage to chromosome Xq28.
>
> Use of the term 'intestinal neuronal dysplasia' is not recommended since it appears non-specific and there is no consensus on diagnostic features.

formed at a later stage. This is known as a staged procedure. Now a number of centers prefer to perform a so-called primary pull-through without the need for a stoma. This procedure is often done laparoscopically. In our experience the results after a primary pull-through are comparable to those after a staged procedure.

Familial visceral neuropathy associated with multiple endocrine neoplasia

The multiple endocrine neoplasia type 2 syndromes may be associated with involvement of the gastrointestinal tract. These include MEN 2A, MEN 2B and isolated medullary thyroid carcinoma.[59,60,61] These conditions are inherited as autosomal dominant traits and are a consequence of mutation of the gene encoding the *RET* tyrosine kinase receptor. In most patients, disorders of gastrointestinal motility are the first manifestations of the disease, but the presentation is variable both in severity and in time, some patients presenting in early infancy (very like Hirschsprung's disease) and others not until adult life. There is nearly always colonic dysfunction present and the most usual presentations are either with chronic constipation, episodes of functional obstruction or mimicking Hirschsprung's disease. In all the patients the authors have studied,[61] evidence of medullary thyroid carcinoma has been present from very early on, either as clumps of malignant cells *in situ* within the thyroid gland or as an overt tumor.

Pathogenesis

MEN 2A and 2B are associated with neuropathic dysmotility as a consequence of the development of either aganglionosis, as in some cases of MEN 2A,[59] or transmural intestinal ganglioneuromatosis, in MEN 2B.[61] In both conditions this may cause severe constipation or episodes of obstruction.

Genetic factors

RET is extremely important in the development of the ENS as *Ret* null knockout mice do not develop neurons within the gut. There is now good evidence to show that *Ret* is not only important for the colonization of the primitive gastrointestinal tract by neural crest cells, but also in the migration of these cells down the length of the gut and their further differentiation.[37] In MEN 2A and isolated medullary thyroid carcinoma there is abnormality of the *RET* gene between codons 619 and 638, the cystine-rich region of the gene, which results in the development of medullary thyroid carcinoma with or without pheochromocytoma.[59] This is thought to be due to changes in the dimerization of RET following ligand binding. In about 5% of patients with MEN 2A, Hirschsprung's disease is also present.[59]

In MEN 2B there are germ-line mutations M918T or A883F of the *RET* proto-oncogene[44] and there is always involvement of the gastrointestinal tract with transmural intestinal ganglioneuromatosis. Eventually, medullary thyroid carcinoma inevitably develops.[61]

Diagnosis

Transmural intestinal ganglioneuromatosis is a serious condition that one should be aware of. The appearance is of a striking proliferation of neural tissue (neurons, supporting cells and nerves), which appears as a thick band of nerve tissue with mature nerve cells embedded. The hyperplastic nerve fibers are accompanied by large ganglionic nodes containing numerous glial cells with a normal or increased quantity of neurons.[61] Ganglioneuroma in the submucosa of a suction rectal biopsy

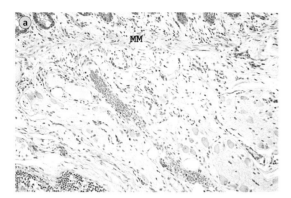 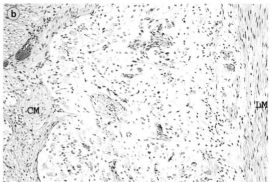

Fig. 5.5 Hematoxylin- and eosin-stained sections showing typical appearances of intestinal ganglioneuromata occupying the entire submucosa (a) and the myenteric plexus (b). MM, muscularis mucosae. CM, circular muscle. LM, longitudinal muscle.

may also be an indication of transmural involvement. This abnormality of the ENS is present along the entire gastrointestinal tract and the hyperplastic neurons may be seen within the mouth or anal canal (Fig. 5.5).

Suspicion of ganglioneuromatosis warrants further screening for medullary carcinoma of the thyroid and pheochromocytoma. Frequently in patients in whom there are only collections of cells *in situ* within the gland, screening investigations such as CT scanning of the thyroid and calcitonin determinations have not been helpful, and molecular investigations to exclude multiple endocrine neoplasia type 2B (MEN 2B) should be undertaken.[61] It is only when there is a considerable mass of C-cells present that the normal screening investigations become positive.

Treatment

Functional intestinal obstruction and intractable constipation in these patients is usually widespread, involving also the small bowel. Ileostomy usually works well, but in our experience closing it results in obstructive symptoms.[61]

Monitoring the calcitonin concentrations and scans for adrenal and thyroid masses is not sufficient. Microscopic medullary thyroid carcinoma can be present without raised calcitonin concentrations even with pentagastrin stimulation or without identifiable masses on imaging. It is for this reason, together with the lack of a satisfactory radiotherapeutic or chemotherapeutic treatment, that prophylactic thyroidectomy[61] is recommended, together with continued surveillance of the adrenal glands for evidence of pheochromocytoma.

Sporadic visceral neuropathies

Neuropathic dysmotility may also be produced by having too few myenteric neurons (hypoganglionosis) as well too many (hyperganglionosis) or none at all (aganglionosis). The conditions that cause these states are nearly always congenital, though both hypoganglionosis and aganglionosis may result from acquired disorders in which there is destruction of neurons. As these conditions are defined by the numbers of neurons present, it is clear that a reliable means of assessing neuronal density is required. Neuronal density is affected by the age of the patient, tissue freshness and intestinal dilatation as well as by the disease process. It is therefore important that a standardized technique for assessing neuronal density is used.[6] A full-thickness sample of intestine at an appropriate site is required, which needs to be greater than 1 cm in length. Preferably, neurons should be counted in sections cut longitudinally along the long axis of the bowel rather than transversely. If sections are cut transversely, they should be at least 30 μm apart to avoid counting each neuron more than once. There are few published studies, especially in children, but Smith[6] reported a mean neuronal density of 3.6 neurons per millimeter for the jejunum, 4.3 per millimeter for the ileum and 7.7 per millimeter for the colon, with no significant difference between transverse and longitudinal sections.

Myenteric hypoganglionosis

Infants affected by this condition usually present as if they have Hirschsprung's disease, but also with recurrent episodes of diffuse functional obstruction and neuropathic dysmotility.[3,62] The cause of the condition is unknown and so far no genetic factors have been identified.

Diagnosis

Baseline data for normal myenteric neuronal density are available in different regions of the gut.[6] Isolated hypoganglionosis is a disorder in which there are reduced numbers of myenteric neurons. The ganglia are small, often containing only one or two neurons, and are far apart from each other. The circular muscle coat appears to be hypo-innervated, with a reduced number of varicosities, as shown by immunostaining for neural markers (e.g. S100, PGP9.5, N-CAM and synaptophysin) or in frozen tissue by assessing acetyl cholinesterase activity. In addition, in the small bowel mucosa fibers are also reduced or absent. The extent to which the bowel is involved may not be easy to determine, since seromuscular biopsies do not contain sufficient length of the plexus for meaningful assessment of the normal density.

Treatment

If an isolated segment of affected gut can be identified then resection is the treatment of choice, with ultimately a definitive pull-through procedure if it is a terminal segment. If the gut is diffusely involved, a decompression ileostomy may reduce the number of episodes of obstruction.

Myenteric hyperganglionosis

Presentation of infants with this condition is very variable, from Hirschsprung-like to simply constipated.[62] The symptoms seem to be due to neuropathic dysmotility.

Genetic factors

It is not know what causes myenteric hyperganglionosis, although Enx (Hox 11L1)-deficient mice develop myenteric neuronal hyperplasia and megacolon.[21]

Diagnosis

Myenteric hyperganglionosis is defined as a disorder in which the myenteric neuronal density is increased.[6] This may be accompanied by other features, such as an increase in fine vertical acetyl cholinesterase-positive fibers in the lamina propria without an increase in the muscularis mucosae. Ectopic neurons may be present in the muscularis propria or lamina propria of the mucosa. Those with mild submucous hyperganglionosis have sometimes been reported to suffer from intestinal neuronal dysplasia, a term which has been used over the last 30 years to describe quantitative and qualitative abnormalities of enteric ganglia.[63,64,65] The term was originally used to describe abnormalities of both the myenteric and the submucous plexus. However, over the last 20 years or so diagnosis has largely been dependent on suction rectal biopsy and, thus, changes in the submucous plexus and the mucosal innervation.[63,64,65] The term has raised confusion and controversy among clinicians and pathologists. It appears to affect all age groups, though it is mostly seen in infants with chronic constipation and was first considered to be a developmental defect of the submucous plexus. Part of the problem has been the lack of agreed criteria and the confusion has been further compounded by the use of the histological description as a clinical diagnosis.[63,64,65] No studies have shown correlation between morphological features of intestinal neuronal dysplasia and symptoms or long-term outcome.[66] Nevertheless, surgical procedures have been recommended on the basis of the histological diagnosis. In one prospective study of rectal biopsies, the inter-observer variation between centers was enormous and close to that which might occur by chance.[67] In this study, 377 biopsies from 108 children aged 4–15 years were assessed by three experienced pathologists for a number of agreed histological features and a final diagnosis.[67] Complete concordance was obtained for the diagnosis of Hirschsprung's disease, but in only 14% of the remainder was there concordance. Assessment of the clinical symptoms 1 year after biopsy furthermore demonstrated that the diagnosis of intestinal neuronal dysplasia had no prognostic value for the outcome in these individuals. It seems, therefore, that 'intestinal neuronal dysplasia' describes neither a specific histological entity nor a clinical entity and remains controversial. Because there is no consistent consensus of the clinicopathological phenotype of intestinal neuronal dysplasia, it is safer to discard this term and describe the exact features encountered in the biopsy. In our opinion, the diagnosis cannot be made on suction rectal biopsies. Myenteric hyperganglionosis exists as an isolated finding, but can also be present in the bowel proximal to an aganglionic segment in Hirschsprung's disease.

Treatment

Patients with myenteric hyperganglionosis behave clinically like patients with Hirschsprung's disease. Resection of the abnormal segment is indicated, provided it is possible to identify the extent of the hyperganglionic segment. Ileostomy works well in these patients, and if the small bowel is not involved ileoanal anastomosis may be possible.

X-linked intestinal neuropathy

This condition was identified in a large Italian kindred in whom affected children presented in the neonatal period with intestinal obstruction, pyloric stenosis, malrotation and a short small intestine.[6,8] It maps to Xq28. The obstruction is due to a neuropathic dysmotility as a consequence of abnormality of myenteric neurons. The neurons have a degenerative appearance, being condensed on ultrastructural examination. They have irregular neurofilaments on silver staining, although care should be exercised in the interpretation of silver staining in babies under 1 year of age,[69] since young babies do not generally have argyrophilic nerve cells. The chromosomal regions linked to the condition is rich in genes, and so far no specific candidate has been identified in these patients. L-1CAM is a neuronal adhesion molecule mapping to Xq28 and is responsible for isolated and syndromic forms of hydrocephalus, but we have been unable to find any mutations in this gene in this kindred.

Miscellaneous neurodevelopmental defects

Some neuropathic disorders of the gut have presented as congenital defects which are poorly understood, yet clearly identified abnormalities of the ENS are present.

Glial cell hyperplasia

This is diagnosed when there appears to be an increase in neural tissue. In these patients, the myenteric plexus is noted to be almost continuous,[3] but there is no hyperganglionosis.

Immaturity of enteric neurons

In children, most myenteric neurons measure 20–23 μm in diameter, occasional neurons measuring 30 μm,[6,65,69] whereas in adults most neurons measure 30 μm and some larger neurons in excess of 40 μm can also be seen. In neonates, most neurons measure 8–15 μm and only rarely are larger neurons detected. Immaturity of myenteric neurons is diagnosed if the neuronal size is inappropriately small for the age of the child.[6,65,69] What causes this arrest in neuronal growth is not known. It is also unclear if some patients improve with time.

References

1   Heneyke S, Smith VV, Spitz L, Milla PJ. Chronic intestinal pseudoobstruction: treatment and long term follow up of 44 patients. *Arch Dis Child* 1999; **81**: 21–7.

2   Milla PJ. Clinical features of intestinal pseudoobstruction in children. In: Kamm M, Lennard Jones JE, eds. *Constipation*. Petersfield: Wrightson, 1994: 251–8.

3   Navarro J, Sonsino E, Boige N *et al*. Visceral neuropathies responsible for chronic intestinal pseudoobstruction syndrome in paediatric practice: analysis of 26 cases. *J Paediatr Gastroenterol Nutr* 1990; **11**: 179–95.

4   Furness JB, Costa M. *The Enteric Nervous System*. Edinburgh: Churchill Livingstone, 1987.

5   Wood JD. Physiology of the enteric nervous system. In: Johnson LR, ed. *Physiology of the Gastrointestinal Tract*, 3rd edn. New York: Raven Press, 1994: 423–82.

6   Smith VV. Intestinal neuronal density in childhood: a baseline for the objective assessment of hypo and hyper aganglionosis. *Paediatr Pathol* 1993; **13**: 225–37.

7   Sanders KM. A case for interstitial cells of Cajal as pace makers and mediators of neurotransmission in the gastrointestinal tract. *Gastroenterology* 1996; **111**: 492–515.

8   Larsen WJ. *Human Embryology*. New York: Churchill-Livingstone, 1993.

9   Haffen K, Kedinger M, Simon-Assmann P. Cell contact dependent regulation of enterocytic differentiation. In: Lebenthal E, ed. *Human Gastrointestinal Development*. New York: Raven Press, 1989: 19–39.

10   Le Douarin NM, Teillet MA. The migration of neural crest cells to the wall of the digestive tract in avian embryo. *J Embryol Exp Morphol* 1973; **30**: 31–48.

11   Manak JR, Scott MP. A class act: conservation of homeo domain protein functions. *Development* 1994 (Suppl.): 61–77.

12   McGuinness W, Krumlauf R. Homeobox genes and axial

patterning. *Cell* 1992; **68**: 283–302.

13   Hunt P, Krumlauf R. Hox codes and positional specification in invertebrate embryonic axis. *Annu Rev Cell Biol* 1992; **8**: 227–56.

14   Kessel M, Gruss P. Murine development control genes. *Science* 1990; **249**: 374–9.

15   Duboule D, Dollae P. The structural and functional organisation of the murine Hox gene family resembles that of Drosophila homeotic genes. *EMBO J* 1989; **8**: 1497–505.

16   Dolle P, Izpisua-Belmonte JC, Bonchonelli E, Deboule D. The Hox 4.8 gene is localised at the '5 prime' extremity of the Hox 4 complex and is expressed in the most posterior parts of the body during development. *Mech Dev* 1991; **36**: 3–13.

17   Wilkinson DG, Bhatt S, Cook M, Bonchonelli E, Krumlauf R. Segmental expression of Hox 2 homeobox containing genes in the developing mouse hind brain. *Nature* 1989; **341**: 405–9.

18   Hunt P, Gulisano M, Cook M *et al.* A distinct Hox code for the branchial region of the vertebrate head. *Nature* 1991; **353**: 861–4.

19   Pitera J, Smith VV, Milla PJ. Normal expression of Hox genes in the developing gastrointestinal tract: a basis for understanding abnormalities in enteric neuromusculature. *Gastroenterology* 1997; **112**: A898.

20   Pitera J, Smith VV, Thorogood P, Milla PJ. Co-ordinated expression of 3' Hox genes during murine embryonal gut development: an enteric Hox code. *Gastroenterology* 1999. (In press.)

21   Shirasawa S, Yunker AM, Roth KA, Brown GA, Orning S, Korsmeyer S. ENX (Hox L11 1) deficient mice develop myenteric neuronal hypoplasia and mega-colon. *Nat Med* 1997; **3**: 646–50.

22   Wolgemuth DJ, Beringer RR, Mostola MP, Brinster RL, Palmiter RD. Transgenic mice over expressing the mouse homeobox containing gene Hox 1.4 exhibit abnormal gut development. *Nature* 1989; **337**: 464–7.

23   Kondo T, Dolle P, Zakany J, Duboule D. Function of posterior Hox D genes in the morphogenesis of the anal sphincter. *Development* 1996; **122**: 2651–9.

24   Ramalho-Santos M, Melton DA, McMahon AP. Hedgehog signals regulate multiple aspects of gastrointestinal development. *Development* 2000; **127**: 2763–72.

25   Roberts DJ, Johnson RL, Burke AC, Nelson CE, Morgan BA, Tabin C. Sonic hedgehog is an endodermal signal inducing Bmp-4 and Hox genes during induction and regionalisation of the chick gut. *Development* 1995; **125**: 2791–801.

26   Powell DW, Mifflin RC, Valentich JD, Crowe SE, Saada JL, West AB. Myofibroblasts. II. Intestinal subepithelial myofibroblasts. *Am J Physiol* 1999; **277** (2Pt1): C183–201.

27   Haffen K, Lacroix B, Kedinger M. Inductive properties of fibroblastic cell cultures derived from rat intestinal mucosa on epithelial differentiation. *Differentiation* 1983; **23**: 226–33.

28   Yntema CL, Hammond WS. The origin of intrinsic ganglia of trunk viscera from vagal neural crest in the chick embryo. *J Comp Neurol* 1954; **101**: 515–41.

29   Peters van de Sanden MGH, Kirby ML, Gittenberger de Groot AC, Tibboel D, Mulder MP, Meijers C. Ablation of various regions within the avian vagal neural crest has differential effects on ganglion formation in the fore, mid and hind gut. *Dev Dyn* 1993; **196**: 183–94.

30   Serbedzija GN, Burgan S, Fraser SE, Broner Fraser M. Vital dye labelling demonstrates a sacral neural crest contribution to the enteric nervous system of chick and mouse embryos. *Development* 1991; **111**: 857–66.

31   Pitera J, Smith VV, Milla PJ. Neurotrophic factors and neural crest cell receptors in the developing murine enteric nervous system. *J Paediatr Gastroenterol Nutr* 1999; **28**: 565.

32   Allan IJ, Newgreen DF. The origin and differentiation of enteric neurons of the intestine of the fowl embryo. *Am J Anat* 1980; **157**: 137–54.

33   Tucker GC, Siment G, Thiery JP. Pathways of avian neural crest cell migration in the developing gut. *Dev Biol* 1986; **116**: 430–50.

34   Pham TD, Gershon MD, Rothman TP. Time of origin of neurons in the murine enteric nervous system sequence in relation to phenotype. *J Comp Neurol* 1991; **314**: 789–98.

35   Fujimoto T, Harter J, Yokoyama S, Mitomi T. A study of the extracellular matrix protein as the migration pathway of neural crest cells in the gut: analysis in human embryos with special reference to the pathogenesis of Hirschsprung's disease. *J Pediatr Surgery* 1989; **24**: 550–6.

36   Trupp M, Arinas E, Fainzibla M, Nilson AS, Sieber VA, Grigoriou M. Peripheral expression and biological activities of GDNF, a new neurotropic factor for avian and mammalian peripheral neurons. *Nature* 1996; **381**: 789–93.

37   Schuchardt A, D'Agati V, Larsson-Blomberg L, Constantini F, Pachnis V. Defects in the kidney and enteric nervous system of mice lacking the tyrosine kinase receptor ret. *Nature* 1994; **367**: 380–3.

38   Kapur RP, Yost C, Palmiter RD. A transgenic model for studying the development of the enteric nervous system in normal and aganglionic mice. *Development* 1992; **116**: 167–75.

39   Hosoda K, Hammer RE, Richardson JA, Baynesh AG, Cheung JC, Giaida A. Targeted and natural pie bald lethal mutations of endothelin B receptor gene produce megacolon associated with spotted coat colour in mice. *Cell* 1994; **79**: 1267–76.

40 Payette RF, Tennyson VM, Pomeranz HD, Pham TD, Rothman TP, Gershon MD. Accumulation of components of basal laminae: association with the failure of neural crest cells to colonise the presumptive aganglionic bowel of LS/LS mutant mice. *Dev Biol* 1988; **125**: 341–60.

41 Sanchez MP, Selos Santiago I, Frezen J, Bin He, Lira SA, Barbacid M. Renal agenesis and the absence of enteric neurons in mice lacking GDNF. *Nature* 1996; **382**: 70–3.

42 Edery P, Lyonnet S, Mulligan LM, Pelet A, Dow E, Abel L. Mutation of the ret proto oncogene in Hirschsprung's disease. *Nature* 1994; **367**: 378–80.

43 Lyonnet S, Bellono A, Pelet A *et al*. A gene for Hirschsprung's disease maps to the proximal long arm of chromosome 10. *Nat Genet* 1993; **4**: 346–50.

44 Eng C, Smith DP, Mulligan LM *et al*. Point mutation within the tyrosine kinase domain of the ret proto oncogene in multiple endocrine neoplasia type 2B and related sporadic tumours. *Hum Mol Genet* 1994; **3**: 237–41.

45 Moore MW, Klein RD, Farinas I *et al*. Renal and neuronal abnormalities in mice lacking GDNF. *Nature* 1996; **382**: 76–9.

46 Fell JM, Smith VV, Milla PJ. Infantile chronic idiopathic intestinal pseudoobstruction: the role of small intestinal manometry as a diagnostic tool and prognostic indicator. *Gut* 1996; **39**: 306–11.

47 Stanghellini V, Camilleri M, Malagelada JR. Chronic idiopathic pseudoobstruction: clinical and intestinal manometric findings. *Gut* 1987; **28**: 5–12,

48 Mayer EA, Schuffler MD, Rotter JI, Hanna P, Mogard M. Familial visceral neuropathy with autosomal dominate transmission. *Gastroenterology* 1986; **91**: 1528–35.

49 Barnett JL, McDonnell WM, Appelman HD, Dobbins WO. Familial visceral neuropathy with neuronal intranuclear inclusions: diagnosis by rectal biopsy. *Gastroenterology* 1992; **102**: 684–91.

50 Faber J, Fich A, Steinberg A *et al*. Familial intestinal pseudoobstruction dominated by a progress neurologic disease at a young age. *Gastroenterology* 1987; **92**: 786–90.

51 Hirschsprung H. Stuhltragheit Neugeborener infolge von Dilatation und Hypertrophie des Colons. *Jarb Kinderheilkd* 1887; **27**: 1–9.

52 Kleinhaus S, Boley SJ, Sheran M, Sieber WK. Hirschsprung's disease. A survey of the members of the surgical section of the American Academy of Pediatrics. *J Pediatr Surg* 1979; **14**: 588–97.

53 Swenson O, Sherman P, Fisher JN. Diagnosis of congenital megacolon: an analysis of 501 patients. *J Pediatr Surg* 1973; **8**: 587–94.

54 Milla PJ. Endothelins, pseudo-obstruction and Hirschsprung's disease. *Gut* 1999; **44**: 148–9.

55 Bolk S, Pelet A, Hofstra R *et al*. A human model for multigenic inheritance: phenotypic expression in Hirschsprung's disease requires both RET gene and a new 9q31 locus. *Proc Natl Acad Sci USA* 2000; **97**: 268–73.

56 Quinn FM, Surana R, Puri P. The influence of trisomy 21 on outcome in children with Hirschsprung's disease. *J Pediatr Surg* 1994; **29**: 781–83.

57 Lake BD, Puri P, Nixon HH, Claireaux AE. Hirschsprung's disease. An appraisal of histochemically demonstrated acetylcholinesterase activity in suction rectal biopsy specimens as an aid to diagnosis. *Arch Pathol Lab Med* 1978; **102**: 244–7.

58 Lavery JC. The surgery of Hirschsprung's disease. *Surg Clin North Am* 1983; **63**: 161–75.

59 Cote CJ, Gaged RF. Lessons learned from the management of a rare genetic career. *N Engl J Med* 2003; **399**: 1566–8.

60 Eng C, Marsh DJ, Robinson BG. Germline RET codon 918 mutation in apparently isolated intestinal ganglioneuromatosis. *J Endocrinol Metab* 1998; **83**: 4191–4.

61 Smith VV, Eng C, Milla PJ. Intestinal ganglioneuromatosis and multiple neoplasia type 2B: implications for treatment. *Gut* 1999; **45**: 143–6.

62 Krishnamurthy S, Heng Y, Shuffler ND. Chronic intestinal pseudoobstruction in infants and children caused by diverse abnormalities of the myenteric plexus. *Gastroenterology* 1993; **104**: 1398–408.

63 Schoffield DE, Yunis EJ. Intestinal neuronal dysplasia. *J Paediatr Gastroenterol Nutr* 1991; **12**: 182–9.

64 Meier-Ruge W, Gambazzi F, Kaufeler RE, Schmid P, Schmidt CP. The neuropathological diagnosis of neuronal intestinal dysplasia (NID B). *Eur J Paediatr Surg* 1993; **4**: 267–73.

65 Smith VV. Isolated intestinal neuronal dysplasia: a descriptive histological pattern or a distinct clinico pathological entity. In: Hadziseli Movic F, Herzog B, eds. *Inflammatory Bowel Disease and Morbus Hirschsprung*. Dordrecht: Kluwer, 1992: 203–14.

66 Cord-Udy CL, Smith VV, Ahmed S, Risdon RA, Milla PJ. An evaluation of the role of suction biopsy in the diagnosis of intestinal neuronal dysplasia. *J Paediatr Gastroenterol Nutr* 1997; **24**: 1–6.

67 Koletzko S, Jesch I, Faus-Kebetaler T *et al*. Rectal biopsy for diagnosis of intestinal neuronal dysplasia in children: a prospective multicentre study on interobserver variation and clinical outcome. *Gut* 1999; **44**: 853–61.

68 Auricchio A, Brancolini V, Casari G *et al*. The locus for a novel syndromic form of intestinal pseudoobstruction maps to XQ28. *Am J Hum Genet* 1996; **58**: 743–9.

69 Smith VV, Milla PJ. Argyrophilia in the developing human myenteric plexus. *Br J Biomed Sci* 1996; **53**: 287–93.

CHAPTER 6

Inflammation

Giovanni Barbara and Roberto De Giorgio

Clinical scenario

The alimentary tract harbors the largest collection of immune cells of the human body and a wide repertoire of functionally distinct classes of neurons, known as the enteric nervous system (ENS). Morphological and functional studies indicate extensive interplay between these two systems (Fig. 6.1). The association between gastrointestinal inflammation and disturbed gut motility and sensory perception has long been recognized. This paradigm applies to common diseases, such as reflux esophagitis, celiac disease, acute infectious gastroenteritis and inflammatory bowel disease (IBD). In addition, evidence is now emerging that immune and inflammatory mechanisms participate in the pathophysiology of a subset of functional bowel disorders. The inflammatory reaction may affect mainly mucosal nerve endings and/or enteric ganglia. Clinical phenotypes which arise in this scenario span a wide spectrum, ranging from mild forms of irritable bowel syndrome (IBS) to end-stage gut failure. Several factors may account for this variability in clinical expression: (i) the etiology (e.g. infective, paraneoplastic); (ii) the patient's genetic background; (iii) the predominant localization of the immune response (mucosal innervation versus enteric ganglia); (iv) the type and severity of immune cells and mediators involved; (v) the duration of the disease and the existence of comorbid conditions (e.g. psychiatric disorders).

This chapter deals with the impact of inflammation and immune activation on functional syndromes characterized by sensorimotor dysfunction, focusing mainly on IBS and enteric neuropathies.

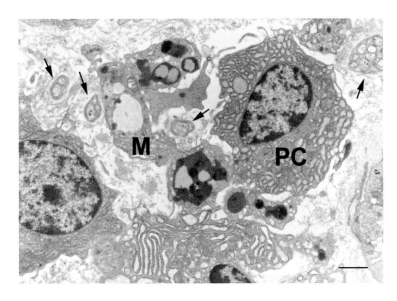

Fig. 6.1 Electron micrograph showing association between nerve fibers (arrows) and immune cells, including a macrophage (M) and a plasma cell (PC), in the colonic mucosa of an IBS patient. Note the proximity (<5 µm) between immune cells and nerve trunks. Calibration bar = 5 µm. Reproduced with permission from reference 73.

Basic mechanisms: inflammation-induced neuroplasticity in the ENS

The ENS is extremely receptive to a variety of stimuli originating from the gut. Enteric neurons are able to elaborate this information into integrated responses which initiate reflex activity controlling motility, epithelial secretion/absorption, blood flow and mucosal immunity. Abnormal stimuli (e.g. infectious, inflammatory and enteroendocrine) may generate long-lasting structural and/or functional phenotypic changes in the enteric neural network. Pioneer studies showed that inflammatory-induced gut sensorimotor dysfunction could be blunted by suppression of the immune/inflammatory reaction, thus demonstrating a cause–effect relationship.[1] Further studies have clarified the relative role played by different inflammatory cells (e.g. T cells, macrophages, mast cells), their mediators (e.g. cytokines, prostanoids, proteases, neuropeptides, neurotrophins) and receptors (e.g. tyrosine kinase receptors, proteinase activated receptors) in several structural and functional aspects of gut sensorimotor function.[2,3] These include effects on the growth and contractile properties of smooth muscle cells, neurotransmitter content and release and related receptor expression, as well as neurophysiological properties of intrinsic (enteric) and extrinsic sensory neurons.[2,3]

Concerning neuroplasticity, recent attention has been focused on nerve growth factor (NGF), a member of a family of tissue-targeted neurotrophic molecules, which exerts a significant role in neuroimmune signaling in the gastrointestinal tract. NGF, released by different cellular sources, including enteroglial cells as well as mast cells and other immunocytes, acts by binding through high-affinity receptors, mainly tyrosine kinase receptor A (TrKA).[3] Typical examples of NGF-induced neuroplastic changes in the gut include the increase in calcitonin gene-related peptide and substance P content in intrinsic and extrinsic nerves, along with the protective effect of this neurotrophic factor in experimental colitis in rats.[4] These data are in agreement with findings indicating that the TrKA gene is markedly upregulated in colonic tissue of patients with IBD.[5]

Animal models have been instrumental in the study of the impact of intestinal inflammation and immune activation on the sensorimotor apparatus of the gut. These studies provide the biological basis for considering intestinal inflammation as a putative mechanism in the pathophysiology of a subset of patients with gut disorders ranging from IBS to chronic intestinal pseudo-obstruction.[2] Accordingly, animal models resembling human functional bowel disorders are now available for research. For example, a postinfective IBS model has been proposed. In selected strains of mice (e.g. NIH Swiss), transient nematode infection evoked intestinal muscle dysfunction which lasted long after the expulsion of the parasite from the gut and resolution of the acute mucosal inflammatory process.[6] These long-term neuromuscular abnormalities were sustained by active synthesis of inflammatory mediators (i.e. cyclooxygenase-2 derived products) within the neuromuscular tissue.[7] Animal models testing the effect of inflammation in gut motor failure include, for example, infection with the nematode *Schistosoma mansoni*[8] and bowel transplantation.[9]

Mucosal inflammation and IBS

In search of a biological basis for IBS

IBS, the most common disorder encountered by gastroenterologists, is responsible for reduced quality of life and a considerable economic burden on society.[10] IBS is characterized by chronic and recurrent symptoms of abdominal pain associated with changes in bowel habit for which there is no identifiable underlying structural basis.[11] Both central and peripheral mechanisms are thought to contribute to IBS symptom perception, including psychosocial factors, abnormal motility and enhanced perception of sensory stimuli arising from the gut wall. Emerging fields of investigation, including genetics, gut infection, immunity, neuroplasticity and endocrinology, support the hypothesis that detectable biochemical or structural changes underlie bowel sensorimotor dysfunction in some IBS patients. The following paragraphs will be restricted to the putative role of immunological changes in the pathophysiology of IBS and will deal only marginally with postinfectious IBS, which is covered in detail in Chapter 15.

Inflammation and IBS: clinical basis

Several studies show low-grade mucosal inflammation:
- conflicting data concerning importance of different cell types;

- increased T cells, mast cells and macrophages reported;
- 10% of patients meeting Rome II criteria for IBS have microscopic colitis; and
- mast cell activation may be important in mediating abdominal pain.

Observations in the clinical setting have provided the rationale for considering gut mucosal immune activation as a putative pathophysiological factor in IBS. Firstly, patients in remission from IBD develop IBS-like symptoms with a prevalence higher than expected.[12,13] Secondly, a low-grade inflammatory response, albeit undetectable macroscopically or with conventional histology, has been shown in the intestinal mucosa of patients with unspecific or postinfective IBS. Nonetheless, conflicting and negative results have also been published. For example, there is no agreement on the type of immunocytes infiltrating the gut mucosa[14–16] and on the presence of increased inflammatory cells in similar regions of the colon.[14–16] Also, one recent study failed to demonstrate any effect of a systemic steroid treatment on symptoms of postinfectious IBS.[17] While we await further investigation in this field, these conflicting results should be viewed in the light of the difficulty in assessing the gastrointestinal immune system and testing the hypothesis of a cause–effect relationship between low-grade mucosal inflammation and symptom generation. Indeed, the gut mucosal immune system is a rather complex structure to study because of its uneven distribution along the longitudinal axis of the alimentary tract and its substantial variability with age[18] and gender.[19] Continuous stimulation by luminal antigens, causing a sort of controlled physiological inflammation, acts as background noise that confounds any clear cut identification of subtle changes in mucosal immunocytes in IBS. Neuroplastic changes, which probably occur after a long-term mucosal inflammatory response, may lead to disappointing results when testing the efficacy of immunosuppressive agents in IBS.[17] Finally, the wide variation in the methods used in this field makes it difficult to compare results obtained by different research groups. All these factors should be taken into account when approaching the literature on this topic.

Mucosal immunopathology and its implications for gut sensorimotor dysfunction

Table 6.1 provides a list of studies investigating the presence of immune activation in IBS. Different independent studies have shown that the intestinal mucosa of IBS patients contains, on average, an increased number of immunocytes.[16,20] These comprise mainly cells of the chronic immune response, such as T cells,[15,16] intraepithelial lymphocytes (IELs)[15] and mast cells.[14–16,21] However, isolated studies suggest that a subgroup of IBS patients may also have a low-grade acute inflammatory infiltrate (i.e. neutrophils) in the colonic mucosa.[15] One study indicates that this low-grade inflammatory response can be detected in roughly three-quarters of IBS patients.[16] Increased inflammatory cells, primarily mast cells, were found to cluster particularly in the terminal ileum or right colon.[14] Based on the inflammatory profile, one study

Table 6.1 Putative causes and consequences of mucosal immune activation in IBS

Clinical setting	Identified and putative causes	Immune activation	Mediators and cellular source	Cellular targets and consequences
Postinfectious IBS	*Campylobacter*, *Salmonella*, *Shigella*, other	T cells, IEL, macrophages	IL-1β (macrophages)	Epithelial cells (↑ permeability, ↑ secretion),
Unspecified IBS	Genetic factors, stress, bile acid malabsorption, abnormal microflora, unrecognized food allergies	Mast cells, T cells (CD25+), IEL, macrophages, neutrophils	Tryptase (mast cells), histamine (mast cells), iNOS (macrophages) ↓ IL-10 (T cells)	ENS (abnormal secretomotor reflexes), primary sensory afferents (visceral hypersensitivity)

ENS, enteric nervous system; IEL, intraepithelial lymphocytes; IL, interleukin; iNOS, inducible nitric oxide synthase.

suggests that IBS patients should be grouped into those (about 50% of patients) with a predominant T-cell (CD3[+]) component and those with additional evidence of increased mast cells and neutrophils (about 40%). Whether these two categories have significant implications for clinical or pathophysiological aspects has yet to be determined. On the other hand, it is interesting to note that about 10% of patients fulfilling the Rome criteria for IBS showed the typical mucosal abnormalities of lymphocytic colitis,[15] indicating that symptom-based criteria alone are insufficient to identify this particular form of organic bowel disease. Postinfectious IBS is an established cause of low-grade inflammation in at least a proportion of IBS patients. In one study, rectal inflammatory cells remained increased in patients who developed chronic IBS symptoms after acute gastroenteritis, whereas these cells normalized in asymptomatic patients.[22] However, recent data in patients with *Campylobacter* infection demonstrate also that asymptomatic patients may not return to normal rectal lamina propria T cells 3 months after infection.[23] Increased rectal IELs have been reported for 3 months, and in some cases up to 1 year, after infection with *Campylobacter*.[23]

The identification of features of immune activation and specific mediator release may be of importance in understanding the mechanisms underlying disturbed neuromotor function in IBS (Table 6.1). Increased expression of CD25, a marker of T-cell activation, has been described recently in the colonic mucosa in IBS.[15] Although this is probably correlated with increased T-cell cytokine production, this has yet to be studied in IBS. On the other hand, increased expression of the proinflammatory cytokine interleukin (IL)-1β has been shown in the rectal mucosa of postinfectious IBS patients.[24] The source of IL-1β in the rectal mucosa in this condition remains undetermined. However, newly recruited calprotectin-positive macrophages are likely candidates.[23] These findings are of importance in the light of the demonstration that impairment of enteric nerve function in the *Trichinella spiralis* model of intestinal inflammation is macrophage-dependent.[25] Furthermore, IL-1β, like other proinflammatory cytokines (e.g. IL-6 and tumor necrosis factor-α), has been implicated in the generation of visceral hyperalgesia, presumably by the direct activation of sensory nerve endings.[26] Macrophages are also an important

source of nitric oxide,[27] which may perturb gastrointestinal function[28] and contribute to prolonged visceral hyperalgesia.[29] Preliminary studies suggest that the inducible isoform of nitric oxide synthase is increased in the colonic mucosa of non-specific IBS, and that its increase is associated with stressful life events.[30]

A number of considerations lead to the hypothesis that mast cells play a role in the altered sensorimotor function observed in patients with IBS.[31] In addition to the increased number of mast cells detectable in the colonic[14,15] and ileal[21] mucosa of IBS patients, mast cells lie in close proximity to mucosal innervation in the human intestine.[32,33] Furthermore, animal studies indicate that mast cell activation increases the excitability of enteric[34,35] and primary afferent neurons,[36] leading to visceral hypersensitivity[37] and abnormal gut motor function.[38] We have recently demonstrated ultrastructural features of increased mast cell activation in the colonic mucosa of IBS patients (Fig. 6.2).[16] Accordingly, mast cells released an increased amount of specific mediators, including tryptase and histamine.[16] It is known that mast cell tryptase, which signals to cells via proteinase-activated receptors (PARs),[39] induces activation of the subtype PAR-2 located on enteric nerves and visceral afferents, evoking neuronal hyperexcitability.[34,35,40] In addition to tryptase, histamine can also activate visceral afferents[36] and enteric neurons[41] binding to histamine-1 (H_1) or H_2 receptors.[42,43] Taken together, these data indicate that tryptase and histamine are candidate mediators for disturbed gut sensorimotor function in IBS.

Correlation between clinical features and immunopathology

A few studies have attempted a correlation between patients' clinical features and immunopathological findings (Table 6.2). The increase in colonic IELs was more pronounced in patients with long-lasting disease (more than 5 years) and in younger patients (under 35 years). These age-dependent changes appeared to be specific for IBS since they were not identified in healthy controls. Conversely, the type of onset of IBS symptoms, i.e. acute (suggestive of an infective origin) versus gradual onset, was not correlated to IEL numbers.[15] One recent study demonstrated that some mucosal immunological features of IBS are gender-dependent. Accordingly, the number of CD8[+] T cells

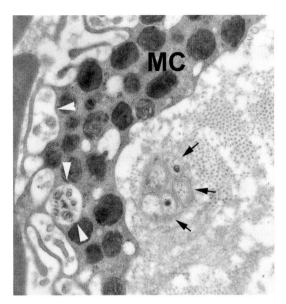

Fig. 6.2 Electron micrograph showing the typical appearance of a degranulating (arrowheads) mast cell (MC) close (<5 μm) to a nerve fiber (arrows) in the colonic mucosa of an IBS patient. Calibration bar = 5 μm. Reproduced with permission from reference 16.

in the colonic mucosa of IBS patients was higher in males than in females. Conversely, the number of mast cells was higher in female than in male patients.[16] These findings are in line with the well-known data showing that the immune system is different in males and females[44] and with the described influence of gonadal steroids in these gender-related differences.[44] This feature is relevant because of the documented gender-related differences in IBS pathophysiology and symptom referral.[45]

Concerning bowel habit, patients with diarrhea-predominant IBS showed an increased number of IELs and CD3[+] T cells compared with patients with constipation-predominant IBS. In contrast, mast cell numbers were higher in constipated IBS patients in one study,[15] whereas they were similarly increased in both constipation- and diarrhea-predominant IBS patients in another study.[16] It is not known why increased mast cells may be involved in such contrasting bowel habit. Although mastocytosis is often accompanied by diarrhea, due to increased neuronal secretomotor function,[46] mast cells may also evoke enteric neuron functional impairment in constipated patients due to

erratic contractile colonic motor activity, which delays colonic transit. Colonic mast cells have also been implicated in the pathophysiology of abdominal pain perception in IBS.[31] In this line, we demonstrated that both severity and frequency of perceived abdominal painful sensations were correlated with the presence of activated mast cells in proximity to nerve endings in the colonic mucosa (Fig. 6.3).[16]

Putative causes of immune activation

Previous infectious enteritis is now a recognized etiological factor in IBS (see Chapter 15) and the cause of immune cell infiltration and activation in the rectal mucosa in at least a subgroup of IBS patients (Table 6.1).[47]

At present there is limited evidence for genetic predisposition to IBS.[48–50] However, large-scale testing showed abnormalities of genes controlling down-regulation (i.e. IL-10 and transforming growth factor-β_1 alleles and genotype frequencies) of inflammation in IBS.[51]

Allergic reactions to foods and to other luminal antigens evoke inflammatory cell infiltration (i.e. mast cells and eosinophils) and activation in the gastrointestinal mucosa.[52,53] Food allergies continue to be a confounding factor in IBS because of the lack of sensitivity and specificity of diagnostic tests.[54]

Stress is believed to contribute to patients' consultations and probably to visceral hypersensitivity and gut motor dysfunction in IBS.[10] It is still debatable whether stress alone is a cause of low-grade inflammation in the

Table 6.2 Association between clinical features and immunopathological findings in IBS

Clinical features	Immune activation
Age (<35 years)	IEL
Gender	
Female	Mast cells
Male	Mast cells, CD8[+] T cells
Disease duration (>5 years)	IEL
Bowel habit	
Diarrhea	IEL, CD3[+], mast cells
Constipation	Mast cells
Abdominal pain	Mast cells in proximity to ENS

IEL, intraepithelial lymphocytes.

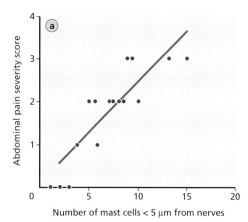
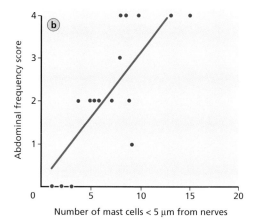

Fig. 6.3 Correlation between severity (a) and frequency (b) of abdominal pain and the number of mast cells per field located within 5 μm of nerves in the colonic mucosa of patients with irritable bowel syndrome ($r = 0.75$, $P = 0.001$ and $r = 0.70$, $P = 0.003$, respectively). Reproduced with permission from reference 16.

bowel. However, stress may contribute to the increased activation of mucosal inflammatory cells, especially mast cells. Stress-induced release of corticotropin-releasing factor (CRF) may be responsible for mast cell activation and mediator release. In support of these data, recent experimental work has shown that acute stress modulates mast cell histamine content in the gastrointestinal tract via IL-1 and CRF release in rats.[55] This is of particular relevance since CRF infusion in IBS patients evokes an exaggerated colonic motor response.[56] Preliminary data suggest that stressful life events are associated with increased inducible nitric oxide synthase expression in colonic biopsies.[30] Furthermore, nerves may also play a role in the activation of mucosal mast cells in IBS. We have demonstrated an increased rate of degranulation of mast cells that are close to colonic nerves in IBS, suggesting that neuropeptides (e.g. substance P, calcitonin gene-related peptide) or NGF may participate in the increased rate of degranulation.[3]

Another putative mechanism that may play a role in low-grade inflammation in IBS relates to bile acid malabsorption, which has been shown to occur in some IBS patients.[57] Bile acids may irritate the ileal and colonic mucosa. It is probable that abnormalities of enteric microflora represent luminal irritants involved in excessive stimulation of gut lymphoid tissue (G Barbara and R De Giorgio, unpublished observations) and play a role in IBS pathogenesis.[58] However, confirmatory studies are awaited.

Inflammatory neuropathies of the enteric nervous system

Pathological and clinical features
In addition to the intrinsic and extrinsic nerves supplying the gastrointestinal mucosa, enteric ganglia may be a target of inflammatory/autoimmune reactions. These forms of enteric neuropathy, also referred to

---

Key points

1 Commonest lesion is inflamation of myenteric plexus.
2 Cellular infiltrate may be lymphocytic or eosinophilic.
3 Associated loss of ganglion cell bodies.

4 Ganglionitis may be primary or secondary to other diseases.
5 Antineuronal antibodies may disrupt normal function by blocking neurotransmission.

as *enteric ganglionitis or plexitis*, are characterized by a dense and composite inflammatory infiltrate of lymphocytes, plasma cells, monocytes and other elements located within myenteric (Auerbach's) and/or submucosal (Meissner's) ganglia/plexuses and/or throughout the axonal processes supplying the alimentary tract.[59–62] Myenteric ganglia appear to be more commonly involved than submucosal ganglia, raising the interesting hypothesis that myenteric neurons express peculiar constitutive antigens that are preferentially targeted by the immune system. Furthermore, the inflammatory/immune infiltrate within enteric ganglia is commonly associated with neuronal degeneration up to complete loss of neurons (i.e. acquired aganglionosis).[63] As a result, the inflammatory/autoimmune injury to the enteric ganglionated plexuses and nerves causes gut dysfunction, including dysmotility and delayed transit, at any level of the gastrointestinal tract. Depending on the segment involved by the inflammatory neuropathy, clinical manifestations range from achalasia (or esophageal and lower esophageal sphincter dysmotility)[64] and gastroparesis[65] up to intestinal pseudo-obstruction, colonic inertia and/or megacolon.[61,63,66–70,71]

Enteric ganglionitis can be classified into primary and secondary forms. The former are also termed 'idiopathic' as the search for underlying disorders responsible for inflammatory changes of the ENS is negative (Table 6.3).[63,65,67,72] The latter, in contrast, can occur in the context of a variety of diseases listed in Table 6.4. Primary and secondary ganglionitis do not appear to differ histopathologically (e.g. inflammatory infiltrate within enteric ganglia) and clinical manifestations (e.g. severe dysmotility syndromes).[73] Both primary and secondary forms of enteric inflammatory neuropathies are rarely encountered in clinical practice. Nevertheless, there is renewed interest for these conditions for at least two reasons: (i) ganglionitis and/or axonitis is a peculiar form because of the selectivity of the immune reaction against the ENS, which opens new perspectives to better understand mechanisms of neurodegeneration; and (ii) early diagnosis of a motility disorder related to an underlying ganglionitis/axonitis is important because it may allow appropriate immunosuppressive treatment, which often results in a significant amelioration of patients' clinical condition.

Table 6.3 Idiopathic enteric ganglionitis: clinical and pathological findings

Dysmotility type	Pathology	Inflammatory infiltrate
Four female patients with CIPO[71]	Lymphoid infiltrate in the lamina propria, muscularis propria and myenteric plexuses; absence of neuromuscular degeneration	Polyclonal T and B lymphocytes
One female and one male patient with CIPO[63]	Enteric ganglionitis (mainly myenteric) with neurodegeneration up to aganglionosis in both cases	Predominance of T cells (with CD4+ and CD8+)
One male patient with gastroparesis[65]	Enteric ganglionitis (mainly myenteric) with neurodegeneration and reduced SP-containing nerves in the muscularis propria	Predominance of T cells (with CD4+ and CD8+)
Two female patients with colonic inertia and megacolon; one male with CIPO[67]	Enteric ganglionitis (mainly myenteric) with neurodegeneration up to aganglionosis in all cases	Predominance of T cells (with CD4+ and CD8+)
Three female patients with CIPO[72]	Enteric ganglionitis (mainly myenteric) without overt neurodegeneration in each case	Predominance of eosinophilic infiltrate

CIPO, chronic intestinal pseudo-obstruction.

Type of disease	Example
Paraneoplastic	Small cell lung carcinoma; lung carcinoid; neuroblastoma; thymoma
Infectious	Chagas' disease; CMV infection
Autoimmune disorders of the CNS	Encephalomyeloneuropathy
Connective tissue disorders	Scleroderma
Immune-mediated disorders of the gastrointestinal tract	IBD (ulcerative colitis and Crohn's disease)

Table 6.4 Diseases associated with enteric ganglionitis. CNS, central nervous system; CMV, cytomegalovirus; IBD, inflammatory bowel disease

Although enteric ganglionitis is a condition usually associated with severe gut disorders, recent findings raise the possibility that ENS inflammation underlies the wide spectrum of gut sensorimotor abnormalities.[31,73,74] In this respect, a minimal inflammatory infiltrate (mainly composed of lymphocytes) was found in the myenteric plexus of full-thickness jejunal specimens collected from patients with severe IBS.[75] Further research in this field is now awaited. Whether the severity of immune response within enteric ganglia or other factors (e.g. the individual genetic background influencing the immune system) are relevant for clinical phenotypes (IBS/functional syndromes versus severe abnormalities of gut motility) remains unresolved.

Cellular mechanisms

Two major histopathological forms of enteric ganglionitis have been described, the lymphocytic and the eosinophilic type. Both these pathological entities have been mainly identified in patients with severe abnormalities of gut motility.

Lymphocytic ganglionitis

The immunohistochemical examination of cases with this type of ganglionitis shows a significant component of CD3[+] T lymphocytes surrounding ganglion cell bodies that are mainly confined within the myenteric plexus (i.e. myenteric lymphocytic ganglionitis). The vast majority of these T cells belong to the T-helper (CD4[+]) and T-cytotoxic/suppressor (CD8[+]) subclasses of lymphocytes and are distributed with a similar ratio (1:1 instead of the normal 2:1) (Fig. 6.4), implying a predominant T-cytotoxic activity that probably targets constitutively present proteins or *de novo*-expressed antigens on the surface of enteric

neurons.[60,63,65,67,71] The presence of a prominent component of T-cytotoxic cells has been also reported by Clark and colleagues in specimens from patients with achalasia related to ganglionitis.[76] The infiltration of T cells detected in cases of lymphocytic ganglionitis is accompanied, although to a lesser extent, by other immunocytes, including CD79α-expressing cells, indicating the presence of mature B lymphocytes.[65,67,71] The role of B lymphocytes is far from being elucidated. However, the evidence of circulating antineuronal antibodies in patients with enteric ganglionitis provides a conceptual basis that supports the idea that these lymphocytes contribute to the immune response by synthesizing and releasing immunoglobulins directed against antigens expressed by enteric neurons (see also below: Humoral mechanisms: antineuronal antibodies). Furthermore, other immunocytes that have been occasionally reported in cases of lymphocytic ganglionitis include CD68[+] cells, whose role, however, is still unclear.

The molecular mechanisms leading to immune cell recruitment within enteric plexuses in cases of lymphocytic ganglionitis are not fully clarified. As we will discuss below, the expression of *de novo* antigens, changes in the molecular structure of proteins brought about by infectious agents, molecular mimicry, and loss of self versus not-self function by the immune system may all be claimed as potential factors triggering an immune/inflammatory response within enteric ganglia. In addition to these putative mechanisms, chemokines, whose expression can be modulated by the inflammatory process during ganglionitis, may play an important role in facilitating the movement of lymphocytes into enteric ganglia. In an attempt to identify a role for chemokines, we investigated

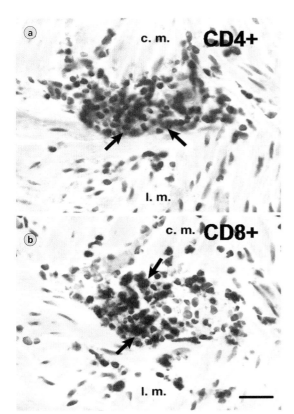

Fig. 6.4 Micrograph showing a dense population of CD4+ (a) and CD8+ (b) T lymphocytes (red-brown color) widely dispersed throughout myenteric neurons (arrows) of the left colon of a 20-year-old man with chronic idiopathic pseudo-obstruction. Alkaline phosphatase anti-alkaline phosphatase immunohistochemistry. Calibration bar = 25 μm. c.m., circular muscle. l.m., longitudinal muscle. Reproduced with permission from reference 67.

the expression of RANTES (regulated upon activation normal T-cell-expressed and secreted), MCP-1 (monocyte chemoattractant protein-1) and MIP-1α, (macrophage inflammatory protein-1α) either in small bowel or colonic specimens obtained from patients with idiopathic lymphocytic ganglionitis, and found that only MIP-1α was detected in immune cells and in neuronal and non-neuronal cells within enteric ganglia.[77] The evidence that MIP-1α is expressed within enteric ganglia supports the concept of active recruitment of immune cells (mainly T lymphocytes) into the enteric neuronal microenvironment in inflammatory neuropathies.[78]

Eosinophilic ganglionitis

This form of ganglionitis has recently been reported in studies in humans and laboratory animals. Schäppi and colleagues were the first to demonstrate an inflammatory neuropathy characterized by a prominent infiltration of eosinophils in enteric ganglia of three children with functional intestinal obstruction.[72] In one of these cases there was intense neuronal expression of IL-5, a molecule able to exert a powerful chemoattractive effect on eosinophils, suggesting active recruitment of these cells into the ENS microenvironment. In contrast to lymphocytic ganglionitis, the eosinophilic form does not appear to be associated with neuronal cell damage, indicating that eosinophils evoke neuronal dysfunction rather than degeneration. In agreement with these observations, we have recently observed a similar histopathological pattern in an adult patient with an Ogilvie's syndrome (or acute colonic pseudo-obstruction) (G Barbara and R De Giorgio, unpublished) (Fig. 6.5).

Data on animal models of gut inflammation confirm the general features of eosinophilic ganglionitis in humans and provide a basis for better understanding of how granulocytes (mainly eosinophils and neutrophils) alter enteric neuron function. Bogers and colleagues infected mice with *Schistosoma mansoni*, a nematode known to evoke mucosal ileitis, granulomas and diffuse inflammation of the neuromuscular layer with eosinophilic and neutrophilic ganglionitis of the myenteric plexus.[79] Like the patients previously described, infected mice bearing eosinophilic ganglionitis did not show significant neurodegeneration, as reflected by the low number of apoptotic neuronal cells found in this experimental model. These data are of considerable importance because they describe one of the few available models of experimental eosinophilic ganglionitis, which may be useful in elucidating the mechanisms leading to enteric neuron dysfunction.

Humoral mechanisms: antineuronal antibodies

In addition to the activation of immunocytes, patients with inflammatory neuropathies develop a significant humoral response with a wide array of circulating antineuronal antibodies. These autoantibodies, which may be identified in cases of idiopathic and secondary (e.g.

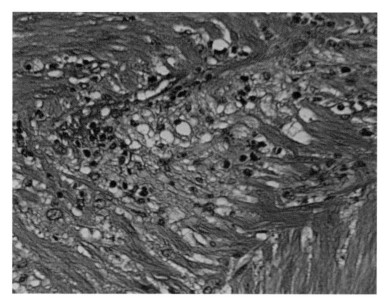

Fig. 6.5 Representative photomicrograph of a case of eosinophilic ganglionitis. The patient was a 60-year-old man operated on for an acute intestinal pseudo-obstruction (Ogilvie's syndrome). Note that the inflammatory infiltrate within the myenteric plexus of the right colon was mainly composed of eosinophilic granulocytes. Hematoxylin–eosin staining. Original magnification, ×200.

paraneoplastic syndrome) lymphocytic ganglionitis, target different antigens expressed by enteric neurons. Whether antineuronal antibodies have a pathogenetic role in ENS damage is still debated (see below). However, their detection is nowadays considered useful in the diagnosis of gut dysmotility associated with underlying ganglionitis.[60,67,69,80] Since enteric ganglia are protected by a blood–enteric barrier, which shares similarities with the blood–brain barrier, it is questionable how circulating antibodies can get into an environment as sheltered as that of the ENS. The answer to this is unknown, although it may be suggested that the activation of the immune system results in disruption of the blood–enteric barrier, which facilitates entry of the immunocytes into the ENS microenvironment. This possibility is supported by the histopathological findings in enteric ganglionitis. Thus, the alteration or loss of the blood–enteric barrier makes it possible that specific antineuronal antibodies may reach their targets.[73]

Antineuronal antibodies are directed against a variety of molecules expressed by central and enteric neurons, including the RNA-binding protein Hu (anti-Hu, also called type-1 antineuronal nuclear antibodies, ANNA-1), Yo protein (an antibody targeting a Purkinje cell cytoplasmic antigen), P/Q- and N-type Ca^{2+} channels, and ganglionic type nicotinic acetylcholine receptors.[81] These antineuronal antibodies can be found in the sera of patients with gut motor disorders associated

with paraneoplastic syndromes, although they can also be identified in cases of idiopathic ganglionitis[63,67] and dysautonomia.[81]

The Hu antibodies, which include immunoglobulin (Ig) G binding several molecules of the Hu family (HuC, HuD, HuR and Hel-N1), are the most common type of antineuronal antibody identified in enteric ganglionitis.[82,83] The Hu antigens are RNA-binding proteins that share sequence homology with the embryonic-lethal abnormal vision (ELAV) proteins of *Drosophila*. The ELAV/Hu proteins have an important role in neuronal development, maintenance and survival,[84] and therefore their inhibition by specific autoantibodies may lead to degeneration and loss in several types of central and peripheral neurons, including the ENS. It has been suggested recently that interaction between IgGs and the Hu system of enteric neurons determines the neuronal degeneration that accompanies gut dysmotility in paraneoplastic syndromes.

In addition to anti-Hu, autoantibodies directed against anti-voltage-gated Ca^{2+} channels (mainly P/Q- and N-type) can be detected in patients with Lambert–Eaton myasthenic syndrome related to small-cell lung carcinoma.[80,85] In addition, the anti-N-type Ca^{2+} channel antibodies may evoke dysfunction of the ENS in patients with paraneoplastic dismotility.[69,80,81]

Antiganglionic acetylcholine receptor antibodies have been identified in patients with idiopathic or secondary (including paraneoplastic syndrome associated with thymomas or small cell lung carcinoma) dysautonomic diseases with gastrointestinal involvement.[86] Vernino and colleagues[86] found antiganglionic acetylcholine receptor antibodies in 16% of patients with dysautonomia, whereas 4% of these cases had autoantibodies blocking receptor function. The titers of these autoantibodies correlated with the severity of autonomic dysfunction, and the decrease or disappearance of the circulating antibodies was associated with the improvement of autonomic function. Interference of these antibodies with nicotinic receptors leads to functional impairment of ENS reflexes, thus contributing to the pathogenesis of gastrointestinal dysmotility and related symptoms.[86]

Anti-Yo antibodies have been identified in patients with paraneoplastic cerebellar degeneration related to gynecological or breast cancer. Anti-Yo antibodies have also been detected in rare cases of paraneoplastic gastrointestinal dysmotility as a manifestation of ovarian carcinoma.[69] The molecular target of these autoantibodies is the Yo antigen, which has recently been redefined as cerebellar-degeneration-related (cdr) protein. The Yo/cdr is a transduction signal protein which inhibits *c-myc* transcriptional activity. Therefore, abrogation of Yo/cdr function may evoke neuronal degeneration via the activation of apoptosis.[87]

In addition to the examples described above, in which circulating antineuronal antibodies with defined molecular targets appear to contribute to neuronal dysfunction, it is likely that antisera directed against neuronal proteins may also occur as a result of neuronal degeneration in patients with enteric ganglionitis.[88,89]

Finally, non-selective, functionally active autoantibodies directed to type-3 muscarinic receptor (M3), which can be expressed by different tissues, including the lacrimal and salivary glands, bladder detrusor and intestinal smooth muscle as well as enteric neurons, have been identified in patients with gastrointestinal symptoms related to scleroderma and Sjögren's syndrome.[85,90]

Functional role of antineuronal antibodies in motility disorders

Antineuronal antibodies may have a direct role in disturbing gastrointestinal motility. Early findings indicated that purified anti-Hu/ANNA-1 antibodies from patients with paraneoplastic dysmotility affected the peristaltic reflex via a selective alteration of the ascending excitatory pathways.[91] Recent data from our laboratory indicated that sera of patients with high titers of anti-Hu antibodies induced apoptosis *in vitro* when exposed either to the SH-Sy5Y neuroblastoma cell line or to isolated myenteric neurons.[92] Apoptosis in both neuroblastoma cells and enteric neurons was associated with the expression of activated pro-apoptotic messengers, including caspase-3 and apaf-1, suggesting that anti-Hu antibodies may affect directly the intrinsic innervation of the gut via mitochondria-dependent or -independent mechanisms. This immune-mediated neuronal dysfunction may contribute to gut motility disorders in several clinical settings, including paraneoplastic syndromes. The evidence that anti-Hu antibodies evokes neuronal apoptosis *in vitro* does not necessarily imply that this event invariably occurs *in vivo*. However, it is conceivable that disruption of the enteric microenvironment, for example as a result of immune cross-reactivity between tumoral antigens and neuronal proteins in paraneoplastic syndromes (see below, Molecular mimicry), may allow autoantibodies to target enteric neurons at any level of the alimentary tract.

Other *in vitro* studies support the concept that antineuronal antibodies are functionally significant. For instance, sera of patients with circulating antibodies reduce the neuromuscular function of rat intestinal muscle strips.[93] Similarly, Goldblatt and colleagues[90] showed that the anti-M3 antibodies found in patients with scleroderma and Sjögren's syndrome are functionally active and responsible for gut dysmotility via direct inhibition of enteric cholinergic neurotransmission. Interestingly, the sera of these patients had no effect on tachykinergic neurotransmission mediated via neurokinin receptors. Both M3 stimulation and neurokinin receptor stimulation were dependent on activation of L-type voltage-gated Ca^{2+} channels, and had specific interaction with muscarinic receptors.[90] Recently, Lennon and colleagues devised an *in vivo* experimental model of acquired neuronal nicotinic acetylcholine receptor disorder in which rabbits immunized against the α_3 subunit develop signs related to severe dysautonomia, with impairment of gastrointestinal motility, dilated pupils with abnormal reflex to light, and urinary bladder dysfunction. These data are of clinical relevance because they emerge as a paradigm for paraneoplastic neurological autoimmunity observed in patients with small-cell lung carcinoma and circulating antibodies to ganglionic nicotinic acetylcholine receptors.[94]

Taken together, these data support the concept that antineuronal antibodies may impair gut motility directly as a consequence of direct abrogation of the function of key molecules, G-protein-coupled receptors and channels.

Putative pathogenetic mechanisms leading to enteric ganglionitis

Several mechanisms are claimed to play a pathogenetic role in enteric ganglionitis (Table 6.5). For the sake of clarity, it is important to point out that these mechanisms apply to the case of lymphocytic ganglionitis, whereas the recruitment of eosinophils into enteric ganglia remains poorly understood. Perhaps each of the mechanisms underlying lymphocytic ganglionitis may be associated with a specific clinical setting. In this context, we suggest that viral antigens expressed by infected enteric neurons may be related to idiopathic cases of ganglionitis; damage of enteric glia is possibly

Table 6.5 Putative mechanisms leading to enteric ganglionitis

Mechanism	Example
De novo expression of antigens in the ENS	Viral infection (herpes virus, cytomegalovirus)
Disruption of ENS microenvironment	Glial cell damage
Molecular mimicry	Immune cross-reactivity to onconeural proteins (e.g. paraneoplastic syndromes) or sequence homology with antigens expressed by exogenous noxae (e.g. *Trypanosoma cruzi*)
Autoimmune aggression to CNS/ENS neurons	Loss of self vs not-self recognition from the immune system

CNS, central nervous system; ENS, enteric nervous system.

associated with the ganglionitis found in some cases of IBD; molecular mimicry is relevant to ganglionitis in paraneoplastic syndromes and in patients affected by Chagas' disease; finally, autoimmunity may target both central and enteric neurons as a result of the loss of immunological tolerance against self-antigens.

De novo expression of antigens in the ENS

This mechanism is based on the ability of some infectious agents (i.e. neurotropic viruses) to have their antigens expressed by infected enteric neurons. The *de novo* expression of viral antigens may elicit an immune response leading to ganglionitis.

Several types of neurotropic viruses have been associated with gut dysmotility through an intraganglionic immune response secondary to the infection of enteric neurons.[95,96] Robertson and colleagues[97] used *in situ* hybridization histochemistry in esophageal specimens of patients with achalasia to test the presence of DNA viruses, including herpes simplex type 1, cytomegalovirus and varicella zoster. Varicella zoster DNA was found in three out of nine of the patients investigated. The DNA of the other two viruses was never detected. The way in which the varicella zoster virus determines neuronal degeneration and loss in the esophagus remains poorly understood. Recently, both latent and lytic infections of varicella zoster have been demonstrated to occur in isolated guinea-pig enteric neurons,[98] implying that this rather common virus may also have a pathogenetic role in inflammatory neuropathies affecting the small bowel. Debinski and colleagues used the polymerase chain reaction to assay viral DNA in specimens of the small and large intestine of 13 patients with chronic idiopathic pseudo-obstruction.[99] Viral DNA was identified in three patients: two were positive for Epstein–Barr virus and one for cytomegalovirus. Interestingly, the case who turned out to be positive for Epstein–Barr virus cDNA in myenteric neurons showed histopathological features of ganglionitis.[99] Finally, Sonsino and colleagues described a case of chronic idiopathic pseudo-obstruction associated with cytomegalovirus infection of the myenteric plexus.[100]

Disruption of ENS microenvironment

As mentioned previously, the ENS is sheltered by a blood–enteric barrier which prevents damage of neural cells by exogenous noxious agents. Glial cells are among the key players in this protective system. Indeed, enteric glia, the astrocyte-like cells wrapping around neural elements of the gut, exert a critical role in ENS maintenance and survival. *In vitro* studies have demonstrated that primary cultures of enteric glial cells are actively stimulated by proinflammatory cytokines, as reflected by *c-fos* mRNA expression,[101] and that these cells can synthesize and release IL-6 after IL-1β stimulation.[102] Remarkably, mice with selective ablation of enteric glia develop severe enteritis with a dense inflammatory infiltrate localized mainly in the mucosa, but also in the muscularis externa.[103,104] The reduction in glial cells is associated with a progressive decrease in the neuronal population.[103,104] According to these results, it is possible to postulate that, at least in some cases, changes in enteric neurons may be secondary to disruption of enteric glia.

Molecular mimicry

Chagas' disease, the parasitic infection induced by *Trypanosoma cruzi*, and paraneoplastic syndromes are disorders in which ganglionitis may occur as a consequence of a molecular mimicry.

The gastrointestinal tract is affected in cases of paraneoplastic syndromes related to small-cell lung carcinoma, thymoma and gynecological and breast tumors.[59,60,69,86,105] The reasons for an immune response directed against the ENS in the context of paraneoplastic syndrome remain largely undefined, although it is likely that onconeural antigens (i.e. proteins shared by tumor cells and enteric neurons) represent the trigger leading to both antineuronal antibody generation and inflammatory/immune infiltrate within enteric ganglia.[82] Typical target molecules of paraneoplastic syndromes with gastrointestinal involvement are the Hu and Yo (or cdr2) proteins, along with transmitter G-protein-coupled receptors and channels (see above, Functional role of antineuronal antibodies in motility disorders).

Trypanosoma cruzi, a parasite transmitted to humans by triatomine insects (beetles of the family Reduviidae, the kissing bugs), is responsible for Chagas' disease, which is an endemic disorder in South America, especially Brazil.[106–108] In addition to cardiac and urinary system involvement, patients with Chagas' disease often demonstrate severe motor dysfunction of the gastrointestinal tract. Gut abnormalities such as achalasia (mega-esophagus), megaduodenum and megacolon and involvement of extrahepatic biliary tract represent possible end-stages of the progressive degeneration and loss of the intrinsic innervation of the digestive system.[106–108]

The underlying enteric ganglionitis is probably the result of molecular mimicry leading to immune cross-reactivity between the parasite and enteric neurons. In particular, the *Trypanosoma cruzi* flagellar antigen Fl-160, a 160-kDa surface protein, mimics a 48-kDa protein expressed by mammalian axons and myenteric neurons.[109] The immune-mediated damage contributes to the complete loss of enteric neurons, leading to acquired aganglionosis, an extreme condition in many ways identical to that documented in idiopathic cases of progressive enteric ganglionitis.

Autoimmune aggression against CNS/ENS neurons

This mechanism has been postulated to occur in cases of CNS involvement (e.g. encephalomyeloneuropathy) with extension to the ENS. Indeed, the interesting report of Horoupian and colleagues dates back to the early 1980s, describing the case of a patient with concomitant disease of the CNS who developed severe gut dysmotility as a consequence of a florid lympho-plasmacellular infiltrate to the enteric ganglia.[110] The presumed pathogenesis was ascribed by the authors to a possible autoimmune disorder that targeted both central and enteric neurons. Since the CNS and ENS share embryological, morphological, neurochemical and functional features,[111–114] it is likely that underlying autoimmune aggression, due to loss of self versus not-self function, may lead to central and enteric neurodegeneration. Further research is need to clarify the occurrence of pure autoimmune mechanisms in patients with enteric ganglionitis.

Conclusions

Increasing evidence indicates the relevance of neuroimmune interactions in the pathogenesis of disturbed sensory and motor function of the gut. This occurs as a result of the effects induced by a number of mediators on the structure and function of the intrinsic and extrinsic sensory neural network. Although the spectrum of clinical conditions related to activation of an inflammatory/immune response is rather wide, a low-grade inflammation targeting nerve processes of the mucosa is usually associated with mild diseases, such as IBS. In contrast, inflammatory-mediated damage of the ENS is more commonly linked to severe disorders characterized by motility failure. Understanding the mechanisms of this neuroimmune crosstalk will help to better define the pathophysiology of these syndromes and foster new pharmacological targets for the better management of patients with gut sensorimotor abnormalities. Evidence of a biological basis underlying at least subsets of functional gastrointestinal disorders is emerging, with basic and clinical implications.

Acknowledgments

The present work was supported by FAR funds from the University of Bologna and the Ministry of University, Research, Science and Technology of Italy. The authors wish to thank Dr Cesare Cremon for his valuable help in preparing the manuscript and his crucial role in collecting and analyzing data derived from our personal work presented in this chapter. We are indebted to Drs Vincenzo Stanghellini and Roberto Corinaldesi for their constant support and encouragement in our research. Finally, we wish to thank Dr Stephen M Collins for his extensive work in this field, which inspired the present chapter.

References

1 Sukhdeo MV, Croll NA. Gut propulsion in mice infected with *Trichinella spiralis*. *J Parasitol* 1981; **67**: 906–10.

2 Collins SM. The immunomodulation of enteric neuromuscular function: implications for motility and inflammatory disorders. *Gastroenterology* 1996; **111**: 1683–99.

3 Sharkey KA, Mawe GM. Neuroimmune and epithelial interactions in intestinal inflammation. *Curr Opin Pharmacol* 2002; **2**: 669–77.

4 Reinshagen M, Rohm H, Steinkamp M *et al*. Protective role of neurotrophins in experimental inflammation of the rat gut. *Gastroenterology* 2000; **119**: 368–76.

5 di Mola FF, Friess H, Zhu ZW *et al*. Nerve growth factor and Trk high affinity receptor (TrkA) gene expression in inflammatory bowel disease. *Gut* 2000; **46**: 670–9.

6 Barbara G, Vallance BA, Collins SM. Persistent intestinal neuromuscular dysfunction after acute nematode infection in mice. *Gastroenterology* 1997; **113**: 1224–32.

7 Barbara G, De Giorgio R, Deng Y, Vallance B, Blennerhassett P, Collins SM. Role of immunologic factors and cyclooxygenase 2 in persistent postinfective enteric muscle dysfunction in mice. *Gastroenterology* 2001; **120**: 1729–36.

8 Moreels TG, De Man JG, Bogers JJ *et al*. Effect of *Schistosoma mansoni*-induced granulomatous inflammation on murine gastrointestinal motility. *Am J Physiol Gastrointest Liver Physiol* 2001; **280**: G1030–42.

9 Heeckt PF, Halfter WM, Schraut WH, Lee KK, Bauer AJ. Small bowel transplantation and chronic rejection alter rat intestinal smooth muscle structure and function. *Surgery* 1993; **114**: 449–56.

10 Camilleri M. Management of the irritable bowel syndrome. *Gastroenterology* 2001; **120**: 652–68.

11 Thompson WG, Longstreth GF, Drossman DA, Heaton KW, Irvine EJ, Muller-Lissner SA. Functional bowel disorders and functional abdominal pain. *Gut* 1999; **45** (Suppl. 2): II43–7.

12 Isgar B, Harman M, Kaye MD, Whorwell PJ. Symptoms of irritable bowel syndrome in ulcerative colitis in remission. *Gut* 1983; **24**: 190–2.

13 Simren M, Axelsson J, Abrahamsson H, Svedlund J, Bjsmsson ES. Symptoms of irritable bowel syndrome in inflammatory bowel disease in remission and relationship to psychological factors [abstract]. *Gastroenterology* 2000; **118**: A702.

14 O'Sullivan M, Clayton N, Breslin NP *et al*. Increased mast cells in the irritable bowel syndrome. *Neurogastroenterol Motil* 2000; **12**: 449–57.

15 Chadwick VS, Chen W, Shu D *et al*. Activation of the mucosal immune system in irritable bowel syndrome. *Gastroenterology* 2002; **122**: 1778–83.

16 Barbara G, Stanghellini V, De Giorgio R *et al*. Activated mast cells in proximity to colonic nerves correlate with abdominal pain in irritable bowel syndrome. *Gastroenterology* 2004; **126**: 693–702.

17 Dunlop SP, Jenkins D, Neal KR *et al*. Randomized, double-blind, placebo-controlled trial of prednisolone in post-infectious irritable bowel syndrome. *Aliment Pharmacol Ther* 2003; **18**: 77–84.

18 Thoreux K, Owen RL, Schmucker DL. Intestinal lymphocyte number, migration and antibody secretion in young and old rats. *Immunology* 2000; **101**: 161–7.

19 Bradesi S, Eutamene H, Theodorou V, Fioramonti J, Bueno L. Effect of ovarian hormones on intestinal mast cell reactivity to substance P. *Life Sci* 2001; **68**: 1047–56.

20 Salzmann JL, Peltier-Koch F, Bloch F, Petite JP, Camilleri JP. Morphometric study of colonic biopsies: a new method

of estimating inflammatory diseases. *Lab Invest* 1989; **60**: 847–51.

21 Weston AP, Biddle WL, Bhatia PS, Miner PB Jr. Terminal ileal mucosal mast cells in irritable bowel syndrome. *Dig Dis Sci* 1993; **38**: 1590–5.

22 Gwee KA, Leong YL, Graham C *et al.* The role of psychological and biological factors in postinfective gut dysfunction. *Gut* 1999; **44**: 400–6.

23 Spiller RC, Jenkins D, Thornley JP *et al.* Increased rectal mucosal enteroendocrine cells, T lymphocytes, and increased gut permeability following acute *Campylobacter* enteritis and in post-dysenteric irritable bowel syndrome. *Gut* 2000; **47**: 804–11.

24 Gwee KA, Collins SM, Read NW *et al.* Increased rectal mucosal expression of interleukin 1beta in recently acquired post-infectious irritable bowel syndrome. *Gut* 2003; **52**: 523–6.

25 Galeazzi F, Haapala EM, van Rooijen N, Vallance BA, Collins SM. Inflammation-induced impairment of enteric nerve function in nematode-infected mice is macrophage dependent. *Am J Physiol Gastrointest Liver Physiol* 2000; **278**: G259–65.

26 Coelho AM, Fioramonti J, Bueno L. Systemic lipopolysaccharide influences rectal sensitivity in rats: role of mast cells, cytokines, and vagus nerve. *Am J Physiol Gastrointest Liver Physiol* 2000; **279**: G781–90.

27 Weinberg JB. Nitric oxide production and nitric oxide synthase type 2 expression by human mononuclear phagocytes: a review. *Mol Med* 1998; **4**: 557–91.

28 Shah V, Lyford G, Gores G, Farrugia G. Nitric oxide in gastrointestinal health and disease. *Gastroenterology* 2004; **126**: 903–13.

29 Coutinho SV, Gebhart GF. A role for spinal nitric oxide in mediating visceral hyperalgesia in the rat. *Gastroenterology* 1999; **116**: 1399–408.

30 O'Sullivan M, Clayton N, Moloney G *et al.* Increased iNOS expression in irritable bowel syndrome (IBS) patients with stress related symptoms [abstract]. *Gastroenterology* 2003; **124**: M1642.

31 Barbara G, De Giorgio R, Stanghellini V, Cremon C, Corinaldesi R. A role for inflammation in irritable bowel syndrome? *Gut* 2002; **51** (Suppl. 1): i41–4.

32 Stead RH, Dixon MF, Bramwell NH, Riddell RH, Bienenstock J. Mast cells are closely apposed to nerves in the human gastrointestinal mucosa. *Gastroenterology* 1989; **97**: 575–85.

33 Stead RH, Tomioka M, Quinonez G, Simon GT, Felten SY, Bienenstock J. Intestinal mucosal mast cells in normal and nematode-infected rat intestines are in intimate contact with peptidergic nerves. *Proc Natl Acad Sci USA* 1987; **84**: 2975–9.

34 Reed DE, Barajas-Lopez C, Cottrell G *et al.* Mast cell tryptase and proteinase-activated receptor 2 induce hyperexcitability of guinea-pig submucosal neurons. *J Physiol* 2003; **547**: 531–42.

35 Gao C, Liu S, Hu HZ *et al.* Serine proteases excite myenteric neurons through protease-activated receptors in guinea pig small intestine. *Gastroenterology* 2002; **123**: 1554–64.

36 Nozdrachev AD, Akoev GN, Filippova LV *et al.* Changes in afferent impulse activity of small intestine mesenteric nerves in response to antigen challenge. *Neuroscience* 1999; **94**: 1339–42.

37 Bueno L, Fioramonti J, Delvaux M, Frexinos J. Mediators and pharmacology of visceral sensitivity: from basic to clinical investigations. *Gastroenterology* 1997; **112**: 1714–43.

38 Castex N, Fioramonti J, Fargeas MJ, More J, Bueno L. Role of 5-HT3 receptors and afferent fibers in the effects of mast cell degranulation on colonic motility in rats. *Gastroenterology* 1994; **107**: 976–84.

39 Macfarlane SR, Seatter MJ, Kanke T, Hunter GD, Plevin R. Proteinase-activated receptors. *Pharmacol Rev* 2001; **53**: 245–82.

40 Coelho AM, Vergnolle N, Guiard B, Fioramonti J, Bueno L. Proteinases and proteinase-activated receptor 2: a possible role to promote visceral hyperalgesia in rats. *Gastroenterology* 2002; **122**: 1035–47.

41 Tamura K, Wood JD. Effects of prolonged exposure to histamine on guinea pig intestinal neurons. *Dig Dis Sci* 1992; **37**: 1084–8.

42 Fu LW, Pan HL, Longhurst JC. Endogenous histamine stimulates chemically sensitive abdominal visceral afferents through H1 receptors. *Am J Physiol* 1997; **273**: H2726–37.

43 Liu S, Hu HZ, Gao N, Gao C *et al.* Neuroimmune interactions in guinea pig stomach and small intestine. *Am J Physiol Gastrointest Liver Physiol* 2003; **284**: G154–64.

44 Schuurs AH, Verheul HA. Effects of gender and sex steroids on the immune response. *J Steroid Biochem* 1990; **35**: 157–72.

45 Chang L, Heitkemper MM. Gender differences in irritable bowel syndrome. *Gastroenterology* 2002; **123**: 1686–701.

46 Wood JD. Neuropathophysiology of irritable bowel syndrome. *J Clin Gastroenterol* 2002; **35**: S11–22.

47 Spiller RC. Postinfectious irritable bowel syndrome. *Gastroenterology* 2003; **124**: 1662–71.

48 Locke GR III, Zinsmeister AR, Talley NJ, Fett SL, Melton LJ III. Familial association in adults with functional gastrointestinal disorders. *Mayo Clin Proc* 2000; **75**: 907–12.

49 Morris-Yates A, Talley NJ, Boyce PM, Nandurkar S, Andrews G. Evidence of a genetic contribution to functional bowel disorder. *Am J Gastroenterol* 1998; **93**: 1311–7.

50 Levy RL, Jones KR, Whitehead WE, Feld SI, Talley NJ, Corey LA. Irritable bowel syndrome in twins: heredity and social learning both contribute to etiology. *Gastroenterology* 2001; **121**: 799–804.

51 Gonsalkorale WM, Perrey C, Pravica V, Whorwell PJ, Hutchinson IV. Interleukin 10 genotypes in irritable bowel syndrome: evidence for an inflammatory component? *Gut* 2003; **52**: 91–3.

52 Maluenda C, Phillips AD, Briddon A, Walker-Smith JA. Quantitative analysis of small intestinal mucosa in cow's milk-sensitive enteropathy. *J Pediatr Gastroenterol Nutr* 1984; **3**: 349–56.

53 Wershil BK, Furuta GT, Wang ZS, Galli SJ. Mast cell-dependent neutrophil and mononuclear cell recruitment in immunoglobulin E-induced gastric reactions in mice. *Gastroenterology* 1996; **110**: 1482–90.

54 Smout A, Azpiroz F, Coremans G et al. Potential pitfalls in the differential diagnosis of irritable bowel syndrome. *Digestion* 2000; **61**: 247–56.

55 Eutamene H, Theodorou V, Fioramonti J, Bueno L. Acute stress modulates the histamine content of mast cells in the gastrointestinal tract through interleukin-1 and corticotropin-releasing factor release in rats. *J Physiol* 2003; **553**: 959–66.

56 Fukudo S, Nomura T, Hongo M. Impact of corticotropin-releasing hormone on gastrointestinal motility and adrenocorticotropic hormone in normal controls and patients with irritable bowel syndrome. *Gut* 1998; **42**: 845–9.

57 Sciarretta G, Fagioli G, Furno A et al. 75Se HCAT test in the detection of bile acid malabsorption in functional diarrhoea and its correlation with small bowel transit. *Gut* 1987; **28**: 970–5.

58 King TS, Elia M, Hunter JO. Abnormal colonic fermentation in irritable bowel syndrome. *Lancet* 1998; **352**: 1187–9.

59 Krishnamurthy S, Schuffler MD. Pathology of neuromuscular disorders of the small intestine and colon. *Gastroenterology* 1987; **93**: 610–39.

60 De Giorgio R, Stanghellini V, Barbara G et al. Primary enteric neuropathies underlying gastrointestinal motor dysfunction. *Scand J Gastroenterol* 2000; **35**: 114–22.

61 Krishnamurthy S, Schuffler MD, Belic L, Schweid AI. An inflammatory axonopathy of the myenteric plexus producing a rapidly progressive intestinal pseudoobstruction. *Gastroenterology* 1986; **90**: 754–8.

62 Wood JD. Neuropathy in the brain-in-the-gut. *Eur J Gastroenterol Hepatol* 2000; **12**: 597–600.

63 Smith VV, Gregson N, Foggensteiner L, Neale G, Milla PJ. Acquired intestinal aganglionosis and circulating autoantibodies without neoplasia or other neural involvement. *Gastroenterology* 1997; **112**: 1366–71.

64 Goldblum JR, Rice TW, Richter JE. Histopathologic features in esophagomyotomy specimens from patients with achalasia. *Gastroenterology* 1996; **111**: 648–54.

65 De Giorgio R, Barbara G, Stanghellini V et al. Idiopathic myenteric ganglionitis underlying intractable vomiting in a young adult. *Eur J Gastroenterol Hepatol* 2000; **12**: 613–16.

66 Schuffler MD, Baird HW, Fleming CR et al. Intestinal pseudo-obstruction as the presenting manifestation of small-cell carcinoma of the lung. A paraneoplastic neuropathy of the gastrointestinal tract. *Ann Intern Med* 1983; **98**: 129–34.

67 De Giorgio R, Barbara G, Stanghellini V et al. Clinical and morphofunctional features of idiopathic myenteric ganglionitis underlying severe intestinal motor dysfunction: a study of three cases. *Am J Gastroenterol* 2002; **97**: 2454–9.

68 Chinn JS, Schuffler MD. Paraneoplastic visceral neuropathy as a cause of severe gastrointestinal motor dysfunction. *Gastroenterology* 1988; **95**: 1279–86.

69 Lee HR, Lennon VA, Camilleri M, Prather CM. Paraneoplastic gastrointestinal motor dysfunction: clinical and laboratory characteristics. *Am J Gastroenterol* 2001; **96**: 373–9.

70 Schobinger-Clement S, Gerber HA, Stallmach T. Autoaggressive inflammation of the myenteric plexus resulting in intestinal pseudoobstruction. *Am J Surg Pathol* 1999; **23**: 602–6.

71 McDonald GB, Schuffler MD, Kadin ME, Tytgat GN. Intestinal pseudoobstruction caused by diffuse lymphoid infiltration of the small intestine. *Gastroenterology* 1985; **89**: 882–9.

72 Schäppi MG, Smith VV, Milla PJ, Lindley KJ. Eosinophilic myenteric ganglionitis is associated with functional intestinal obstruction. *Gut* 2003; **52**: 752–5.

73 De Giorgio R, Guerrini S, Barbara G et al. Inflammatory neuropathies of the enteric nervous system. *Gastroenterology* 2004; **126**: 1873–83.

74 De Giorgio R, Camilleri M. Human enteric neuropathies: morphology and molecular pathology. *Neurogastroenterol Motil* 2004. (In press.)

75 Tornblom H, Lindberg G, Nyberg B, Veress B. Full-thickness biopsy of the jejunum reveals inflammation and enteric neuropathy in irritable bowel syndrome. *Gastroenterology* 2002; **123**: 1972–9.

76 Clark SB, Rice TW, Tubbs RR, Richter JE, Goldblum JR. The nature of the myenteric infiltrate in achalasia: an immunohistochemical analysis. *Am J Surg Pathol* 2000; **24**: 1153–8.

77 De Giorgio R, Barbara G, Pulsatelli L et al. Chemokine expression and lymphocyte subsets in patients with idiopathic myenteric ganglionitis [abstract]. *Gastroenterology* 2000; **118**: A630.

78 Baggiolini M. Chemokines and leukocyte traffic. *Nature* 1998; **392**: 565–8.

79 Bogers J, Moreels T, De Man J *et al. Schistosoma mansoni* infection causing diffuse enteric inflammation and damage of the enteric nervous system in the mouse small intestine. *Neurogastroenterol Motil* 2000; **12**: 431–40.

80 Lennon VA. Calcium channel and related paraneoplastic disease autoantibodies. In: Peter, JB, Shoenfeld Y, eds. *Textbook of Autoantibodies.* Amsterdam: Elsevier Science, 1996: 139–47.

81 Vincent A, Dalton P, Clover L, Palace J, Lang B. Antibodies to neuronal targets in neurological and psychiatric diseases. *Ann N Y Acad Sci* 2003; **992**: 48–55.

82 Dropcho EJ. Remote neurologic manifestations of cancer. *Neurol Clin* 2002; **20**: 85–122.

83 Benyahia B, Liblau R, Merle-Beral H, Tourani JM, Dalmau J, Delattre JY. Cell-mediated autoimmunity in paraneoplastic neurological syndromes with anti-Hu antibodies. *Ann Neurol* 1999; **45**: 162–7.

84 Wakamatsu Y, Weston JA. Sequential expression and role of Hu RNA-binding proteins during neurogenesis. *Development* 1997; **124**: 3449–60.

85 Waterman SA. Autonomic dysfunction in Lambert–Eaton myasthenic syndrome. *Clin Auton Res* 2001; **11**: 145–54.

86 Vernino S, Low PA, Fealey RD, Stewart JD, Farrugia G, Lennon VA. Autoantibodies to ganglionic acetylcholine receptors in autoimmune autonomic neuropathies. *N Engl J Med* 2000; **343**: 847–55.

87 Okano HJ, Park WY, Corradi JP, Darnell RB. The cytoplasmic Purkinje onconeural antigen cdr2 down-regulates c-Myc function: implications for neuronal and tumor cell survival. *Genes Dev* 1999; **13**: 2087–97.

88 Moses PL, Ellis LM, Anees MR, Ho W, Rothstein RI, Meddings JB, Sharkey KA, Mawe GM. Antineuronal antibodies in idiopathic achalasia and gastro-oesophageal reflux disease. *Gut* 2003; **52**: 629–36.

89 Volta U, De Giorgio R, Petrolini N *et al.* Clinical findings and anti-neuronal antibodies in coeliac disease with neurological disorders. *Scand J Gastroenterol* 2002; **37**: 1276–81.

90 Goldblatt F, Gordon TP, Waterman SA. Antibody-mediated gastrointestinal dysmotility in scleroderma. *Gastroenterology* 2002; **123**: 1144–50.

91 Caras SD, McCallum HR, Brashear HR, Smith TK. The effect of human antineuronal antibodies on the ascending excitatory reflex and peristalsis in isolated guinea pig ileum: 'Is the paraneoplastic syndrome a motor neuron disorder?' [abstract]. *Gastroenterology* 1996; **110**: A643.

92 De Giorgio R, Bovara M, Barbara G *et al.* Anti-HuD-induced neuronal apoptosis underlying paraneoplastic gut dysmotility. *Gastroenterology* 2003; **125**: 70–9.

93 Eaker EY, Kuldau JG, Verne GN, Ross SO, Sallustio JE. Myenteric neuronal antibodies in scleroderma: passive transfer evokes alterations in intestinal myoelectric activity in a rat model. *J Lab Clin Med* 1999; **133**: 551–6.

94 Lennon VA, Ermilov LG, Szurszewski JH, Vernino S. Immunization with neuronal nicotinic acetylcholine receptor induces neurological autoimmune disease. *J Clin Invest* 2003; **111**: 907–13.

95 Vassallo M, Camilleri M, Caron BL, Low PA. Gastrointestinal motor dysfunction in acquired selective cholinergic dysautonomia associated with infectious mononucleosis. *Gastroenterology* 1991; **100**: 252–8.

96 Chang AE, Young NA, Reddick RL *et al.* Small bowel obstruction as a complication of disseminated varicella-zoster infection. *Surgery* 1978; **83**: 371–4.

97 Robertson CS, Martin BA, Atkinson M. Varicella-zoster virus DNA in the oesophageal myenteric plexus in achalasia. *Gut* 1993; **34**: 299–302.

98 Chen JJ, Gershon AA, Li ZS, Lungu O, Gershon MD. Latent and lytic infection of isolated guinea pig enteric ganglia by varicella zoster virus. *J Med Virol* 2003; **70** (Suppl. 1): S71–8.

99 Debinski HS, Kamm MA, Talbot IC, Khan G, Kangro HO, Jeffries DJ. DNA viruses in the pathogenesis of sporadic chronic idiopathic intestinal pseudo-obstruction. *Gut* 1997; **41**: 100–6.

100 Sonsino E, Mouy R, Foucaud P, Cezard JP, Aigrain Y, Bocquet L, Navarro J. Intestinal pseudoobstruction related to cytomegalovirus infection of myenteric plexus. *N Engl J Med* 1984; **311**: 196–7.

101 Ruhl A, Trotter J, Stremmel W. Isolation of enteric glia and establishment of transformed enteroglial cell lines from the myenteric plexus of adult rat. *Neurogastroenterol Motil* 2001; **13**: 95–106.

102 Ruhl A, Franzke S, Collins SM, Stremmel W. Interleukin-6 expression and regulation in rat enteric glial cells. *Am J Physiol Gastrointest Liver Physiol* 2001; **280**: G1163–71.

103 Bush TG, Puvanachandra N, Horner CH *et al.* Leukocyte infiltration, neuronal degeneration, and neurite outgrowth after ablation of scar-forming, reactive astrocytes in adult transgenic mice. *Neuron* 1999; **23**: 297–308.

104 Bush TG, Savidge TC, Freeman TC *et al.* Fulminant jejuno-ileitis following ablation of enteric glia in adult transgenic mice. *Cell* 1998; **93**: 189–201.

105 Pande R, Leis AA. Myasthenia gravis, thymoma, intestinal pseudo-obstruction, and neuronal nicotinic acetylcholine receptor antibody. *Muscle Nerve* 1999; **22**: 1600–2.

106 Meneghelli UG. Chagas' disease: a model of denervation in the study of digestive tract motility. *Braz J Med Biol Res* 1985; **18**: 255–64.

107 Chamond N, Coatnoan N, Minoprio P. Immunotherapy of

Trypanosoma cruzi infections. *Curr Drug Targets Immune Endocr Metab Disord* 2002; **2**: 247–54.

108 Williams-Blangero S, VandeBerg JL, Blangero J, Correa-Oliveira R. Genetic epidemiology of *Trypanosoma cruzi* infection and Chagas' disease. *Front Biosci* 2003; **8**: e337–45.

109 Van Voorhis WC, Schlekewy L, Trong HL. Molecular mimicry by *Trypanosoma cruzi*: the F1-160 epitope that mimics mammalian nerve can be mapped to a 12-amino acid peptide. *Proc Natl Acad Sci USA* 1991; **88**: 5993–7.

110 Horoupian DS, Kim Y. Encephalomyeloneuropathy with ganglionitis of the myenteric plexuses in the absence of cancer. *Ann Neurol* 1982; **11**: 628–32.

111 Gershon MD, Kirchgessner AL, Wade PR. Functional anatomy of the enteric nervous system. In: Johnson LR, ed. *Physiology of the Gastrointestinal Tract*. New York: Raven Press, 1994: 381–422.

112 Furness JB, Costa M. *The Enteric Nervous System*. Edinburgh: Churchill-Livingstone, 1987.

113 Furness JB, Bornstein JC. The enteric nervous system and its extrinsic connections. In: Yamada T, ed. *Textbook of Gastroenterology*. New York: Lippincott, 1991: 2–24.

114 Wood JD. Neural and humoral regulation of gastrointestinal motility. In: Schuster MM, Crowell MD, Koch KL, eds. *Gastrointestinal Motility in Health and Disease*. Hamilton: B.C. Decker, 2002: 19–42.

CHAPTER 7

Stress and the Gut: Central Influences

Heng Y Wong and Lin Chang

Introduction

Stress is an inevitable component of life that threatens an organism's state of well-being. From a teleological viewpoint, the ability to respond appropriately to stress underpins the ability of an organism to adapt to its environment and survive. Examples include the ability to respond quickly to the threat of a predator, which determines an animal's survival and is the basis of the 'fight or flight' response; the rapid expulsion of noxious visceral contents, which aids in the removal of an internal stressor; and stress-induced arousal as an adaptive mechanism that allows an organism to detect subtle changes in a hostile environment. However, in many functional disorders it is the inappropriate reaction to stressors that gives rise to pathological states.

Stress encompasses a diverse range of stimuli and may be physical or psychological. Physical stress acts peripherally and may be external (exteroceptive), as in the case of somatic pain, or internal (interoceptive),

---

Key points

1 The emotional motor system (EMS) comprises the amygdala, hypothalamus and periaqueductal gray.
2 The EMS is a central network involved in the coordination of autonomic, neuroendocrine and pain modulatory outputs to the gut in response to physical and psychological stressors.
3 Psychological stress, particularly early life stress, may play a role in an individual's susceptibility to developing functional gastrointestinal disorders (FGID) by altering the subsequent expression of noradrenergic and serotonergic systems, and the hypothalamic–pituitary–adrenal axis.
4 Physical and/or psychological stress also plays a role in the exacerbation of symptoms in FGID.
5 Activation of central stress circuits within the EMS contributes to stress-enhanced visceral hyperalgesia, gut motility and mucosal inflammation.

6 Physical and psychological stress can enhance gut pain perception, motility and immune function in health and in FGID.
7 Altered activation of central stress circuits, particularly in the periaqueductal gray and anterior cingulate cortex, may play a role in the pathophysiology of FGID.
8 The effects of stress on the gut are mediated by a number of neurotransmitters, including norepinephrine, serotonin and corticotropin releasing factor.
9 Non-gastrointestinal chronic stress-sensitive pain disorders often coexist with FGID and may share common alterations of central stress circuits.
10 Subregions of an anatomically defined area of the brain (e.g. anterior cingulate cortex) may be very different functionally, and care must be taken in interpreting functional brain imaging studies.

as in the example of an endotoxin in or trauma to the gastrointestinal tract. On the other hand, psychological stress, considered a form of exteroceptive stress, mediates its effects centrally.

The central influence of stress on the gastrointestinal tract is manifold. Firstly, the central perception of a visceral event in the gastrointestinal tract and the central control of motor activity and inflammation are modulated by both physical and psychological stressors. It is important to differentiate between acute and chronic stress. Although individuals with functional gastrointestinal disorders (FGID) may respond abnormally to an acute stressor, it is sustained or chronic stressors that lead to long-lasting alterations of central stress circuits. Secondly, early stressful life events are increasingly recognized to be a risk factor for the development of FGID. Lastly, shared central effects of stress may explain similarities in the clinical features of FGID and other chronic pain disorders such as fibromyalgia and interstitial cystitis.

This chapter will focus primarily on central stress circuits, the role of stress in the susceptibility and development of FGID, stress-induced modulation of gastrointestinal function (sensory, motor and inflammatory) and the effect of stress on other chronic pain disorders.

Central stress circuitry: emotional motor system

Any discussion of the central effects of stress on the gastrointestinal tract mandates a description of the emotional motor system (EMS), a network of structures in the brain that are hypothesized to integrate the autonomic, neuroendocrine and pain modulatory responses (including those of the gastrointestinal tract) to central stressors associated with anger, anxiety and other emotions (Fig. 7.1). The EMS conceptualizes a neurobiological basis of stress sensitivity in FGID.[1,2]

The EMS comprises the amygdala, hypothalamus and periaqueductal gray (PAG), and receives input from visceral and somatic afferents as well as cortical structures, particularly subregions of the anterior cingulate cortex (ACC) and medial prefrontal cortex. Inputs from the prefrontal cortex are primarily inhibitory. There are three parallel outputs of the EMS, the autonomic, neuroendocrine and pain modulatory systems, and these are mediated by the pontomedullary

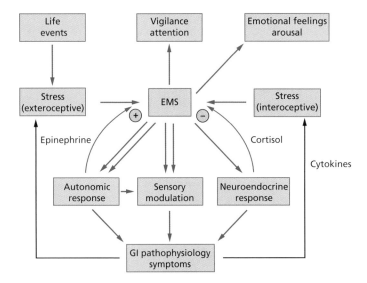

Fig. 7.1 The functional role of the emotional motor system (EMS). The EMS receives and integrates inputs from both exteroceptive and interoceptive stressors, and its major outputs to the peripheral are the autonomic, sensory modulatory and neuroendocrine responses. Feedback from the gastrointestinal (GI) tract occurs via neuroendocrine as well as visceral afferent mechanisms. An important output of the EMS to the forebrain occurs via the ascending noradrenergic system and mediates vigilance attention and arousal. From Mayer EA, Naliboff BD, Chang L, Coutinho SV. Stress and the gastrointestinal tract. V. Stress and irritable bowel syndrome. *Am J Physiol Gastrointest Liver Physiol* 2001; **280**: G519–24. Reproduced with permission from the American Physiological Society.

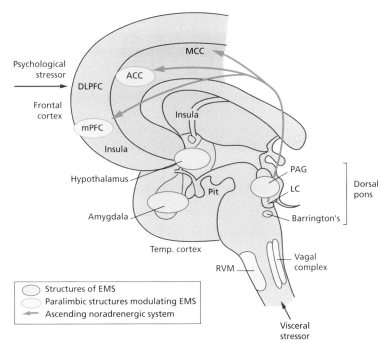

Fig. 7.2 Components of the emotional motor system (EMS), together with closely associated paralimbic structures and ascending noradrenergic system from the LC. ACC, anterior cingulate cortex; MCC, mid-cingulate cortex; mPFC, medial prefrontal cortex; DLPFC, dorsolateral prefrontal cortex; PAG, periaqueductal gray; LC, locus ceruleus; RVM, rostroventral medulla; Pit, pituitary gland; Temp. cortex, temporal cortex.

nuclei (e.g. locus ceruleus, Barrington's complex and raphe nuclei), the hypothalamic–pituitary–adrenal (HPA) axis and the PAG (Fig. 7.2).

The locus ceruleus (LC) is the main source of norepinephrine in the brain and provides norepinephrine input to the EMS and corticolimbic structures via the ascending noradrenergic pathway.[3] This is thought to provide the neurophysiological correlate of arousal that occurs in situations of acute stress, such as that experienced when one is awoken in the middle of the night by the need to micturate, or by the sound of an unwelcome intruder. Corticotropin releasing factor (CRF) is another key neuroendocrine hormone in the stress responsiveness of the EMS. It mediates many of the peripheral effects of stress, and at the same time has been reported to mediate stress-related behavioral responses via CRF_1 receptors in the forebrain.[4]

Multiple feedback loops exist between the EMS and structures providing input and output to the EMS. An important example is the interaction between the LC and the paraventricular nucleus (PVN), a subregion of the hypothalamus. Activation of the LC results in increased CRF release from the PVN, and CRF in turn stimulates the LC complex, thereby establishing a posi-

tive feedback loop.[1] Positive feedback loops in isolation are potentially unstable, and negative feedback mechanisms, such as the inhibitory effect of cortisol on the LC and PVN, provide stability to this system. However, under pathological conditions of chronic stress, the negative feedback mechanisms may break down and down-regulation of glucocorticoid receptors occur in certain regions of the brain, including the LC and PVN.[5] The resulting hyperactivity of the main components of the central stress response, the HPA axis and the sympathetic nervous system (SNS), is thought to manifest as hypervigilance and may also have other central and peripheral effects that account for many of the clinical features of FGID. Furthermore, early life stress is thought to effect changes in the HPA axis and LC, thus potentially making an individual more vulnerable to developing functional disorders (see below).

Alterations in EMS structures such as the amygdala and PAG may be important clinically in irritable bowel syndrome (IBS). For example, positron emission tomography (PET) studies evaluating regional cerebral blood flow report greater activation of the dorsal pons in the region of the PAG in healthy control subjects but greater activation of the dorsal ACC in IBS subjects in response to rectal distension.[6] Furthermore, deactivations of the amygdala have been demonstrated to mediate antinociceptive effects in response to aversive visceral stimuli.[7] Similarly, decreased prefrontal cortex activity has been reported in post-traumatic stress disorder and depression, which are conditions that frequently coexist with IBS. These similarities suggest that these commonly overlapping disorders may share similar underlying central pathophysiological mechanisms characterized by greater activation of limbic and paralimbic brain regions (including the amygdala and ACC) which are part of the EMS and which may result in facilitation of the perceptual response to a visceral stimulus.

Classically, descriptions of the various brain regions are based primarily on anatomical and cytoarchitectural characteristics (e.g. Brodmann areas). However, it is important to note that functional roles may not correlate with the anatomically distinct areas. It is possible for subregions within an anatomically defined area to subserve entirely different functions. For example, the ventral and dorsal subdivisions of the ACC have been demonstrated to mediate different functions. Some of the conflicting results from functional brain imaging studies arose because the subdivisions of classically described areas were not taken into account. Care must therefore be exercised in interpreting the results of such studies.

The role of stress in FGID

The association of psychological stress with the presence of bowel symptoms (e.g. nausea and vomiting, diarrhea) in healthy individuals is a widely appreciated phenomenon, and has been reported in a questionnaire-based study.[8] This finding appears to be accentuated in and considered a hallmark of FGID. Stress and psychological factors appear to play a major role in the initial development and subsequent exacerbation of FGID (Fig. 7.3). Numerous studies indicate that IBS patients report more lifetime and daily stressful events, including abuse, compared with medical comparison groups or healthy controls.[1,9,10]

Stress and susceptibility to FGID

It has been postulated that, in the predisposed individual, sustained stress can alter central stress responsiveness and increase vulnerability to the development of FGID. IBS patients report more lifetime stressful events, including severe abuse history[11] and early childhood adverse events, than controls.[12] Similarly, adverse childhood stressors may predispose individuals to developing functional dyspepsia and heartburn as sexual abuse in childhood has been reported to be associated with these disorders.[12] It is currently assumed that early life stress may interact with genetic predisposition to determine the vulnerability of an individual to developing functional or affective disorders.

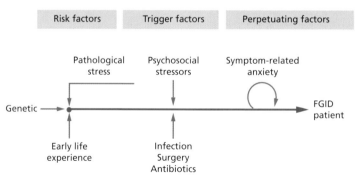

Fig. 7.3 The role of stress in the development and symptom exacerbation of FGID. In individuals with pre-existing susceptibility (genetic programming, early life stressors), chronic and sustained stressors may trigger the onset of FGID. Subsequent stress may lead to symptom exacerbation and perpetuation of the underlying pathology. From Mayer EA, Naliboff BD, Chang L, Coutinho SV. Stress and the gastrointestinal tract. V. Stress and irritable bowel syndrome. *Am J Physiol Gastrointest Liver Physiol* 2001; **280**: G519–24. Reproduced with permission from the American Physiological Society.

The role of early life stress has been tested in rodent models in which pups subjected to neonatal maternal deprivation subsequently develop into adults that display features of IBS, i.e. stress-induced increase in colonic motility, visceral hyperalgesia, somatic hypoalgesia and increased intestinal permeability when exposed to an acute stressor.[2] These effects of neonatal stress on the adult phenotype were abolished by infusion of an intraperitoneal CRF antagonist, implicating a role of the HPA axis in the pathophysiology of IBS.

The effects of early life stress may be mediated by alterations in the HPA axis and norepinephrine pathways of the EMS. In rodent models of early life stress (e.g. maternal separation), changes in HPA responsiveness to stress have been reported and may be secondary to decreased expression of glucocorticoid receptors in the hypothalamus, hippocampus and frontal cortex.[13] This has been replicated in human studies, in which the presence of childhood stress predicts the level of cerebrospinal fluid (CSF) CRF (see below).[14] Early life stress from maternal separation has also been reported to lead to decreased expression of the inhibitory presynaptic α_2-adrenergic receptor, but not the excitatory postsynaptic α_1-adrenergic receptor in the LC.[13] As the LC is closely associated with CRF-secreting neurons of the PVN, alterations of α_2-adrenergic receptors can modulate concomitant changes of the HPA axis. The presence of parallel neonatal stress-sensitive mechanisms would allow fine-tuning of the animal's overall response to stress.

In addition, the serotonergic system may be modified by early life stress. Prolonged maternal separation in neonatal rats has been reported to result in the development of stress-sensitive rats which have decreased 5-HT_{1B} mRNA compared with stress-resistant rats in the dorsal raphe nucleus, a major source of serotonergic projections to the forebrain.[15] There is also some evidence of reduced sensitivity of excitatory α_1-adrenergic receptors in the dorsal raphe nucleus and inhibitory presynaptic 5-HT_{1A} receptors in the frontal cortex following maternal separation.[16]

The consequences of early life stress on the central nervous system are further complicated by the differential effects of timing on the specific alterations. For example, in non-human primates, exposure to neonatal stress at 10–12 weeks of age led to increases in CSF CRF later in adulthood, while stressors at 18–20 weeks caused decreases in CSF CRF levels. In humans, preschool stress (0–5 years of age) correlated positively with CSF CRF in adulthood, whereas the correlation was negative when the stress occurred in the preteen years (6–13 years of age).[14]

Stress and the onset and exacerbation of FGID symptoms

Chronic life stressors frequently lead to exacerbation of symptoms in functional gastrointestinal disorders. Stressful events are more likely to lead to abdominal pain and change in stool pattern in IBS patients than healthy controls and stress has been correlated with the numbers of bowel symptoms, disability days and physician visits.[11] Furthermore, the presence of sustained psychological stressors before, during or after episodes of bacterial gastroenteritis increases the probability of patients developing postinfectious IBS (PI-IBS). With regard to other FGID, the onset of pain in functional abdominal pain syndrome (FAPS) is frequently associated with stressful events, such as the demise of a relative, spouse or other important figure, and previous aversive events, such as physical or sexual abuse, are frequently seen in FAPS.[17] It has been reported in a population-based study that 64% of patients with gastro-esophageal reflux disease (GERD) had exacerbation of symptoms with stress, and GERD patients who are chronically anxious and exposed to long periods of stress are more likely to exhibit stress-induced symptoms exacerbation.[1] Several studies reported an association between stress and functional dyspepsia,[18,19] while such an association has not been demonstrated in other studies.[20]

Effects of stress on gastrointestinal function

Visceral perception

Visceral perception of an interoceptive (or internal) stressor is modulated by concomitant exteroceptive (or external) stress and may be the neurophysiological correlate of stress-related exacerbation of abdominal pain/discomfort. For example, in healthy subjects the application of an aversive stimulus (cold water stress) was reported to reduce the perceptive and pain thresholds to esophageal balloon dilatation.[21]

A large proportion of patients with FGID have hypersensitivity to interoceptive stressors such as balloon inflation or peristaltic contractions. Extensive literature supports the notion that 50–70% of IBS patients have lower perceptual thresholds for pain and discomfort in response to rectal or colonic balloon distension.[11] When other measures of enhanced pain perception (subjective ratings and viscerosomatic referral) were grouped with discomfort thresholds during rectal balloon distension, 94% of IBS patients showed evidence of visceral hypersensitivity.[22] Visceral hypersensitivity has also been demonstrated in 34–65% of patients with functional dyspepsia.[23,24] Using combined measurements of pain perception, 87% of functional dyspepsia patients had visceral hypersensitivity, although this study was performed in a relatively small number of patients.[23]

The modulation of visceral sensation by exteroceptive stress is greater in subjects with FGID than in healthy individuals. Auditory stress has been associated with enhanced perception of rectal distension in IBS patients.[25] However, significant stress-induced changes in visceral perception were not demonstrated in healthy subjects. In another study, stress applied to the sigmoid colon by repetitive noxious distensions induced rectal hypersensitivity in IBS subjects but not controls.[26] The modulation of visceral sensation by stress may be relevant therapeutically, as treatment of IBS with the tricyclic antidepressant amitriptyline resulted in reduced rectal pain perception only in the presence of concurrent acoustic stress and not relaxing music.[27]

Central mechanisms

There has been considerable debate on the localization of visceral hypersensitivity (e.g. peripheral versus central) in FGID but there is good evidence to support predominant central mechanisms. Firstly, IBS subjects have an increased viscerosomatic referral area in response to colonic distension compared with controls. This suggests that visceral hypersensitivity does not occur solely in the primary visceral afferents and occurs at least in second-order neurons in the dorsal horn of the spinal cord or cephalad. Secondly, the insula is considered to function as the viscerosensory cortex, but PET studies showed no difference in insula activity in response to rectosigmoid distension in IBS patients and healthy controls.[6] Moreover, IBS subjects showed increased activity in the dorsal ACC and de-

creased activity in the ventral (perigenual) ACC as well as the PAG.[6] The ventral subdivisions of the ACC and PAG are thought to be integral parts of the subcortical pain modulation systems, while the dorsal subdivision of the ACC may be associated with attentional and emotional modulation of pain.[28] This suggests that the enhanced perception of visceral stressors may be due to altered attentional/emotional modulation of the afferent input and deficient cortical activation of pain inhibitory systems. This is in accordance with classical theories of pain in which both sensory and affective/cognitive components play important roles in the experience of pain.

The clinical relevance of the central mechanisms of visceral hypersensitivity is reflected in the medications proven to be effective in the treatment of FGID. Centrally acting medications, such as tricyclic antidepressants, have been shown in large randomized placebo controlled trials to be effective visceral analgesic agents in FGID.[29] Alosetron is a selective 5-HT_3 antagonist that is effective in relieving abdominal pain or discomfort and urgency, and in normalizing bowel habits in female patients with diarrhea-predominant IBS. Until recently, it was assumed that alosetron mediated its effects via peripheral 5-HT_3 receptors on enteric neurons, but recent evidence suggests that it also decreases activity in frontal and limbic structures, including the amygdala, infragenual cingulate cortex and medial orbitofrontal cortex, which are considered to be involved in the modulation of pain and the autonomic nervous system.[30]

What are the neurophysiological correlates of stress-induced visceral hyperalgesia? There is some evidence that activation of the SNS plays a role in modulating visceral sensitivity. Firstly, the LC/norepinephrine system is activated during fear and acute stress, and acute stress-induced increases in norepinephrine have been reported in the amygdala, hippocampus and prefrontal cortex.[31] Secondly, the perception of duodenal distension in healthy subjects was enhanced by sympathetic activation that was induced experimentally by negative pressure on the lower body.[32] Interestingly, the perception of somatic sensation was not enhanced during sympathetic activation, which is consistent with the observation that hypersensitivity in IBS subjects is limited to visceral and not somatic structures. Lastly, there is a substantial projection from the Barrington's nucleus/LC complex to the PAG, a key region involved in endogenous pain inhibition.[3]

Activation of central noradrenergic pathways can modulate activity in cortical areas via the ascending noradrenergic system. Norepinephrine has been shown to augment evoked activity while decreasing spontaneous activity of the same neuron, thereby enhancing the signal-to-noise ratio in target organs. Such enhancement of inputs has been reported in several LC target areas, such as the cerebral cortex, hippocampus, thalamus and midbrain.[33] In healthy subjects, the anticipatory response to aversive rectal stimuli resulted in widespread activation of the cortex (ventral part of ACC, supraorbital) and brainstem (PAG, thalamus).[6] In contrast, IBS patients overall had much smaller and less widespread changes, with the exception of greater activation of the dorsal ACC,[6] which was similarly reported by Mertz *et al*[34] in a functional magnetic resonance imaging study comparing brain activation patterns in IBS patients and healthy controls in response to rectal distension. This is consistent with enhanced central norepinephrine activity in IBS, as similar patterns of activation have been demonstrated in post-traumatic stress disorder subjects, in whom there is much evidence of heightened central norepinephrine activity.[31]

Taken together, the evidence suggests that the EMS mediates the modulation of visceral perception to exteroceptive stress, and may therefore play an important role in stress-induced symptom exacerbation in FGID. The modulation of visceral perception by psychological stress is consistent with the clinical observation that psychotropic agents and psychological therapies are effective in FGID. Moreover, physicians are well acquainted with the beneficial and often remarkable placebo effect in patients with FGID, with up to 70% of IBS patients reporting symptomatic improvement with placebo. A recent PET study reported that symptom improvement with placebo in IBS patients was associated with activation of the orbitofrontal cortex and deactivation of the dorsal ACC.[35]

Gastrointestinal motility

In addition to the modulation of visceral perception, acute stress can also alter gastrointestinal motility. In healthy subjects, both dichotic listening challenges and cold pressor tests have been reported to increase esophageal motility. Acute stress has also been reported to alter gastric antral motility[36] and duodenal phase-2 motor activity in healthy subjects.[37] Anger has been reported to increase colonic motility in healthy subjects.[38]

The effect of stress on gastrointestinal motility has also been observed in IBS subjects but is quantitatively different from that in healthy controls. Duodenal phase-2 motor activity was decreased in both IBS subjects and controls during acute psychological stress, but the effect was less marked in IBS patients.[37] In addition, an anger-provoking psychological stressor led to significantly greater colonic motility in IBS subjects compared with healthy control subjects.[38]

Stress-induced colonic motility in rats may be mediated by α_2-adrenoceptors as the α_2-antagonist yohimbine inhibits stress-induced defecation but not castor oil-induced diarrhea.[39] In addition, the serotonergic system may play a role, as 5-HT$_{1A}$ agonists were reported to inhibit stress-induced fecal excretion specifically and not 5-HT-induced fecal excretion.[40]

Central mechanisms

The EMS is thought to mediate the effects of acute stress on gastrointestinal motility via the peripheral effects of the autonomic nervous system. Barrington's nucleus (Fig. 7.4) is pivotal in this respect and merits further discussion. It comprises a cluster of neuronal cell bodies that is adjacent to and closely associated with the LC to the extent that, in some animals, no clear distinction can be made between the LC and the equivalent of Barrington's nucleus. In addition, Barrington's nucleus has reciprocal connections with lumbosacral preganglionic parasympathetic neurons (responsible for motor activity in the distal colon and bladder), the dorsal motor nucleus of the vagus (DMV) (responsible for motor activity in the proximal gut) and other supraspinal areas, such as the bed nucleus of the stria terminalis, the hypothalamus and corticolimbic structures.[3] Barrington's nucleus comprises a heterogeneous population of neurons that express many different neurotransmitters, such as CRF and excitatory amino acids. A large percentage of these neurons co-localize with glucocorticoid receptors, indicating the possibility that the stress responsiveness of these neurons occurs via the HPA axis. This is supported by the observation that the central application

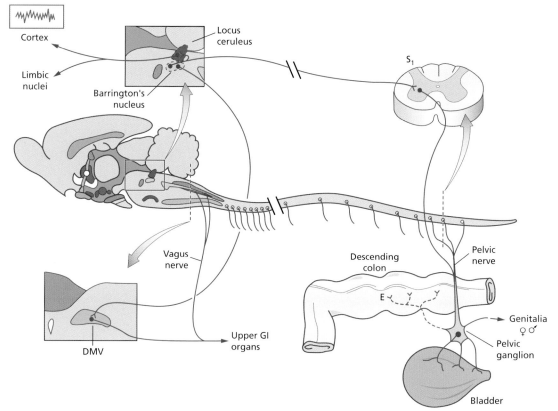

Fig. 7.4 Barrington's nucleus and its extensive ascending and descending projections. Reprinted from Valentino RJ, Miselis RR, Pavcovich LA. Pontine regulation of pelvic viscera: pharmacological target for pelvic visceral dysfunctions. *Trends in Pharmacological Sciences* **20**: 253–60. Copyright 1999, with permission from Elsevier. Modified from Pavcovich LA, Yang M, Miselis RR, Valentino RJ. Novel role for the pontine micturition center, Barrington's nucleus: evidence for coordination of colonic and forebrain activity. *Brain Research* **784**: 355–61. Copyright 1998, with permission from Elsevier.

of CRF mimics stress-induced increases in colonic motility and is inhibited by CRF antagonists. Moreover, acute stress was shown to upregulate CRF expression in Barrington's nucleus and it reduced LC sensitivity to CRF in animal models.[3] Hence, Barrington's nucleus is well poised, with its direct output to the distal colon, indirect output to the proximal gastrointestinal tract (via the DMV) and stress-sensitive mechanisms, to mediate the effects of acute stress on gastrointestinal motility. Current functional imaging techniques do not have the spatial resolution to detect changes in structures as small as Barrington's nucleus, but it is hoped that, with future refinements in technology, its role in mediating stress-related responses can be fully characterized.

Inflammation of the gastrointestinal tract

There is evidence that central stress can influence immune or inflammatory responses in the gastrointestinal tract. This has been demonstrated for both healthy individuals and patients with organic disease. In medical students taking examinations, the immune response to a hepatitis B vaccine was affected by the level of stress and social support. In the gastrointestinal tract, mast cell degranulation is induced by cold pain stress in healthy subjects.[41]

The importance of psychological stress in influencing mucosal inflammation in gastrointestinal disorders is illustrated in postinfective (PI)-IBS, in which the probability of developing PI-IBS is related to the presence of concurrent psychological stressors at the time of gastrointestinal infection. Mucosal abnormalities such as increased permeability, intraepithelial lymphocytes and enteroendocrine cells have also been reported in PI-IBS. Other evidence comes from the observation that major stressful events were significantly associated with subsequent exacerbation of inflammatory bowel disease.[42,43]

Central mechanisms

The effect of central stress on inflammation occurs largely through the HPA axis and the autonomic nervous system. The anti-inflammatory effects of the HPA axis are mediated by circulating glucocorticoids, while the autonomic nervous system, particularly the SNS, influences immune function via epinephrine secreted by the adrenal medulla, or by direct innervation of primary and secondary lymphoid organs, where noradrenergic nerve terminals interact directly with immune cells.[44] Catecholamines and glucocorticoids have been demonstrated to shift the mucosal immune system towards a T-helper type-2 response.[45] The interaction between the central nervous system and mucosal inflammation is bidirectional, as interleukin 6 stimulates the release of CRF.

Other chronic stress-sensitive pain disorders

IBS is frequently associated with other chronic stress-sensitive pain disorders, such as fibromyalgia and interstitial cystitis. There is evidence that similar alterations in central stress circuits may account for the frequent co-existence of these disorders. PET studies performed in fibromyalgia patients during somatic stimuli showed increased ACC activity similar to that seen during rectal distension in IBS subjects. In another study, IBS subjects had greater activation of the dorsal aspect of the ACC in response to rectal distension compared with IBS subjects with fibromyalgia. On the other hand, IBS subjects with fibromyalgia rated chronic somatic pain more intensely than their abdominal pain, and correspondingly their dorsal ACC showed more activity in response to somatic pain compared with IBS subjects.[46] Whilst common patterns of dorsal ACC activity may account for the similarities between IBS and fibromyalgia, the different sites of hyperalgesia could

conceivably be due to subtle alterations in attention to specific afferent outputs from different target organs. However, further studies are needed to clarify this hypothesis. This model may also explain the change in symptoms of IBS to those of functional dyspepsia and vice versa over time that is seen in clinical practice.

In subjects with interstitial cystitis, there is also evidence of alterations in the main components of the central stress response, the HPA axis and the SNS. Symptoms correlated with morning salivary cortisol levels and both the adrenocorticotropic hormone and the norepinephrine response to central CRF were significantly different from controls. It has been demonstrated that cats with interstitial cystitis have increased central sympathetic activity, as their LC had greater levels of tyrosine hydroxylase, the rate-limiting enzyme in catecholamine synthesis, compared with cats without interstitial cystitis.[47] The efferent connections of Barrington's complex to both the distal colon and the bladder provide a common neuroanatomical pathway for the concomitant dysregulation of colonic and bladder function[3] in IBS and interstitial cystitis, respectively.

Conclusion

Central circuits in the EMS and its associated structures play a key role in regulating the stress responsiveness of the gastrointestinal tract in terms of sensory, motor and inflammation function. Early-life stress may be associated with greater vulnerability to the development of FGID as well as other functional or affective disorders via long-term changes in the HPA axis and the norepinephrine system, which are the main components of the central stress response. However, sustained physical and psychological stress experienced later in life appear to be associated with the onset and/or exacerbation of FGID. Moreover, alterations in the central stress response may explain the overlap of FGID with chronic stress-sensitive pain disorders.

Acknowledgments

We wish to thank Cathy Liu for her technical assistance in the preparation of this manuscript. Dr Chang is supported by NIH grants R01 AR46122-01 and P50 DK64539.

References

1 Mayer EA. The neurobiology of stress and gastrointestinal disease. *Gut* 2000; **47**: 861–9.

2 Mayer EA, Collins SM. Evolving pathophysiologic models of functional gastrointestinal disorders. *Gastroenterology* 2002; **122**: 2032–48.

3 Valentino RJ, Miselis RR, Pavcovich LA. Pontine regulation of pelvic viscera: pharmacological target for pelvic visceral dysfunctions. *Trends Pharmacol Sci* 1999; **20**: 253–60.

4 Mayer EA, Fanselow MS. Dissecting the components of the central response to stress. *Nat Neurosci* 2003; **6**: 1011–12.

5 Makino S, Hashimoto K, Gold PW. Multiple feedback mechanisms activating corticotropin-releasing hormone system in the brain during stress. *Pharmacol Biochem Behav* 2002; **73**: 147–58.

6 Naliboff BD, Derbyshire SW, Munakata J et al. Cerebral activation in patients with irritable bowel syndrome and control subjects during rectosigmoid stimulation. *Psychosom Med* 2001; **63**: 365–75.

7 Berman SM, Suyenobu B, Gordon W, Mandelkern M, Naliboff B, Mayer EA. Evidence for antinociceptive deactivation of the amygdala in functional GI disorders. *Gastroenterology* 2002; **122**: A313.

8 Whitehead WE, Crowell MD, Robinson JC, Heller BR, Schuster MM. Effects of stressful life events on bowel symptoms: subjects with irritable bowel syndrome compared with subjects without bowel dysfunction. *Gut* 1992; **33**: 825–30.

9 Drossman DA, Leserman J, Nachman G et al. Sexual and physical abuse in women with functional or organic gastrointestinal disorders. *Ann Intern Med* 1990; **113**: 828–33.

10 Mayer EA, Craske M, Naliboff BD. Depression, anxiety, and the gastrointestinal system. *J Clin Psychiatry* 2001; **62** (Suppl. 8): 28–36.

11 Drossman DA, Camilleri M, Mayer EA, Whitehead WE. AGA technical review on irritable bowel syndrome. *Gastroenterology* 2002; **123**: 2108–31.

12 Talley NJ, Fett SL, Zinsmeister AR, Melton LJ. Gastrointestinal tract symptoms and self-reported abuse: a population-based study. *Gastroenterology* 1994; **107**: 1040–9.

13 Liu D, Caldji C, Sharma S, Plotsky PM, Meaney MJ. Influence of neonatal rearing conditions on stress-induced adrenocorticotropin responses and norepinephrine release in the hypothalamic paraventricular nucleus. *J Neuroendocrinol* 2000; **12**: 5–12.

14 Carpenter LL, Tyrka AR, McDougle CJ et al. Cerebrospinal fluid corticotropin-releasing factor and perceived early-life stress in depressed patients and healthy control subjects. *Neuropsychopharmacology* 2004; **4**: 777-84.

15 Neumaier JF, Edwards E, Plotsky PM. 5-HT(1B) mRNA regulation in two animal models of altered stress reactivity. *Biol Psychiatry* 2002; **51**: 902–8.

16 Gartside SE, Johnson DA, Leitch MM, Troakes C, Ingram CD. Early life adversity programs changes in central 5-HT neuronal function in adulthood. *Eur J Neurosci* 2003; **17**: 2401–8.

17 Drossman DA. Chronic functional abdominal pain. *Am J Gastroenterol* 1996; **91**: 2270–81.

18 Haug TT, Wilhelmsen I, Berstad A, Ursin H. Life events and stress in patients with functional dyspepsia compared with patients with duodenal ulcer and healthy controls. *Scand J Gastroenterol* 1995; **30**: 524–30.

19 Bennett E, Beaurepaire J, Langeluddecke P, Kellow J, Tennant C. Life stress and non-ulcer dyspepsia: a case-control study. *J Psychosom Res* 1991; **35**: 579–90.

20 Talley NJ, Piper DW. Major life event stress and dyspepsia of unknown cause: a case control study. *Gut* 1986; **27**: 127–34.

21 Galeazzi F, Luca MG, Lanaro D et al. Esophageal hyperalgesia in patients with ulcerative colitis: role of experimental stress. *Am J Gastroenterol* 2001; **96**: 2590–5.

22 Mertz H, Naliboff B, Munakata J, Niazi N, Mayer EA. Altered rectal perception is a biological marker of patients with irritable bowel syndrome. *Gastroenterology* 1995; **109**: 40–52.

23 Mertz H, Fullerton S, Naliboff B, Mayer EA. Symptoms and visceral perception in severe functional and organic dyspepsia. *Gut* 1998; **42**: 814–22.

24 Tack J, Caenepeel P, Fischler B, Piessevaux H, Janssens J. Symptoms associated with hypersensitivity to gastric distention in functional dyspepsia. *Gastroenterology* 2001; **121**: 526–35.

25 Dickhaus B, Mayer EA, Firooz N et al. Irritable bowel syndrome patients show enhanced modulation of visceral perception by auditory stress. *Am J Gastroenterol* 2003; **98**: 135–43.

26 Munakata J, Naliboff B, Harraf F et al. Repetitive sigmoid stimulation induces rectal hyperalgesia in patients with irritable bowel syndrome. *Gastroenterology* 1997; **112**: 55–63.

27 Mertz H, Pickens D, Morgan V. Amitriptyline reduces activation of anterior cingulate cortex in irritable bowel syndrome patients during rectal pain. *Gastroenterology* 2003; **124**: A47.

28 Petrovic P, Ingvar M. Imaging cognitive modulation of pain processing. *Pain* 2002; **95**: 1–5.

29 Drossman DA, Toner BB, Whitehead WE et al. Cognitive-behavioral therapy versus education and desipramine versus placebo for moderate to severe functional bowel

disorders. *Gastroenterology* 2003; **125**: 19–31.

30 Mayer EA, Berman S, Derbyshire SW *et al*. The effect of the 5-HT3 receptor antagonist, alosetron, on brain responses to visceral stimulation in irritable bowel syndrome patients. *Aliment Pharmacol Ther* 2002; **16**: 1357–66.

31 Southwick SM, Bremner JD, Rasmusson A, Morgan CA 3rd, Arnsten A, Charney DS. Role of norepinephrine in the pathophysiology and treatment of posttraumatic stress disorder. *Biol Psychiatry* 1999; **46**: 1192–204.

32 Iovino P, Azpiroz F, Domingo E, Malagelada JR. The sympathetic nervous system modulates perception and reflex responses to gut distention in humans. *Gastroenterology* 1995; **108**: 680–6.

33 Aston-Jones G, Rajkowski J, Cohen J. Role of locus ceruleus in attention and behavioral flexibility. *Biol Psychiatry* 1999; **46**: 1309–20.

34 Mertz H, Morgan V, Tanner G *et al*. Regional cerebral activation in irritable bowel syndrome and control subjects with painful and nonpainful rectal distention. *Gastroenterology* 2000; **118**: 842–8.

35 Lieberman MD, Jarcho JM, Berman S *et al*. The neural correlates of placebo effects: A disruption account. *Neuroimage* 2004; **22**: 447–55.

36 Welgan P, Meshkinpour H, Ma L. Role of anger in antral motor activity in irritable bowel syndrome. *Dig Dis Sci* 2000; **45**: 248–51.

37 Kellow JE, Langeluddecke PM, Eckersley GM, Jones MP, Tennant CC. Effects of acute psychologic stress on small-intestinal motility in health and the irritable bowel syndrome. *Scand J Gastroenterol* 1992; **27**: 53–8.

38 Welgan P, Meshkinpour H, Beeler M. Effect of anger on colon motor and myoelectric activity in irritable bowel syndrome. *Gastroenterology* 1988; **94**: 1150–6.

39 Yamamoto O, Niida H, Tajima K *et al*. Effect of alpha-2 adrenoceptor antagonists on colonic function in rats. *Neurogastroenterol Motil* 2000; **12**: 249–55.

40 Abe M, Saito K. Reduction of wrap restraint stress-induced defecation by MKC-242, a novel benzodioxan derivative, via 5-HT1A-receptor agonist action in rats. *Jpn J Pharmacol* 1998; **77**: 211–17.

41 Santos J, Saperas E, Nogueiras C *et al*. Release of mast cell mediators into the jejunum by cold pain stress in humans. *Gastroenterology* 1998; **114**: 640–8.

42 Duffy LC, Zielezny MA, Marshall JR *et al*. Relevance of major stress events as an indicator of disease activity prevalence in inflammatory bowel disease. *Behav Med* 1991; **17**: 101–10.

43 Levenstein S, Prantera C, Varvo V *et al*. Psychological stress and disease activity in ulcerative colitis: a multidimensional cross-sectional study. *Am J Gastroenterol* 1994; **89**: 1219–25.

44 Padgett DA, Glaser R. How stress influences the immune response. *Trends Immunol* 2003; **24**: 444–8.

45 Chrousos GP. Stress, chronic inflammation, and emotional and physical well-being: concurrent effects and chronic sequelae. *J Allergy Clin Immunol* 2000; **106** (Suppl.): S275–91.

46 Chang L, Berman S, Mayer EA *et al*. Brain responses to visceral and somatic stimuli in patients with irritable bowel syndrome with and without fibromyalgia. *Am J Gastroenterol* 2003; **98**: 1354–61.

47 Reche Junior A, Buffington CA. Increased tyrosine hydroxylase immunoreactivity in the locus ceruleus of cats with interstitial cystitis. *J Urol* 1998; **159**: 1045–8.

CHAPTER 8

Stress and the Gut: Peripheral Influences

Mulugeta Million and Yvette Taché

This chapter addresses:

- the biochemical coding of stress as it relates to corticotropin releasing factor (CRF);
- the patterns of gut motor alterations in response to stress;
- the peripheral autonomic pathways involved in stress-related motility changes;

- new insight into the role of central and peripheral CRF signaling pathways in stress-related inhibition of gastric transit and stimulation of colon motor and epithelial function;
- the role of CRF receptors in stress-related modulation of viscerosensibility.

Introduction

Stress represents a real or perceived threat to homeostasis, from within or outside, that translates to endocrine, behavioral, immune and autonomic responses, including alterations of the gastrointestinal function. For over a century now, the central nervous system has been recognized for its ability to modulate gastrointestinal functions. The butterflies that we feel in our gut during strong emotions exemplify the impact of the brain on the gut. Despite the early clinical investigations by Cabanis, Beaumont and then Cannon, demonstrating that emotional stress influences gastric function, neurosciences and gastroenterology developed as separate fields for many years. The last two decades have witnessed, however, an explosive growth in interdisciplinary research related to brain–gut interactions. Understanding of these interconnected systems is emerging, particularly in relation with mechanisms subserving stress-related alterations in gut function. The autonomic nervous system, which is divided into three major components – the parasympathetic, the sympathetic and the enteric nervous system (ENS) – provides a network for the rapid influence of stress on the gastrointestinal tract.

Biochemical coding of the stress response

Selye's pioneer contribution in the 1930s was to establish the concept of stress as a qualitative commonality of the endocrine (adrenal enlargement), gastric (ulcer formation) and immune (thymus involution) responses induced by a wide variety of 'nocuous agents'. Subsequent testing of this concept proved Selye's hypothesis, overall, to be qualitatively valid, although direct measurements of endocrine and sympathetic activities revealed quantitative differences in the patterns of circulating adrenocorticotropic hormone (ACTH) and epinephrine/norepinephrine changes depending upon the stressful stimuli.[1]

A major step forward in the understanding of the biological coding of stress came from the isolation of the 41-amino acid peptide corticotropin releasing

Activation of brain CRF$_1$ receptor

The activation of brain CRF$_1$ receptor is now viewed as a major mechanism that initiates the repertoire of endocrine (HPA activation), behavioral (arousal, anxiety/depression), autonomic (sympathetic activation) and visceral (cardiovascular and gastrointestinal) limbs of the stress response (Fig. 8.1).[2]

factor (CRF) by Vale and collaborators in the early 1980s. Soon after the characterization of CRF as one of the major stimulants of the hypothalamic–pituitary–adrenal (HPA) axis during stress, anatomical studies revealed the widespread distribution of CRF immunoreactivity in brain areas outside those primarily involved in the control of pituitary hormone secretion. Simultaneously, a number of studies showed that CRF injected into the brain is capable of reproducing many stress-like effects independently of the activation of the HPA (Fig. 8.1). These investigations supported the notion that CRF in the brain may be a key component of the multifaceted stress response. Subsequently, novel mammalian CRF-related peptides, urocortin 1, urocortin 2 and urocortin 3, and two cloned G protein-coupled receptors, CRF$_1$ and CRF$_2$, with distinct affinity for CRF family ligands, were discovered (Fig. 8.1). CRF displays higher affinity for the CRF$_1$ than for the CRF$_2$ receptor, urocortin 1 has equal affinity for both subtypes, while urocortins 2 and 3 are selective ligands for the CRF$_2$ receptor. Additionally, potent, selective CRF$_1$ antagonists and, more recently, CRF$_2$ receptor antagonists have been developed and transgenic CRF deficient or overexpressing mice have been generated.[2] These pharmacological tools and animal models are instrumental in advancing our understanding of the role of CRF pathways in the orchestration of the bodily stress response and the pathophysiology resulting from dysregulation of the CRF system.[3,4]

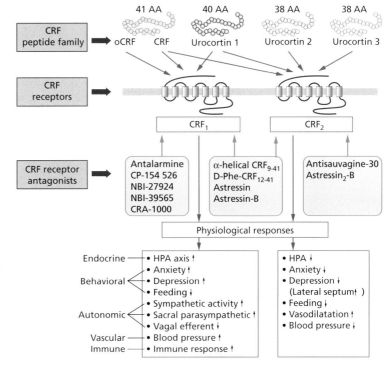

Fig. 8.1 Schematic representation of the mammalian CRF-related peptides, CRF receptors, CRF receptor antagonists and their physiological responses. Ovine CRF binds preferentially to CRF$_1$ receptor, whereas CRF and urocortin (Ucn) 1 bind to both CRF receptor subtypes, although with different affinities. Ucn 2 and 3 bind selectively to CRF$_2$ receptors. The activation of the CRF$_1$ receptors induces a wide range of endocrine, behavioral, immunological, autonomic and visceral effects mimicking stress-like responses, while the activation of CRF$_2$ dampens these endocrine, behavioral and cardiovascular responses. (oCRF: ovine CRF; AA: amino acid; HPA: hypothalamic-pituitary-adrenal axis)

Stress responses in the gut

Most psychological and physical stressors inhibit motion and transit in the upper gut while stimulating them in the lower gut. Differences between the upper and lower gut in the motility response to stress are primarily due to differences in innervation and the local neural and chemical mediators involved.

Only recently, the role of CRF_2 receptors has been examined with the advent of selective CRF_2 receptor antagonists and CRF_2 knockout mice.[2] Evidence indicates that these receptors may be important in dampening stress sensitivity, although controversy exists whether CRF_2 functions to enhance or impede the anxiety-like behaviors induced by stress.[2] The biological actions of CRF and CRF-related ligands and the overactivity of CRF-CRF_1 pathways in various clinical conditions, including anxiety/depression, have spurred interest in potential uses of small CRF_1 antagonist molecules that are active orally and cross the blood–brain barrier (Fig. 8.1).[3,4]

Patterns of gastrointestinal motor alterations induced by stress

The vulnerability of the gastrointestinal tract to physical, emotional or chemical aversive stimuli has been demonstrated both in clinical and experimental settings.

In the esophagus, an association between esophageal symptoms and behavioral abnormalities has been reported. Earlier studies showed that 84% of patients with contraction abnormality of the esophagus had psychiatric diagnoses compared with 31% of those with normal motility. Dichotic listening tasks increase resting pressure in the upper esophageal sphincter of healthy volunteers. However, existing evidence indicates that the upper esophageal response to stress in normal subjects is stimulus-specific and small in magnitude, and does not translate into symptoms. Psychological stress also induces only minor effects on esophageal muscle and lower esophageal sphincters.[5]

In the stomach, different acute stressors inhibit gastric motility and emptying across species (Table 8.1). In humans, psychological (fear, stressful tests) and physical (cold-pain immersion, intense exercise) stressors cause a profound delay in gastric emptying of caloric and acaloric meals, through inhibition of gastric contractility and/or coordination. Likewise, in experimental animals, a variety of stressors such as restraint stress, operant avoidance, radiation, acoustic stimulation, hemorrhage, swim stress, abdominal or cranial surgery, anesthetics, immune challenges and fear inhibit gastric motion and emptying of nutrient or non-nutrient meals (Table 8.1). However, the pattern of the gastric motility change is influenced by the duration and type of stressor, test meal and species.[6,7] For instance, acute exposure to cold stress in rats and mice causes gastric transit acceleration, the stimulus-specificity of the response lying in the activation of brain medullary thyrotropin-releasing hormone, which produces pronounced gastric vagal activation.[8]

In the small intestine, studies in humans show that cold-pain stress or active coping stress inhibits orocecal transit. Acute psychological stress suppresses the duodenal phase II migrating motor complex. In rats, transit in the small intestine is also inhibited by acute exposure to wrap restraint, cold water swimming or ether, whereas phase III myoelectric activity is replaced by irregular phase II activity (Table 8.2).

In the human large intestine, the pattern of change in motility in response to various stressors is mainly stimulatory (Table 8.2). Likewise, in experimental animals acute water avoidance, conditioned fear to inescapable foot shocks, tail shock, loud noise, open-field testing, restraint at room temperature and cold environment and immune challenge decrease colonic transit time, induce defecation and diarrhea, and increase colonic myoelectric spike activity.[9]

Stress and the autonomic nervous system of the gut

The autonomic nervous system is the efferent limb mediating the effects of stress on gastrointestinal function. It is reciprocally connected with the brain CRF/urocortin 1 system and transmits central signals

Table 8.1 Patterns of gastric transit alterations induced by various stressors in humans and experimental animals (Cal, caloric; iv, intravenous; ic, intracisternal; liq, liquid)

Stressors	Species	Meal	Effect
Fear, anger	Human	Cal	Delay
Preoperative anxiety	Human	Liq non cal	Delay
Physical stress, severe	Human	Water	Delay
Physical stress, mild	Human	Water	Accelerated
Shock avoidance task	Human	–	Gastric dysrhythmia
Cold immersion	Human	Cal	Delay (~70%)
Operant avoidance	Monkey	Water	Delay
Acoustic	Dog	Cal	Delay (45–50%)
Novel environment	Dog	Cal	Delay (50%)
Handling or noise	Guinea-pig	Non cal	Delay
Restraint	Rat	Liq non cal	Delay
Cold restraint	Rat	Liq non cal	Accelerate/Delay
Interleukin-1β, iv	Rat	Liq non cal	Delay (up to 80%)
Interleukin-1β, ic	Rat	Liq non cal	Delay (up to 90%)
Surgery	Rat/mice	Liq non cal	Delay
Cold	Mice	Milk	Accelerate
Frequent handling	Mice	Liq non cal & cal	Delay (~54%)

to the ENS and effector cells. A voluminous literature describes the activation of brain CRF gene expression and autonomic centers under various conditions of stress. From detailed mapping using Fos immunohistochemistry as a marker of neuronal activation, distinct patterns of brain neuronal activation have emerged depending upon the systemic versus physico-psychological nature of the stressors.[10]

Parasympathetic nervous system

The parasympathetic innervation of the gastrointestinal tract is provided mainly by the vagal fibers arising from cell bodies located in the dorsal motor nucleus of the vagus (DMN) (Fig. 8.2). The injection of CRF into the cerebrospinal fluid inhibits the activity of DMN neurons and there is a decrease in vagal efferent activity recorded in the gastric branch in anesthetized rats. The end target of vagal fibers is the myenteric ganglia. Individual vagal efferent axons ramify widely to produce extensive collaterals that envelop virtually all gastric myenteric neurons as well as the submucous plexus, although to a lesser extent in the latter. The hepatic and gastric branches innervate nearly 70% of the myenteric neurons in the duodenum. In the distal small intestine and proximal colon, the pattern of the vagal efferent network derives exclusively from the celiac branches

Table 8.2 Patterns of small and large bowel transit and motility in responses to various stressors in human and experimental animals (representative studies)

Stressor	Species	Small intestine	Large intestine
Mental stress	Human	↓ Transit (52%)	N/A
Cold stress	Human	↓ Transit	↑ Spike frquency (~160%)
Anger/excitement	Human	N/A	↑ Motility index
Active coping stress	Human	↓ Transit (~30%)	N/A
Social intruder	Monkey	N/A	↑ Defecation
Immobilization	Dog	↑ Motility index	N/A
Cold restraint	Rat	N/A	↑ Defecation (62%)
Restraint	Rat	↓ Transit	↑ Defecation
Conditioned fear	Rat	N/A	↑ Spike burst (82%)
Water avoidance	Rat	N/A	↑ Defecation (8-fold)
Morphine withdrawal	Rat	N/A	Diarrhea
Restraint	Mice	N/A	↑ Defecation (5-fold)

N/A, not applicable.

Mechanism of stress responses

Collectively, the evidence so far supports the notion that activation of CRF receptors in the brain mediates the dual actions of stress on parasympathetic outflow to the gut. This is inhibitory in the upper gut, acting through the decrease in gastric vagal efferent activity, and stimulatory in the lower gut (colon), acting through the activation of SPN.[8]

---

and resembles that of the stomach, but with a much lower density.

The parasympathetic input to the colon originates from cell bodies located in the sacral intermediolateral column (sacral parasympathetic nucleus, SPN). The efferent axons travel within the pelvic nerve and innervate the pelvic plexus, and postganglionic fibers project to the ENS of the distal colon and rectum (Fig. 8.2). The SPN is synaptically linked to central autonomic circuits through bulbospinal pathways. These include the direct efferent projections from Barrington's nucleus (formerly known as the pontine micturition center) containing numerous CRF-immunoreactive neurons, the subceruleus nucleus and the interconnected locus ceruleus (LC) (Fig. 8.1).[11] Paired animal models (inbred Fischer and Lewis rats), selected for their high and low CRF response in the paraventricular nucleus (PVN) of the hypothalamus, respectively, when exposed to various stressors, show differential activation of SPN after water avoidance stress.

The neurochemical identity of vagal fibers and myenteric neurons receiving vagal input has been characterized recently. Parasympathetic nerves commonly synthesize and release acetylcholine, adenosine 5′-triphosphate (ATP), nitric oxide (NO) and vasoactive intestinal peptide (VIP). Vagal preganglionic fibers end on serotonin-, VIP-, NO-, gastrin-releasing peptide (GRP)- and GRP/VIP-containing myenteric neurons in gastric myenteric ganglia. Using antibody against the splice variant of the acetylcholine transferase (pChAT) expressed selectively in the peripheral nervous system, 60–70% of the myenteric neurons in the gastrointestinal tract were shown to be pChAT-positive and surrounded by pChAT-containing fibers.[12] These findings demonstrated the prominent cholinergic vagal innervation of the ENS.[8] How the various stressors influence parasympathetic transmitter release within the gut and what type of myenteric neurons, in addition to cholinergic neurons, are mainly affected by alterations in parasympathetic outflow during stress remain to be defined.

Sympathetic nervous system

The main neurotransmitters/neuromodulators of post-ganglionic sympathetic innervation of the gastrointestinal tract are norepinephrine, ATP and neuropeptide Y (NPY). Opioid peptides are also widely distributed in the sympathetic neurons, where their role is mainly to exert a prejunctional inhibitory influence. The release or co-release of these substances upon sympathetic stimulation varies depending on the tissue and the parameters of stimulation. For instance, low frequency and short bursts favor ATP release, while longer stimulation favors the adrenergic component, and NPY is released in response to high-frequency, intermittent bursts of stimulation.[13] The sympathetic nervous system also interacts with sensory motor and vagal nerves that are in close proximity; NPY, norepinephrine and opiate exert a prejunctional inhibitory influence on cholinergic neurotransmission.[13]

The CRF system in the PVN and the sympathetic nervous system are anatomically and functionally interrelated and regulate each other's functions. This is exemplified by the connections between the CRF-containing neurons in the PVN and the LC (A6 catecholaminergic neurons) in the brainstem. Water avoidance and restraint as well as central injection of CRF induce a CRF_1 receptor-mediated increase in the activity of A6 neurons and elevate circulating levels of epinephrine and, more prominently, norepinephrine.[14,15] Spontaneous hypertensive rats display high activation of neurons and CRF gene expression in the PVN and Barrington's nucleus/LC, correlated with hyperstimulation of sympathetic nervous system activity after restraint stress compared with normotensive rats. Hence, the increase in CRF gene expression in hypothalamic and pontine/brainstem centers is generally viewed as a major factor that governs the activation of catecholamine release in the blood after stress exposure.[15]

The sympathetic nervous system also transmits neural signals to the immune system through dense innervation of both primary and secondary lymphoid organs

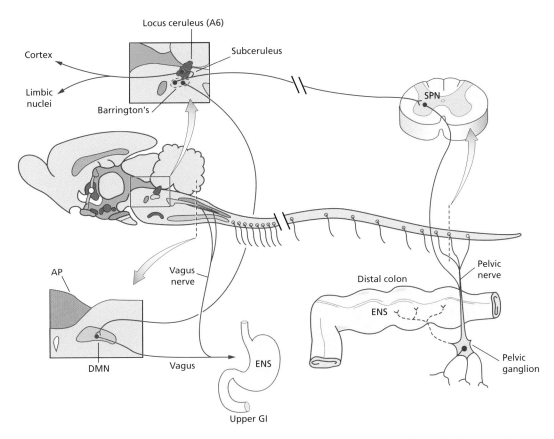

Fig. 8.2. Pontine and medullary parasympathetic efferent innervation of the gastrointestinal tract in rats. Efferent fibers from Barrington's complex project to the dorsal motor neurons (DMN) in the brainstem and the sacral parasympathetic nucleus (SPN). Axons from DMN provide vagal innervation to the stomach and small intestine and, to a lesser extent, to the cecum and proximal colon. The end target of vagal efferent fibers is the enteric nervous system (ENS). Efferent output from the SPN projects primarily through the pelvic nerve to the pelvic ganglia, and postganglionic fibers innervate the ENS in the distal colon. Stress activates the locus ceruleus/Barrington's complex, which has a unique ability to modulate the two major parasympathetic preganglionic nucleus innervations to the gut. Barrington's nucleus, by its reciprocal connections with the locus ceruleus, can also be influenced by or influence the noradrenergic neurons in the locus ceruleus projecting to the forebrain. Adapted from reference 11.

and through postganglionic sympathetic neurons. In particular, stress degranulates colonic mucosal mast cells through sympathetic and muscarinic-dependent pathways, leading to stress-related alterations in colonic epithelial cell function.[16] When activated, the sympathetic nervous system also causes systemic release of interleukin-1β and tumor necrosis factor α. In keeping with the crosstalk between the immune and neuroendocrine systems, interleukin-1β activates the brain CRF pathways leading to the activation of the sympathetic nervous system.[17] This may provide the biochemical basis for the sustained visceral manifestations of stress.

CRF signaling pathways and autonomic-dependent inhibition of gastric and small intestinal motor function

Several studies have shown that CRF receptor antagonists injected centrally prevent the inhibition of gastric emptying induced by various types of stressors, including physico-psychological (restraint, forced swimming), immunological (central or peripheral injection of interleukin-1β), visceral (trephination, abdominal surgery) and chemical (central injection of CRF) stressors.[9] With regard to the delayed gastric emptying induced by surgery, a role of CRF_1 receptors was established in mice with deletion of the CRF_1 receptor gene. CRF_1 knockout mice did not develop postoperative gastric ileus.[18] By contrast, restraint stress-induced delayed gastric emptying was not altered by selective CRF_1 antagonist but was blocked by CRF_2 antagonists.[19] The CRF receptor subtype involved in delayed gastric emptying induced by various stressors needs to be further characterized. Central CRF receptors are also involved in restraint stress-induced inhibition of small intestinal transit, although less information is available.[9]

The increases in ACTH, corticosteroid and β-endorphin secretion induced by the brain CRF activation during restraint stress do not play a role in mediating the inhibition of gastric and small intestinal transit. The increased circulating levels of these hormones had no effect on gastric transit. Moreover, hypophysectomy or adrenalectomy did not alter the delayed gastric and intestinal transit induced by restraint.[6,20] The rapid onset of changes in gastric motility in response to various stressors favors a direct, neurally mediated mechanism that involves mainly the decrease in vagal outflow to the upper gut as well as modulation of the vago-vagal reflex. However, there is also evidence for a role of sympathetic pathways in specific stressors and central urocortin₁-induced inhibition of gastric emptying.[20,21] There is still very little known regarding the enteric mechanisms translating the changes in autonomic nervous system activity into altered gastric emptying and small intestinal transit.

CRF signaling pathways and autonomic-dependent stimulation of colonic motor and epithelial function

Central CRF signaling pathways

Preclinical studies have shown that a number of selective CRF_1 antagonists (CP-154,526, CRA-1000, NBI-35965, and NBI-27914) blunt the stimulation of colonic motor function induced by various stressors in rodents and monkeys.[9,22,23] Water avoidance, restraint and central injection of CRF, which mimics stress effects on the colon, are models of psychological/physical stress that are used extensively to establish the underlying peripheral mechanisms leading to colonic motor stimulation.[9] While the activation of the HPA axis and

sympathetic/adrenomedullary systems represents the classical peripheral limbs of the endocrine and immune stress responses, respectively, central CRF- and restraint stress-induced stimulation of colonic motor function do not involve these pathways. This is shown by the fact that hypophysectomy, adrenalectomy, noradrenergic blockade and neurotensin and opiate antagonists failed to prevent central CRF- and restraint stress-induced colonic motor stimulation.[16,20] The colonic motor response to these stimuli was reduced by vagotomy and completely prevented by pharmacological blockade of cholinergic nicotinic transmission in autonomic ganglia and by the peripheral administration of muscarinic, CRF, neurokinin-1 (NK-1) and 5-HT₃ receptor antagonists.[23] Fischer rats, which display high hypothalamic CRF in response to various stressors, have greater activation of neurons in the SPN that correlates with greater colonic motor stimulation when exposed to water avoidance stress compared with the hypothalamic CRF-deficient Lewis rats.[23] These experimental data suggest that restraint and water avoidance stress activate colonic motor function through increased sacral parasympathetic cholinergic outflow. Stress also engages local mechanisms involving interplay of released CRF and/or urocortin 1 activating CRF_1 receptors, serotonin activating 5-HT₃ receptors, and substance P acting on NK-1 receptors. Stress activates the pontine Barrington's nucleus, which has direct projections to SPN and forms excitatory synapses on these neurons. The activated Barrington's nucleus also projects to the lateral aspect of the DMN of the vagus, which contains preganglionic neurons innervating the ascending and transverse colon. CRF acting through CRF_1 receptors serves as a modulator of these pathways under stress conditions.[11] These findings provide an anatomical substrate for the stress-induced CRF_1 receptor-mediated cholinergic activation of colonic function, largely through excitatory input to SPN (Fig. 8.2).

Stress-induced intestinal barrier dysfunction in both experimental animals and humans is prevented by atropine, suggesting the importance of peripheral cholinergic mechanisms.[24] Reports from various groups have highlighted the importance of mast cells in colonic mucosal alterations induced by stress (restraint, environmental stress and intracerebroventricular injection of CRF) viz, increase in mucin, prostaglandin E_2, histamine and ion secretion, and the permeability and translocation of macromolecules.[24] The stress-related degranulation of colonic mast cells is prevented by ganglionic, muscarinic and noradrenergic blockade, implicating the activation of both the sacral parasympathetic and the sympathetic pathways, while the pituitary–adrenal endocrine response does not play a role.[16,25]

Peripheral CRF signaling pathways

Consistent reports have established that peripheral administration of CRF and urocortin 1 in several animal species produces stress-like actions in the colon that have relevance to the peripheral mechanisms through which stress influences colonic motor and epithelial function. These peptides, injected peripherally, induce high-amplitude colonic contractions, reduction of large intestine and distal colonic transit time, defecation and, at the highest doses, watery diarrhea in rats and mice.[23] In humans, the stimulation of colonic motility index by intravenous injection of CRF is more pronounced in irritable bowel syndrome (IBS) patients than in healthy volunteers. The actions of CRF and urocortin 1 on the colonic response in experimental animals are mediated by CRF_1 receptors, as shown by the ability of a selective CRF_1 antagonist, but not a selective CRF_2 antagonist, to block the response (Fig. 8.3). Conclusive evidence of CRF_1 mediation was gained by the use of the selective CRF_2 agonists urocortin 2 and urocortin 3, which failed to influence distal colonic transit or defecation in rats and mice when injected peripherally.[19,23] Ganglionic blockade did not alter the stimulation of colonic transit by peripheral injection of CRF, unlike central administration, ruling out mediation by a gut-brain reflex. The increase in peristaltic activity produced in an isolated rat distal colon preparation *in vitro* in response to local injection of CRF established a local site within the colon.[22] CRF is likely to act in the ENS. Intraperitoneal injection of CRF activates cholinergic myenteric neurons in the colon. This is prevented by peripheral injection of peptide CRF antagonists and selective CRF_1 antagonists (Fig. 8.3).[22] The detection of CRF_1 receptors in colonic myenteric and submucosal neurons in the rat provides anatomical support for a direct action on colonic enteric neurons.[23] In addition, possible effects of CRF on interstitial cells of Cajal or

through mediators released by mast cell degranulation induced by CRF were ruled out, as shown by the unchanged colonic motor response in mast cell-deficient Kit^W/Kit^{W-v} mice.[26]

Other studies have demonstrated that peripheral CRF also exerts stress-like effects on several components of the intestinal barrier function, as shown by the degranulation of mucosal mast cells, stimulation of colonic mucin, prostaglandin E_2 and ion secretion, and the increase in paracellular and transcellular permeability to ions, and protein translocation. *In vitro* studies also confirm a local action of CRF to increase distal colonic permeability (Fig. 8.3).[22,24–26]

The colonic epithelial and motor alterations delineated by peripheral administration of CRF are among the peripheral mechanisms through which stress alters colonic function. Ionic secretion and defective epithelial barrier function induced by cold restraint and water avoidance stress are blocked by peripheral administration of peptide CRF antagonists. Restraint-induced stimulation of colonic transit, defecation, increased motility, colonic mucosal mast cell degranulation and prostaglandin E_2 secretion are prevented or dampened by peripheral injection of peptide CRF receptor antagonists that act peripherally (Fig. 8.3).[22,24–26] The mechanisms whereby stress recruits the peripheral pool of CRF and/or urocortin 1 to activate peripheral CRF_1 receptors resulting in colonic motor and epithelial changes are still unsettled. Urocortin 1 is present in the sympathetic nervous system, colonic myenteric neurons and submucosal myenteric plexus as well as in enterochromaffin cells and lamina propria macrophages in rats and humans.[22,23]

Stress and viscerosensitivity

Patients with IBS exhibit enhanced perception of visceral events (visceral hypersensitivity), enhanced motor responses of the distal colon to stress and food ingestion (gastrocolic reflex) and altered autonomic and neuroendocrine responses to stress.[27]

In experimental studies of visceral nociception involving male rats, acute (restraint or water avoidance) or chronic (neonatal maternal separation or colonic irritation) stress increased pain responses to colorectal distension (CRD).[23] Colonic hypersensitivity to CRD and novel stress as well as enhanced visceral pain

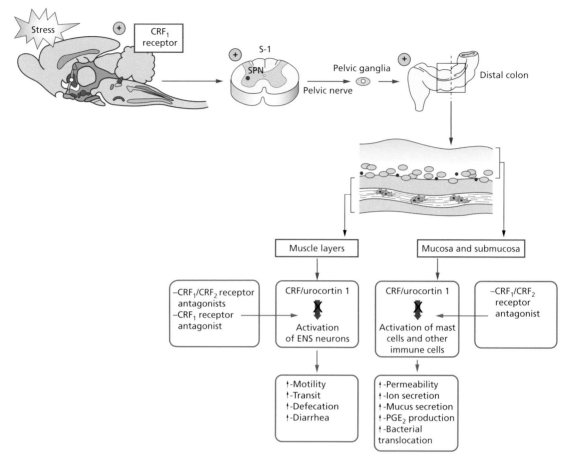

Fig. 8.3 Schematic illustration of pathways involved in stress-related stimulation of colonic motor and epithelial functions. Stress activates CRF–CRF$_1$ signaling pathways in the brain linked with hypothalamic (paraventricular) and pontine (Barrington's and locus ceruleus) nuclei, which stimulate the sacral parasympathetic nucleus (SPN) and subsequently the enteric nervous system (ENS) through postganglionic pelvic projections. There is a postulated release of local CRF ligands in the colon that activates the ENS through CRF$_1$ receptors and the mucosal mast cells through a CRF receptor subtype that is yet to be characterized. The peripheral CRF$_1$-mediated activation of the ENS leads to stimulation of colonic motor function, while that of mast cells results in alterations in the mucosal barrier and secretory functions.

perception in genetically anxiety prone rat strains are well documented.[29] The mechanisms and pathways of stress-induced visceral hypersensitivity are not yet fully understood. Evidence indicates the role of CRF$_1$ receptor in acute stress-induced visceral hypersensitivity to CRF distension.[23] In maternally separated Long Evans male rats, peripheral administration of the non-peptide CRF$_1$ antagonist NBI-35965 blocked acute psychological stress-induced visceral hyperalgesia to CRD (30) (Fig. 8.4). Furthermore, the delayed colonic sensitization (24 hours) following a single acute water avoidance stress session was also prevented by pretreatment with the selective CRF$_1$ antagonist CP-154,126 in male Wistar rats.[31] This study in male Wistar rats has also shown that the delayed colonic hypersensitivity developed following mild psychological stress is prevented by the selective NK-1 antagonist SR140333, but not by peripheral chemical sympathectomy.[31] These data suggest that activation of the CRF/CRF$_1$ and SP/NK-1 systems operates in series in stress-induced hypersensitivity, whereas peripheral norepinephrine and NPY do not play a role in the sensitization. In healthy humans, intravenous

Pathophysiology of IBS

Although the pathophysiology of IBS is not well understood, considerable evidence supports a role of chronic stress in the onset and/or exacerbation of symptoms.[28]

administration of ovine CRF, a preferential CRF_1 receptor agonist, lowered the thresholds for sensation of the urge to defecate and of discomfort in response to CRD.[23] These data suggest that activation of peripheral CRF receptors could modulate visceral pain response through the mechanisms discussed above in relation to mast cell degranulation and changes in colonic permeability, secretion and motility.

In humans, postinfectious IBS tends to occur in patients with psychological profiles similar to those observed in IBS patients and in whom there is a higher incidence of stressful life events just before exposure to the infection.[28] Stress has also been implicated as a modulator of colonic inflammation, as the principal stress response mediator, CRF, exerts a local proinflammatory role through the CRF_1 receptors.[32] In an animal model of postinfectious IBS, visceral hypersensitivity and altered colonic motility in response to stress after subsidence of inflammation is reported. More recently, activation of mast cells in proximity to colonic nerves has been found to correlate with abdominal pain in IBS.[33] These observations link stress and local inflam-

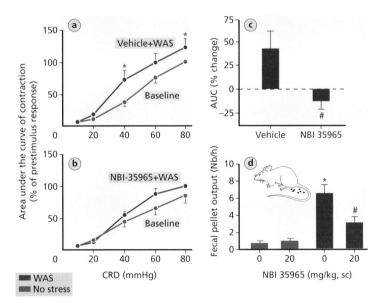

Fig. 8.4. Blockade of water avoidance stress-induced increased stimulation of colonic motor function and visceral pain in response to colorectal distension (CRD) by the CRF_1 receptor antagonist NBI 35965 in conscious rats. (a and b) Visceromotor response (VMR) to graded intensities of phasic CRD. VMR during the control period (before stress) and after 60 minutes of water avoidance stress. (a) Rats were injected with the vehicle (subcutaneously) 60 minutes before the onset of the stress session. (b) Rats were injected with NBI 35965 (20 mg/kg subcutaneously) 60 minutes before the onset of the stress session. Values in panels a and b were normalized. (c) Percentage change in the area under the VMR curve after water avoidance stress compared with the control period in rats treated with NBI 35965 or vehicle. (d) NBI 35965 attenuated water avoidance stress-induced colonic motor response. NBI 35965 was injected subcutaneously (sc) 60 minutes before the onset of the stress session (60 minutes). Values are mean ± SEM of fecal pellet output over 1 hour. In panels a–c, *$P < 0.05$ versus baseline response; #$P < 0.05$ versus vehicle-treated group. In panel d, *$P < 0.05$ versus saline (0); #$P < 0.05$ versus all other groups. Adapted from reference 30.

CRF$_1$ receptor as a target

The central and peripheral CRF$_1$ receptor-dependent stimulation of colonic motor and secretory function, alteration of barrier permeability and hyperalgesia involved in the colonic response to stress indicate that the CRF$_1$ receptor may be an appealing target to alleviate the symptoms of IBS.[23]

---

mation as part of the putative pathogenetic mechanisms in at least a subset of IBS patients, but further elucidation is needed.

Conclusion

The biochemical coding of stress and its involvement in stress-related alterations of gut function, with a primary role of activation of central and peripheral CRF$_1$ receptors, is being unraveled. However, the interplay between the central and peripheral networks and the mechanisms of action of local mediators are still to be determined. Preclinical evidence suggests that acute stress activates central CRF$_1$ receptors, leading to the stimulation of sacral parasympathetic outflow, which recruits peripheral CRF/urocortin 1. These CRF ligands activate peripheral CRF$_1$ receptors located on colonic myenteric neurons, contributing to the propulsive colonic motor response to stress (Fig. 8.3). In addition, peripheral CRF signaling pathways cause degranulation of colonic mucosal mast cells, which results in a mast cell-dependent increase in epithelial secretion of mucin, prostaglandin E$_2$ and ions, together with enhanced transepithelial protein transport of antigenic properties (Fig. 8.3). In animals, acute stress-induced visceral hypersensitivity/hyperalgesia involves central, presumably CRF$_1$, receptors and probably NK-1 receptor activation. How activation of the central CRF system translates into visceral hypersensitivity requires further study. However, the sympathetic system does not seem to be involved in the acute stress-induced colonic hypersensitivity to distension and may be related to increased sacral parasympathetic outflow.

Acknowledgments

The authors' work was supported by the NIH RO1 grants DK-33061, DK-57236, Center grant DK-41301 (Animal Core), DK57238-01A1S1 and P50 AR049550 and VA Merit Award.

References

1   Kopin IJ. Definition of stress and sympathetic responses. *Ann N Y Acad Sci* 2004; **771**: 19–30.

2   Bale TL, Vale WW. CRF and CRF receptor: role in stress responsivity and other behaviors. *Annu Rev Pharmacol Toxicol* 2004; **44**: 5255–57.

3   Grammatopoulos DK, Chrousos GP. Functional characteristics of CRH receptors and potential clinical applications of CRH-receptor antagonists. *Trends Endocrinol Metab* 2002; **13**: 436–44.

4   Keck ME, Holsboer F. Hyperactivity of CRH neuronal circuits as a target for therapeutic interventions in affective disorders. *Peptides* 2001; **22**: 835–44.

5   Cook IJS. The influence of psychological stress on esophageal motility. In: Buéno L, Collins S, Junien JL, eds. *Stress and Digestive Motility*. London: John Libbey, 2004: 71–3.

6   Taché Y. Stress-induced alterations of gastric emptying. In: Bueno L, Collins S, Junien JL, eds. *Stress and Digestive Motility*. Montrouge: John Libbey Eurotext, 1989: 1231–32.

7   Enck P, Holtmann G. Stress and gastrointestinal motility in animals: a review of the literature. *J Gastrointest Motil* 1992; **1**: 83–90.

8   Taché Y. The parasympathetic nervous system in the pathophysiology of the gastrointestinal tract. In: Bolis CL, Licinio J, Govoni S, eds. *Handbook of Autonomic Nervous System in Health and Diseases*. New York: Marcel Dekker, 2002: 463–503.

9   Taché Y, Martinez V, Million M, Wang L. Stress and the gastrointestinal tract. III. Stress-related alterations of gut motor function: role of brain corticotropin-releasing factor receptors. *Am J Physiol* 2001; **280**: G173–7.

10 Senba E, Ueyama T. Stress-induced expression of immediate early genes in the brain and peripheral organs of the rat. *Neurosci Res* 1997; **29**: 183–207.

11 Valentino RJ, Miselis RR, Pavcovich LA. Pontine regulation of pelvic viscera: pharmacological target for pelvic visceral dysfunctions. *Trends Pharmacol Sci* 1999; **20**: 2532–60.

12 Nakajima K, Tooyama I, Yasuhara O, Aimi Y, Kimura H. Immunohistochemical demonstration of choline acetyltrans-

ferase of a peripheral type (pChAT) in the enteric nervous system of rats. *J Chem Neuroanat* 2000; **18**: 31–40.

13 Burnstock G. Structural and chemical organization of the autonomic neuroeffector system. In: Bolis CL, Licinio J, Govoni S, eds. *Handbook of Autonomic Nervous System in Health and Diseases.* New York: Marcel Dekker, 2002: 1–53.

14 Jezova D, Ochedalski T, Glickman M, Kiss A, Aguilera G. Central corticotropin-releasing hormone receptors modulate hypothalamic–pituitary–adrenocortical and sympathoadrenal activity during stress. *Neuroscience* 1999; **94**: 797–802.

15 Brown MR, Fisher LA. Corticotropin-releasing factor: effects on the autonomic nervous system and visceral systems. *Fed Proc* 1985; **44**: 2432–48.

16 Pothoulakis C, Castagliuolo I, Leeman SE. Neuroimmune mechanisms of intestinal responses to stress. Role of corticotropin-releasing factor and neurotensin. *Ann N Y Acad Sci* 1998; **840**: 635–48.

17 Turnbull AV, Lee S, Rivier C. Mechanisms of hypothalamic–pituitary–adrenal axis stimulation by immune signals in the adult rat. *Ann N Y Acad Sci* 1998; **840**: 434–43.

18 Luckey A, Wang L, Jamieson PM *et al.* Corticotropin-releasing factor receptor 1-deficient mice do not develop postoperative gastric ileus. *Gastroenterology* 2003; **125**: 6546–59.

19 Million M, Maillot C, Saunders PR, Rivier J, Vale W, Taché Y. Human urocortin II, a new CRF-related peptide, displays selective CRF2-mediated action on gastric transit in rats. *Am J Physiol* 2002; **282**: G34–40.

20 Taché Y, Martinez V, Million M, Rivier J. Corticotropin-releasing factor and the brain–gut motor response to stress. *Can J Gastroenterol* 1999; **13** (Suppl. A): 18A–25A.

21 Lenz HJ. Neurohumoral pathways mediating stress-induced changes in rat gastrointestinal transit. *Gastroenterology* 1989; **97**: 216–18.

22 Taché Y, Perdue MH. Role of peripheral CRF signaling pathways in stress-related alterations of gut motility and mucosal function. *Neurogastroenterol Motil* 2004; **16** (Suppl. 1): 137–42.

23 Taché Y, Martinez V, Wang L, Million M. CRF1 receptor signaling pathways are involved in stress-related alterations of colonic function and viscerosensitivity: implications for irritable bowel syndrome. *Br J Pharmacol* 2004; **141**: 1321–30.

24 Soderholm JD, Perdue MH. II. Stress and intestinal barrier function. *Am J Physiol Gastrointest Liver Physiol* 2001; **280**: G7–13.

25 Santos J, Saunders PR, Hanssen NPM *et al.* Corticotropin-releasing hormone mimics stress-induced rat colonic epithelial pathophysiology in the rat. *Am J Physiol* 1999; **277**: G391–9.

26 Castagliuolo I, Wershil BK, Karalis K, Pasha A, Nikulasson ST, Pothoulakis C. Colonic mucin release in response to immobilization stress is mast cell dependent. *Am J Physiol* 1998; **274**: G1094–100.

27 Talley NJ, Spiller R. Irritable bowel syndrome: a little understood organic bowel disease? *Lancet* 2002; **360**: 5555–64.

28 Jones J, Boorman J, Cann P *et al.* British Society of Gastroenterology guidelines for the management of the irritable bowel syndrome. *Gut* 2000; **47** (Suppl. 2): ii1–19.

29 Mayer EA, Naliboff BD, Chang L, Coutinho SV. Stress and the gastrointestinal tract. V. Stress and irritable bowel syndrome. *Am J Physiol Gastrointest Liver Physiol* 2001; **280**: G519–24.

30 Million M, Grigoriadis DE, Sullivan S *et al.* A novel water-soluble selective CRF1 receptor antagonist, NBI 35965, blunts stress-induced visceral hyperalgesia and colonic motor function in rats. *Brain Res* 2003; **985**: 32–42.

31 Schwetz I, Bradesi S, McRoberts JA *et al.* Delayed stress-induced colonic hypersensitivity in male Wistar rats: role of neurokinin-1 and corticotropin releasing factor-1 receptors. *Am J Physiol Gastrointest Liver Physiol* 2004; **286**: G683–91.

32 Webster EL, Torpy DJ, Elenkov IJ, Chrousos GP. Corticotropin-releasing hormone and inflammation. *Ann N Y Acad Sci* 1998; **840**: 21–32.

33 Barbara G, Stanghellini V, De Giorgio R *et al.* Activated mast cells in proximity to colonic nerves correlate with abdominal pain in irritable bowel syndrome. *Gastroenterology* 2004; **126**: 693–702.

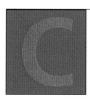

SECTION C

Pathophysiology and Treatment of Human Diseases

CHAPTER 9

Esophageal Disorders

Peter J Kahrilas and Ikuo Hirano

Introduction

Sir Thomas Willis is credited with the first description of a patient with achalasia in 1674. Einhorn in 1888 hypothesized that the disease was due to the absence of opening of the cardia. Over the past three centuries achalasia has emerged as an important model by which to understand the pathophysiology and therapy of motility disorders originating from defects of the enteric nervous system. It is the most extensively studied and readily treatable gastrointestinal motor disorder. This chapter reviews current concepts in achalasia, with emphasis on the pathophysiology and etiology of the disease. Specific secondary etiologies of achalasia are reviewed that provide insight into mechanisms responsible for the neurodegeneration that characterizes the disorder. Diffuse esophageal spasm, nutcracker esophagus and functional chest pain of presumed esophageal origin are also discussed, although there is limited evidence pointing to an enteric neural defect in these disorders.

Pathophysiology of achalasia

Normal esophageal motor physiology

The lower esophageal sphincter (LES) remains toni-cally contracted, working in concert with the crural diaphragm to form a barrier to the reflux of gastric contents. The LES relaxes in response to a variety of stimuli, including swallowing (primary peristalsis), esophageal distension (secondary peristalsis) and gastric distension (transient lower esophageal relaxation). The resting pressure of the lower esophageal sphincter is maintained by both myogenic and neurogenic contributions, whereas LES relaxation occurs in response to neurogenic factors. *Myogenic* tone of the LES refers to the intrinsic property of the smooth muscle in this region to remain contracted in the absence of external neural or hormonal influences. Studies in animals have demonstrated differences in the contractile mechanism and contractile protein isoforms in the LES compared with the esophageal body.[6,110] Such biochemical differences may explain the different contractile properties of these two muscle types. *Neurogenic* factors refer to the effects of the autonomic and enteric nervous systems on the smooth muscle of the LES. Basal release of excitatory neurotransmitters, including acetylcholine and inhibitory neurotransmitters, including nitric oxide, modulate the resting pressure of the LES. Nitric oxide is the primary mediator of relaxation of the lower esophageal sphincter.

Achalasia: presentation and pathology

1 Achalasia is characterized by impaired relaxation of the lower esophageal sphincter.

2 Most cases also have impaired peristalsis.

3 Myenteric ganglion cell numbers are reduced or absent.

4 Both autoimmune and neurotropic viral etiologies have been implicated in the pathogenesis.

5 Pharmacological studies suggest selective loss of inhibitory nitrergic neurons.

6 Achalasia may be secondary to a wide range of other disorders, including genetic defects, infectious diseases and cancer.

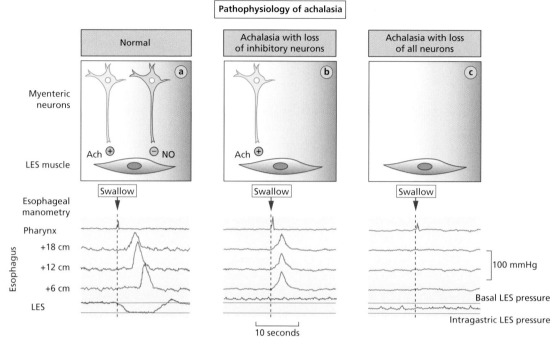

Fig. 9.1 Pathophysiology of idiopathic achalasia. (a) The normal condition, in which excitatory, cholinergic (ACh) motor neurons innervate the smooth muscle cells of the lower esophageal sphincter and contribute to the genesis of basal pressure of the lower esophageal sphincter (LESP). Inhibitory, nitric oxide (NO) motor neurons also act on the lower esophageal sphincter (LES) to produce the relaxation that accompanies a swallow. (b) Achalasia resulting from the loss of inhibitory neurons. In this situation, the absence of NO motor neurons results in an elevation in the basal LESP and absence of swallow-induced relaxation of the LES. Esophageal aperistalsis is defined by simultaneous esophageal body contractions. (c) Achalasia with complete loss of myenteric neurons. Here, the basal LESP is below normal because of the absence of excitatory neurons, and swallow-induced relaxation is absent because of the lack of inhibitory neurons. Esophageal aperistalsis is defined by the absence of esophageal body contractions.

Motility of the esophageal body is characterized by peristalsis, sequential contractions that propel liquids or solids from the cervical esophagus through the lower esophageal sphincter. Peristalsis of the smooth muscle portion of the esophagus is under the direct control of inhibitory and excitatory neurotransmitters arising from motor neurons of the myenteric plexus (Fig. 9.1a). Primary esophageal peristalsis consists of a period of inhibition followed by an excitation phase. The period of inhibition increases in duration from the proximal to the distal aspect of the esophageal body, a phenomenon known as the latency gradient, and is mediated by the inhibitory neurotransmitter nitric oxide. Selective antagonism of nitric oxide eliminates the latency gradient, resulting in simultaneous contractions of the esophagus.[130] Contractile esophageal activity is mediated by excitatory neurotransmitters such as acetylcholine. Administration of an anticholinergic agent such as atropine results in marked reductions in esophageal contractile amplitude. In addition, an excitatory effect is evident in the distal aspects of the esophageal body that is non-cholinergic and is linked to the preceding inhibition, which is mediated by nitric oxide.

Pathology and pathophysiology of achalasia

Pathological studies in achalasia have reproducibly demonstrated the marked paucity and, in many instances, the absence of neurons from the myenteric plexus (Fig. 9.2).[12,21,43,101,123] Illustrative of this is the recent study by Goldblum and colleagues, in which complete absence of

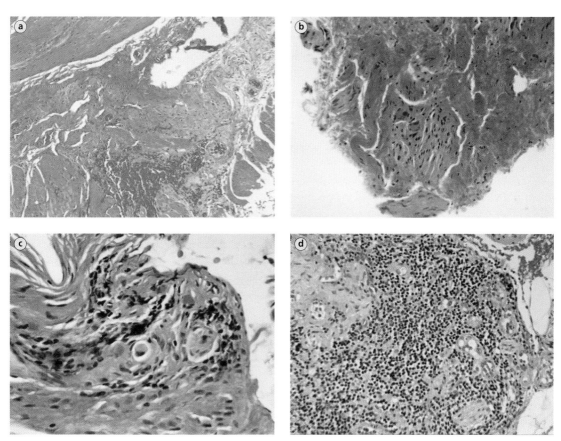

Fig. 9.2 Histopathology of achalasia. (a) Normal myenteric plexus demonstrating multiple ganglion cells and minimal lymphocytic infiltration. (b) Mild myenteric inflammation. Ganglion cells can be identified. (c) Moderate myenteric inflammation with lymphocytic infiltrate. Ganglion cells are absent. (d) Severe myenteric inflammation with lymphocytes densely clustered within the myenteric plexus. Ganglion cells are absent.

myenteric ganglion cells was demonstrated in 64% and marked diminution in 36% of the esophagi of 42 patients with achalasia who underwent esophagectomy.[89] Recent studies have examined muscle biopsies from achalasia patients treated with Heller myotomy and presumably having an earlier stage of disease. These studies detected intact ganglion cells in achalasia patients who had preservation of esophageal contractile activity.[43] Furthermore, a number of physiological studies have uncovered an intact cholinergic innervation to the esophagus. The evidence for the preserved cholinergic innervation to the LES comes from several studies. An *in vitro* study by Trounce in 1957 demonstrated contractions of muscle strips from achalasia patients in response to a combination of the acetylcholinesterase inhibitor eserine and the

ganglionic agonist nicotine.[114] The acetylcholinesterase inhibitor edrophonium chloride was later shown to increase LES pressure significantly in patients with achalasia.[19] These findings suggest that at least some postganglionic cholinergic nerve endings remain intact. Further evidence in this regard came from a study looking at the effects of the anticholinergic agent atropine in patients with achalasia.[52] This study demonstrated a 30–60% reduction in LES pressure with atropine in patients with achalasia. A similar reduction was found in a control group of healthy volunteers. Of note, however, is the fact that the residual pressure after atropine was significantly higher in the achalasia patients (17 mmHg) than in the normal subjects (5 mmHg). Recently, botulinum toxin has been introduced as a novel treatment for achalasia.

Botulinum toxin acts to inhibit the release of acetylcholine from cholinergic nerve endings. Most studies using botulinum toxin have found a significant symptomatic response rate. However, objective measures of response, including LES pressure and esophageal emptying, were less and in some studies not significantly different from baseline values.[80,119] Similar to the studies using atropine, significant residual LES pressure was observed following botulinum toxin; 25 mmHg in a study by Pasricha and 20 mmHg in a more recent study by Cuilliere and colleagues.[22] Therefore, studies using atropine and botulinum toxin both support the concept of preservation of cholinergic nerves in patients with achalasia. Furthermore, they have provided evidence for a significant, non-cholinergic component of LES basal pressure. It is likely that this residual pressure represents the myogenic contribution to LES tone.

Preservation of the excitatory, cholinergic innervation to the esophagus implies that the neuronal loss that characterizes achalasia may be selective for the inhibitory neurons. Dodds and colleagues provided indirect evidence for this through the use of cholecystokinin, which has direct excitatory effects on smooth muscle as well as indirect inhibitory effects via postganglionic inhibitory neurons. In patients with achalasia, cholecystokinin induced LES contraction as opposed to the relaxation seen in control subjects, thereby providing evidence for impaired postganglionic inhibitory nerves.[29] More recent evidence comes from *in vitro* studies looking at the responses of preparations of LES specimens from patients with achalasia. Muscles strips of the LES from normal subjects characteristically relax in response to electrical field stimulation through the activation of inhibitory neurons containing nitric oxide.[111,129] Paradoxically, LES strips from achalasia patients were found to contract in response to electrical field stimulation.[111] Such findings can be readily explained by the absence of inhibitory neurons and presence of excitatory neurons.

Direct evidence to support the concept of inhibitory neuronal loss came from immunohistochemical studies demonstrating the absence of vasoactive intestinal polypeptide nerves and nitric oxide synthase in LES specimens from patients with achalasia.[2,50,71] In fact, a number of recent experimental studies have shown that selective blockade of the inhibitory arm of the enteric innervation of the esophagus produces a manometric picture that closely mimics that of achalasia. Studies in both experimental animals and human subjects have shown that inhibition of nitric oxide synthase increases the resting tone of the LES and nearly abolishes LES relaxation.[63,74,75,129] In the esophageal body, inhibition of nitric oxide synthase results in loss of the normal latency gradient manifest as simultaneous esophageal body contractions. The overall motility pattern of an aperistaltic esophageal body and non-relaxing, hypertensive sphincter mimics the motility pattern of the vigorous form of achalasia that is characterized by aperistaltic esophageal body contractions of normal amplitude (Fig. 9.3b). It lends credence to the model of achalasia that incorporates the selective loss of inhibitory enteric neural function (Fig. 9.1b).

Pathological studies that have examined esophageal resection specimens from achalasia patients undergoing esophagectomy probably select patients with longstanding or end-stage disease. The complete aganglionosis demonstrated in the majority of such patients may represent an end-result of ongoing myenteric inflammation. Such descriptions support a second model of achalasia in which both the excitatory, cholinergic neurons and inhibitory, nitric oxide neurons are absent (Fig. 9.1c). Under such circumstances, the functional obstruction of the gastro-esophageal junction is caused by the residual myogenic tone of the LES. Complete absence of esophageal peristaltic activity is the result of the absence of enteric neural control.

While the nitric oxide-containing neurons may be lost in achalasia, the pathways by which nitric oxide functions remain intact in achalasia. This is evidenced by the efficacy of exogenously administered nitrates that act as nitric oxide donors in the treatment of achalasia. Furthermore, a recent study by Bortolotti *et al.*[9] demonstrated a significant decrease in LES pressure following administration of sildenafil (Viagra). Sildenafil is an inhibitor of phosphodiesterase type 5 that breaks down cyclic GMP stimulated by nitric oxide. The efficacy of sildenafil in achalasia supports the integrity of the nitric oxide second messenger system in the smooth muscle of the LES in achalasia.

Animal models of achalasia

Several animal models have been developed that have provided insight into the pathophysiology of achalasia and the means by which to test novel therapies.

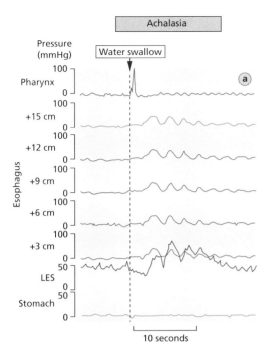

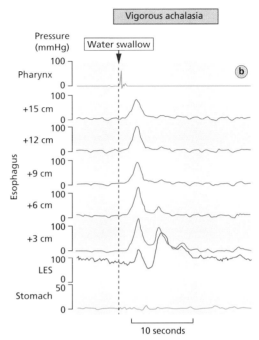

Fig. 9.3 Esophageal manometric findings in achalasia. (a) This figure illustrates the findings in classic achalasia with esophageal body aperistalsis with low-amplitude simultaneous esophageal body contractions, and failed relaxation of the lower esophageal sphincter. (b) This figure is from a patient with vigorous achalasia demonstrating robust, simultaneous esophageal body contractions and failed relaxation of a hypertensive lower esophageal sphincter.

The simplest model involves the surgical creation of a mechanical obstruction of the gastro-esophageal junction. Little and colleagues created a feline model by fixing a 1 cm Gore-Tex band around the gastro-esophageal junction.[66] With this model, basal LES pressure increased slightly and a mild but significant impairment of deglutitive relaxation was achieved. Simultaneous esophageal body contractions were demonstrated in 0% of animals preoperatively compared with 85% at 4 weeks, and esophageal body contractile amplitudes decreased by 30%. Although esophageal dilatation was demonstrated, no significant increase in thickness of the muscularis was demonstrated. The manometric changes were reversible after removal of the band. Using a pressure cuff that applied variable degrees of obstruction of the gastro-esophageal junction in cats, Mittal and colleagues demonstrated that the esophageal body amplitudes and propagation were variably affected by both the degree of distal obstruction and bolus volume.[72] A similar model was created in the opossum by Tung and colleagues.[20,116,117] Esopha-geal dilatation and an increase in thickness of the muscularis was demonstrated. Histological studies in these animals demonstrated hypertrophy of individual smooth muscle cells at both 4- and 8-week postoperative time points as well as some morphological changes in the myenteric ganglia.[117] *In vitro* muscle strip studies demonstrated reduced hyperpolarization in response to electrical stimulation in the hypertrophied muscle compared with controls, suggesting a possible mechanism for the simultaneous contractions. A recent study examined the effects of more complete esophageal obstruction in the opossum that resulted in significant elevation in LES basal pressure and marked reduction in deglutitive relaxation from 99% to 28%. Degeneration of 5–20% of myenteric ganglion cells 2 weeks after gastro-esophageal junction banding and 50–65% of myenteric ganglion cells at up to 6 weeks after operation were demonstrated.[60] In most animals, peristaltic function failed to recover after removal of the band. These experimental models lend credence to the possibility that esophageal aperistalsis can be secondary to distal esophageal obstruction as an alternative to a primary result of enteric neuropathy of the esophageal body.

Surgical vagotomy has also been examined as a model for achalasia. An achalasia-like syndrome was produced in dogs following electrolytic lesions of the medulla and bilateral vagotomy.[48,49] However, the manometric and histological findings varied from those observed in achalasia patients, and this led to another investigation of the effects of cervical vagotomy in primates.[7] In this study, only two of the seven monkeys developed a radiographic and manometric picture consistent with achalasia. Interestingly, most animals demonstrated a significant reduction in the number of esophageal myenteric ganglion cells. Transection or cooling of the vagus nerve has also been shown to abolish primary peristalsis but leave secondary peristaltic function intact in the opossum.[64,82] These animal models demonstrate that vagotomy does not consistently produce an achalasia-like picture. Moreover, significant and lasting dysphagia is uncommonly observed following surgical vagotomy in man. In a study of 96 patients who had undergone proximal gastric vagotomy for ulcer disease, only five patients developed transient, albeit severe, dysphagia with delayed transit of barium and incomplete LES relaxation.[46]

Gaumnitz and colleagues produced a model of achalasia in the opossum by injecting the gastro-esophageal junction with a cationic surfactant that resulted in chemical dennervation.[39] While these animals manometrically resembled achalasia with hypertension and failed relaxation of the LES, further study is needed to delineate whether the effects of the chemical injury are specific for enteric neurons rather than the result of a mechanical obstruction due to injury of other structures in the gastro-esophageal junction. If this model were substantiated, examination for secondary changes to the autonomic nervous system would be of great interest.

Most recently, genetically engineered mice with targeted disruption of the gene encoding the neuronal form of nitric oxide synthase have been studied.[100] Hypertension of the LES was demonstrated as well as marked impairment of swallow-induced LES relaxation. The phenotype of this knockout mouse was dominated by marked gastric distension indicative of the importance of nitric oxide in gastric motility. The

absence of significant esophageal dilatation may be explained by the predominance of striated muscle in the tubular esophagus of the mouse. Nevertheless, this model lends credence to the importance of inhibitory myenteric neural innervation in the pathogenesis of achalasia.

Sensory function in achalasia

Although the pathophysiology of motor dysfunction has been investigated extensively, little is known about the integrity of esophageal sensory function in achalasia. Afferent innervation of the esophagus and conscious perception of sensation depends on vagal and spinal afferent fibers communicating with the central nervous system.[36,40,45] Degeneration of the central, autonomic or enteric nervous systems could lead to impaired visceral sensation in achalasia. Circumstantial evidence for such a functional impairment comes from the observation that patients with achalasia are poorly cognizant of retained food in the esophagus and esophageal distension. Furthermore, uncontrolled studies have reported that achalasia patients have diminished perception of acid reflux events both before and after treatment of their achalasia.[98]

A limited number of investigations have examined esophageal sensation in achalasia. Two previous studies have evaluated visceral sensitivity using intra-esophageal balloon distension.[34,81] Both studies found impairment of sensation in achalasia patients. However, these studies employed fixed-volume, latex balloons. As a result of the technique, the amount of pressure stimulus applied to the esophageal wall varied depending upon the degree of dilatation present secondary to the underlying disease state. Therefore, this method is of limited validity in achalasia patients, in whom esophageal dilatation is common. Rate and colleagues reported diminished esophageal sensory responses to electrical stimulation in a cohort of patients with varied esophageal motility disorders that included achalasia.[88] Brackbill and colleagues recently investigated sensory function in achalasia by the use of a barostat device that maintains a constant pressure stimulus independent of luminal diameter.[10] This study demonstrated significant differences in esophageal mechanosensitivity in achalasia patients who reported higher thresholds for painful, distension-induced sensation than in healthy controls. The same study also demonstrated decreased chemosensitivity in patients with achalasia using a modified Bernstein test. These studies support the concept of impaired esophageal sensitivity in achalasia but do not identify whether the defect occurs at the level of the central, autonomic or enteric nervous system.

In contrast to the diminished esophageal visceral sensitivity, chest pain does occur in patients with achalasia and has been reported in 17–63% of patients. The mechanism for chest pain is unclear and it is likely that more than one mechanism is involved. Proposed etiologies include secondary or tertiary esophageal contractions, esophageal distension by retained food, and esophageal irritation by retained medications, food, and bacterial or fungal overgrowth. Inflammation within the esophageal myenteric plexus could also be involved. A recent prospective study, however, found no association between the occurrence of chest pain and either manometric or radiographic abnormalities. In the same study, patients with chest pain were noted to be younger and had a shorter duration of symptoms compared with patients without pain, suggesting that esophageal visceral pain may be less common with increasing neurodegeneration.[32] Many patients with achalasia report a history of episodes of intense substernal chest pain that improve or resolve over the course of their disease. Interestingly, treatment of achalasia had little impact on the reporting of chest pain, despite relief of dysphagia. A conflicting retrospective study reported chest pain in 44% of patients with achalasia undergoing Heller myotomy but no association between chest pain and either age or duration of symptoms.[84] In addition, chest pain resolved in 84% of patients after Heller myotomy. Despite the retrospective nature of the study, this report does suggest that the etiology of chest pain in achalasia is likely to be heterogeneous. It is likely that varied etiologies for chest pain account for the variations in both its prevalence and its response to therapy.

Etiopathogenesis

Primary achalasia

The etiology of primary achalasia remains unknown, although several hypotheses have been put forth, including viral pathogens, autoimmunity and neurodegeneration. Each hypothesis seeks to account for the loss of ganglia from the esophageal myenteric plexus,

but it is likely that the various mechanisms proposed do not operate independently.

A number of studies have implicated viral agents in the pathogenesis of achalasia. An infectious etiology seems plausible in the light of the uniform age distribution of the incident cases of achalasia. A preliminary report noted a statistically significant increase in antibody titers against measles virus in patients with achalasia compared with controls.[55] While this study has not been substantiated, another study using DNA hybridization techniques found evidence of varicellazoster virus in three of nine myotomy specimens from patients with achalasia but none of 20 control specimens.[92] DNA probes for cytomegalovirus and herpes simplex type I were negative in both achalasics and controls. The herpes virus family was specifically targeted in this study, because of its neurotropic nature. Furthermore, the predilection of the herpes viruses for squamous epithelium as opposed to columnar epithelium makes this an attractive hypothesis. Such tissue selectivity could explain why achalasia involves only the esophagus while sparing the remainder of the gastrointestinal tract. More recent studies using more advanced methods, including polymerase chain reaction techniques, however, failed to detect the presence of measles, herpes or human papilloma viruses in myotomy specimens of patients with achalasia.[8,76,107] These negative studies do not exclude the possibility that the etiology of achalasia is either an alternative viral species or resolved viral infection with disappearance of the inciting viral pathogen from the host tissue. Supporting this possibility is a recent study demonstrating immunoreactivity of inflammatory cells from patients with achalasia in response to viral antigens despite the inability of the investigators to detect the virus in tissue samples.[13]

Early descriptions of inflammatory infiltration of the affected regions of the esophagus in achalasia led to speculation about an autoimmune etiology. Inflammatory infiltration of the myenteric plexus was present in 100% of specimens from a histological analysis of 42 achalasia esophagectomy specimens.[89] Immunohistochemical staining characterized the infiltrative cells as T cells positive for CD3 and CD8.[16] A significant eosinophilic infiltration has been demonstrated in some patients with achalasia.[112] An association between achalasia and class II histocompatibility antigens has been described, specifically identifying a higher genotypic frequency of the HLA-DQw1, DQA1*0101, DQA1*103, DQB1*0602 and DQB1*0603 alleles in achalasia patients than in controls.[26,94,121,126] Class II antigen expression on myenteric neurons could be targeted as foreign antigen. Storch and colleagues demonstrated antibodies against myenteric plexus in the serum of 37 of 58 patients with achalasia but in only four of 54 healthy controls.[108] This study also failed to detect antibodies in the serum of patients with Hirschsprung's disease or esophageal cancer and in only one out of 11 patients with peptic esophagitis. A second study detected serum antibodies against myenteric neurons in seven of 18 achalasia patients but not in healthy controls or reflux patients.[122] The patients' antibodies bound to neurons in enteric plexuses from tissue sections of both the esophagus and the intestine of rats. However, since the defect in primary achalasia is quite specific to the esophagus, the significance of a circulating antibody that targets not only esophageal but also intestinal neurons is unclear. In another recent study, positive immunostaining of the myenteric plexus of the esophagus and ileum of the guinea-pig and mouse were detected in serum samples of 23 out of 45 achalasia patients. However, a similar degree of immunostaining was demonstrated in the serum of eight out of 16 patients with gastro-esophageal reflux disease. This suggests that the antineuronal antibodies detected may represent a non-specific or secondary phenomenon that does not play a causative role in the pathogenesis of achalasia.[73]

Neurodegeneration is a third proposed etiology for primary achalasia. Loss of neurons within the dorsal vagal motor nucleus and degenerative changes of the vagal nerve fibers have been noted.[12,61] Experimental lesions of the brainstem and vagus nerves in animal models (see below) can produce esophageal motility abnormalities that resemble achalasia. Such findings led investigators to speculate that the site of primary involvement in achalasia was in the dorsal motor nucleus and vagus nerve, and that the myenteric abnormalities were secondary. However, most pathological studies have found that the predominant abnormalities are within the myenteric plexus, with marked diminution or complete absence of ganglion cells and intense inflammatory infiltration of the myenteric plexus.[43,101] Neural inflammation has not been described in other

parts of the autonomic or central nervous system of achalasia patients, arguing against these being the primary site of denervation. Furthermore, defects in vagal innervation would be expected to lead to prominent clinical abnormalities outside the esophagus, including gastric emptying disorders, which are not commonly seen in achalasia. A number of studies have looked for autonomic effects on gastric physiology but have provided inconsistent results.[3,31] Significant abnormalities in esophageal function are uncommon clinical manifestations in patients who have had vagal transections. Additional evidence to support the neurodegenerative hypothesis comes from the description of Lewy bodies, intracytoplasmic inclusions characteristically found in Parkinson's disease, in the myenteric plexus and dorsal motor nucleus of achalasia patients.[85] It is likely that the neurodegenerative changes in achalasia are secondary to viral- or autoimmune-mediated destruction of the enteric ganglia.

Secondary achalasia

A number of disorders can result in a clinical presentation that manometrically and radiographically resembles primary achalasia (Table 9.1). Secondary achalasia can occur in a form that is restricted to the esophagus or is part of a generalized motility disorder affecting other parts of the gastrointestinal tract.[45] These secondary forms provide important insights into the pathophysiology of achalasia.

Allgrove first reported the triple A or Allgrove's syndrome in 1978, when he described two pairs of siblings presenting with achalasia, alacrima and adrenal insufficiency. Subsequent studies have characterized the disorder as an autosomal recessive disease with additional features that include peripheral neuropathy, autonomic neuropathy and mental retardation. Most cases have presented in children younger than 10 years, with morbidity being due to hypoglycemia and dysphagia. Pathological studies have demonstrated the absence of ganglion cells in the esophagus as well as atrophy of the adrenal cortical zona fasciculata and reticularis, and both axonal degeneration and nerve fiber loss in peripheral nerves. A study reported linkage of the gene for triple A syndrome to chromosome 12q13.[124] Tullio-Pelet and colleagues reported mutations in a novel gene (*AAAS*) encoding a regulatory protein referred to as ALADIN (for alacri-

Table 9.1 Secondary forms of achalasia.

Achalasia
Allgrove's syndrome (AAA syndrome)
Hereditary cerebellar ataxia
Familial achalasia
Sjögren's syndrome
Sarcoidosis
Post-vagotomy
Post-fundoplication
Autoimmune polyglandular syndrome type II

Achalasia with generalized motility disorder
MEN IIb (Sipple's syndrome)
Neurofibromatosis (von Recklinghausen's disease)
Chagas' disease (*Trypanosoma cruzi*)
Paraneoplastic syndrome (anti-Hu antibody)
Parkinson's disease
Amyloidosis
Fabry's disease
Hereditary cerebellar ataxia
Achalasia with associated Hirschsprung's disease
Hereditary hollow visceral myopathy

Achalasia secondary to cancer (pseudoachalasia)
Squamous cell carcinoma of the esophagus
Adenocarcinoma of the esophagus
Gastric adenocarcinoma
Lung carcinoma
Leiomyoma
Lymphoma
Breast adenocarcinoma
Hepatocellular carcinoma
Reticulum cell sarcoma
Lymphangioma
Metastatic renal cell carcinoma
Mesothelioma
Metastatic prostate carcinoma
Pancreatic adenocarcinoma

ma–achalasia–adrenal insufficiency neurological disorder).[115] The ALADIN protein is believed to function in the normal development of both the peripheral and the central nervous system. It has been proposed that the ALADIN protein is involved in the regulation of nucleocytoplasmic transport, which is essential for the maintenance and development of specific tissues, including the esophageal myenteric plexus. Thus, Allgrove's syndrome, like Hirschsprung's disease, appears to be a genetic disorder leading to tissue-specific defects of the enteric nervous system. An intriguing report noted coexistent Hirschsprung's disease and achalasia in two male siblings. Both siblings were diagnosed shortly after birth with achalasia requiring cardiomyotomy and both were subsequently diagnosed with Hirschsprung's disease, with pathology of the rectum showing absent ganglion cells.[59]

Achalasia can also occur among the motility disorders affecting multiple regions of the gastrointestinal tract. Esophageal dysmotility and achalasia have been described as part of multiple endocrine neoplasia type 2B[41] and von Recklinghausen's neurofibromatosis.[38] Unlike the pathological finding of aganglionosis that characterizes primary achalasia and most forms of secondary achalasia, these two disorders have hyperganglionosis or neuronal dysplasia of the myenteric plexus of the gastrointestinal tract. Recent molecular genetic studies have provided major advances in the understanding of multiple endocrine neoplasia. Over 90% of patients with multiple endocrine neoplasia type 2 (MEN-2) have been found to have mutations in the *RET* proto-oncogene.[35] This gene is located on chromosome 10q11.2 and encodes a receptor tyrosine kinase expressed on neural crest cells. The medullary thyroid carcinoma, pheochromocytoma, mucosal neuromas and gastrointestinal neuronal dysplasia which develop as part of MEN-2 can be explained by the fact that these tissues are all derived from the neural crest during fetal development. Other hereditary forms of achalasia with associated generalized gastrointestinal motility disorders have been described and await molecular genetic characterization.[45]

Chagas' disease is a parasitic infection caused by *Trypanosoma cruzi* and is endemic to regions of Central and South America and Mexico. *T. cruzi* is transmitted from person to person by blood-sucking triatomine (reduviid) insects, and 10–30% of infected individuals develop a chronic infection that presents years or even decades after initial infection. Any portion of the gastrointestinal tract can be involved, but the esophagus is most commonly affected, and in this case secondary achalasia occurs in 7–10% of chronically infected individuals. Recently, antibodies directed at targets within the myenteric plexus have been demonstrated in patients with Chagas' disease and achalasia.[42] Circulating IgG antibodies recognizing the M_2-muscarinic acetylcholine receptor were detected in a series of patients with achalasia secondary to Chagas' disease at much greater frequencies than found in Chagas patients without achalasia, patients with idiopathic achalasia, and healthy controls. These investigators further demonstrated functional effects of the antibody as an *in vitro*, muscarinic agonist-like activity on isolated rat esophageal muscle strips. The significance of this antibody in the clinical presentation of achalasia in Chagas' disease is unclear, since the pathogenesis still involves destruction of the myenteric neurons. Moreover, Dantas has reported greater impairment of the cholinergic pathway in patients with achalasia secondary to Chagas' disease compared with patients with idiopathic achalasia and healthy controls.[24]

Cancer is an important cause of secondary achalasia. It can produce achalasia or an achalasia like picture by one of three mechanisms. The first and most common is by direct mechanical obstruction of the distal esophagus. This is referred to as 'pseudoachalasia' and has been described with a number of cancers (Table 9.1). Neoplastic cells can also invade the submucosa of the lower esophageal sphincter and thereby disrupt the myenteric neurons, resulting in an achalasia-like picture that can be missed on endoscopic examination. Finally, tumors remote from the distal esophagus can cause achalasia through a paraneoplastic syndrome.[15] This is an autoimmune response in which the tumor expresses a neuronal antigen that the host recognizes as non-self. Activated T cells and plasma cell antibodies directed at the antigen act to retard the growth of the tumor but react with portions of the nervous system outside the blood–brain barrier.[25] Anti-Hu (also known as type I antineuronal nuclear autoantibodies or ANNA-1) recognize proteins expressed in cancer tissue and in neurons of the central, peripheral, autonomic and enteric nervous systems.[67] The paraneoplastic syndrome is most commonly seen with small cell lung cancer but has also been described in neuroblastoma and prostate cancer patients. The gastrointestinal manifestations associated with the anti-Hu paraneoplastic syndrome include achalasia, gastroparesis and intestinal pseudo-obstruction. Encephalomyelitis, sensory neuropathy and cerebellar degeneration have also been described. Importantly, the gastrointestinal manifestations can often precede the diagnosis of the cancer and the presence of the paraneoplastic response may portend a better prognosis.[65] Rare cases have been described with intestinal aganglionosis and anti-Hu antibodies in the absence of neoplasm.[102]

Diagnosis of achalasia

Achalasia occurs with an incidence of approximately 1:100 000, with an equal gender distribution.[69] It occurs at all ages but the incidence tends to increase after the seventh decade. Dysphagia is the predominant symptom and is typically accompanied by regurgitation. Additional symptoms include weight loss, nocturnal aspiration and chest pain. Paradoxically, heartburn is reported by some patients and may be due to bacterial fermentation of retained food in the esophagus, poor clearance of even small amounts of acid refluxate, or other non-acid mechanisms of chest pain that are reported as heartburn. Several reports exist of patients referred for refractory heartburn and surgical fundoplication who are prospectively or retrospectively found to have achalasia.

Upper endoscopy is often the first test used to evaluate patients with suspected achalasia and may detect esophageal dilatation with retained saliva or food. However, in a series of newly diagnosed patients with achalasia, upper endoscopies were reported as normal in 44%.[53] A barium esophagram can be highly suggestive of the diagnosis of achalasia, particularly when there is the combination of esophageal dilatation with retained food and barium and a smooth, tapered constriction of the gastro-esophageal junction (Fig. 9.4). However, in the same series as that mentioned above, the diagnosis of achalasia was suggested in only 64% of barium examinations. Quantitative assessment of the degree of esophageal emptying of barium over time may increase the diagnostic sensitivity of the esophagram for achalasia and serves as a valuable means by which to follow the patient's response to therapy (Fig. 9.4).[27,118] In the light of the limited sensitivity of endoscopy and barium studies, the test with the greatest sensitivity in the diagnosis of achalasia is esophageal manometry. The defining manometric features of achalasia are aperistalsis of the distal esophagus and incomplete or absent LES relaxation (Fig. 9.3a). Additional supportive features include a hypertensive lower esophageal sphincter and low-amplitude esophageal body contractions. High-resolution manometry combined with topographic analysis is an emerging technique that offers potential advantages over conventional esophageal manometry.[105] Although it is an emerging method for

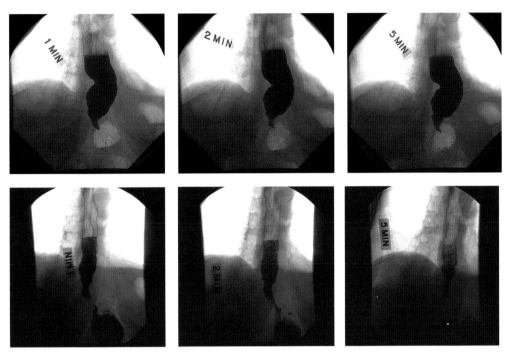

Fig. 9.4 Timed barium swallow. Following the ingestion of a fixed volume of barium, sequential radiographs are taken at 1, 2 and 5 minutes. The upper three panels demonstrate lack of emptying, with a fixed column of barium persisting at 5 minutes. The lower three panels demonstrate the same patient after therapy with pneumatic dilation. An improvement in emptying and degree of esophageal dilatation is shown.

investigative purposes, the advantages of high-resolution manometry with topography over conventional manometry for clinical practice are undefined. Figure 9.5 illustrates a contour plot topographic analysis of a patient with achalasia.

While manometry is accepted as the gold standard for making the diagnosis of achalasia, heterogeneity does exist in the manometric presentation.[50] The most commonly recognized variant of achalasia is known as 'vigorous achalasia', variably defined by the presence of normal to high-amplitude esophageal body contractions in the presence of a non-relaxing LES (Fig. 9.3b). While vigorous achalasia may represent an early stage of achalasia, studies have failed to demonstrate differences in terms of clinical presentation in such patients, including the duration of disease or the occurrence of chest pain. Endoscopic injections of botulinum toxin into the LES have been reported to be more effective in patients with vigorous achalasia, supporting the integrity of the cholinergic neurons in the myenteric plexus in such patients.[79] Additional manometric variants of achalasia include rare individuals with intact peristalsis through the majority of the esophageal body and with preservation of either deglutitive or transient LES relaxation.[50,58] In these cases, the diagnosis of achalasia was substantiated by demonstrating degeneration of myenteric neurons and by observing the clinical response to myotomy. The significance of defining these variants of achalasia lies in the recognition that these sometimes confusing manometric findings are still consistent with achalasia when combined with additional clinical data supportive of the diagnosis.

Therapy of achalasia

Treatment options for idiopathic achalasia include pharmacological therapy, endoscopic botulinum toxin injection, endoscopic pneumatic dilation, and surgical myotomy (Table 9.2).[104] All forms of therapy seek to reduce the LES pressure to allow improved esophageal emptying by gravity, since the esophageal peristaltic pump is typically impaired. Pharmacological therapy

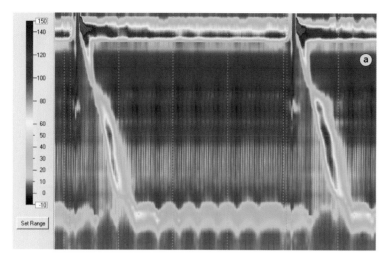

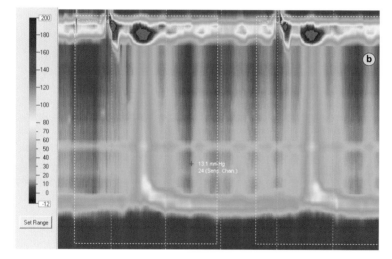

Fig. 9.5. Contour plot topographic analysis of esophageal motility in achalasia. Topographic analysis is a method of axial data interpolation derived from computerized plotting of data from multiple, closely spaced, solid-state recording transducers. The interpolated pressure information is plotted as a two-dimensional contour plot in which pressure amplitude is coded by color. (a) A normal esophageal study with propagation of the peristaltic wave and relaxation of the LES. The upper esophageal sphincter is also depicted at the top of the panel, demonstrating a higher basal pressure and shorter relaxation phase. (b) A study from a patient with achalasia with complete esophageal aperistalsis and incomplete relaxation of the hypertensive lower esophageal sphincter. Although there is partial inhibition of the LES, the relaxation pressures exceed 40 mmHg. An esophagogastric pressure gradient is evident in the distal esophagus.

employs the use of smooth muscle relaxants, such as calcium channel antagonists, nitrates and anticholinergic agents. Given the marked esophageal retention that characterizes achalasia, pharmacological therapy should be delivered by the sublingual route. Small, randomized controlled trials using sublingual nifedipine and isorbide dinitrate have demonstrated a significant reduction in LES pressure and symptom relief. However, the long-term effectiveness of medical therapy has generally been limited by both side-effects and an efficacy that is less than that of the more invasive therapies.

Pasricha and colleagues introduced botulinum toxin injection in 1995 as a novel therapy for achalasia.[79,80] Studies by several investigators have now demonstrated significant symptom benefit in approximately two-thirds of patients treated with botulinum toxin injection into the lower esophageal sphincter. The mechanism of action is via the prevention of the release of acetylcholine from neurons within the myenteric plexus. However, long-term studies using botulinum toxin have shown the need for repeated injections to maintain symptom relief. Highlighting the limitations of this therapy is the report of Vaezi and colleagues of a randomized con-

Table 9.2 Therapy of achalasia.

Therapy	Without further therapy			Repeat treatment	
	Total n	Weighted mean response (p̂) ± SE[†]	Weighted mean follow-up	n	Weighted mean response (p̂) ± SE[†]
Botulinum toxin[61,103,118,124]	221	35 ± 17%	1.3 yr	63	49 ± 26%
Pneumatic dilatation[103]	1276	72 ± 26%	4.9 yr	269	80 ± 42%
Heller myotomy					
Thoracotomy[103]	1221	84 ± 20%	5 yr	Scant data	
Laparotomy[103]	732	85 ± 18%	7.6 yr	Scant data	
Laparoscopy[28,53,82,92,103,105,127]	365	91 ± 13%	1.4 yr	4.1% converted to open	

$$^\dagger \hat{p} = \frac{n_1 p_1 \quad n_2 p_2 \quad n_x p_x}{n_1 \quad n_2 \quad n_x} \quad SE(\hat{p}) = \sqrt{\frac{p_1(1 \quad p_1)}{n_1} \quad \frac{p_2(1 \quad p_2)}{n_2} \quad \frac{p_x(1 \quad p_x)}{n_3}}$$

Adapted from reference 104.

trolled trial of botulinum toxin and pneumatic dilation in 42 patients with achalasia.[119] At the 12-month follow-up, 70% of the pneumatic dilation and only 32% of the botulinum toxin patients were in symptomatic remission. Of greater concern was the finding that, while providing symptom relief, botulinum toxin failed to reduce LES pressure significantly or to reduce barium retention on a quantitative barium swallow. Given the limitations of both pharmacological therapy and botulinum toxin for achalasia, such treatments are generally reserved for patients who are poor candidates for more definitive interventions or as temporizing measures while awaiting such treatment. Additionally, the temporary effects of botulinum toxin make its use appealing in patients in whom the diagnosis of achalasia is questionable.

First-line therapy of achalasia is best achieved by either endoscopic pneumatic dilation or surgical my-otomy. Pneumatic dilation provides symptom relief in approximately 70–80% of patients. Larger balloon diameters provide greater response rates but also increase the risk of perforation, which is generally less than 5%. Recent long-term observational studies have reported that the effectiveness of pneumatic dilation decreases significantly over time, with less than 40% of patients in remission after five years.[33] Surgical myotomy was first performed via thoracotomy by Heller in 1913. The operation can be performed either thoracoscopically or laparoscopically with much shorter lengths of hospitalization (1–3 days in most series) compared with the open procedures. Success using the laparoscopic approach is approximately 90% in most series.[14,83] Retrospective studies and one randomized trial report a superior outcome in patients treated surgically compared with those treated with pneumatic dilation. Fur-

---

Treatment of achalasia

1 Botulinum toxin injection into the LES is successful in under 50% with need for repeated treatments.
2 Pneumatic dilatation achieves greater success at 70% with a low perforation complication rate. Long-term follow-up studies, however, have reported success in less than 40% after five years.
3 Laparoscopic Heller myotomy is probably superior to both the above, with a success rate of around 90%. However, randomized controlled trials comparing endoscopic and laparoscopic therapy are lacking.

thermore, perforations that occur as a result of pneu-matic dilation require repair via open thoracotomy, necessitating a much longer recovery period compared with an elective laparoscopic surgical approach. Available local expertise is an important consideration in the choice of initial therapy for achalasia.

Complications of achalasia

The primary complications of achalasia are related to the functional obstruction rendered by the non-relaxing LES. These include progressive malnutrition and aspiration. Aspiration can be a substantial cause of morbidity, with patients at risk of postprandial and nocturnal coughing and aspiration. Uncommon but important secondary complications of achalasia include the formation of epiphrenic diverticula and esophageal cancer. Epiphrenic diverticula are commonly associated with esophageal motility disorders, presumably as a result of increased intraluminal pressures, and are most commonly detected in the distal esophagus immediately proximal to the LES. Esophageal cancer is also seen with increased frequency in patients with idiopathic achalasia (Fig. 9.6). Most commonly, the cancers that develop are squamous cell carcinomas, although adenocarcinomas are also reported. A large cohort study from Sweden found a 16-fold increased risk of esophageal cancer during years 1–24 after initial diagnosis.[95,127] Cancers detected in the first year after diagnosis of achalasia were excluded to eliminate prevalent cancers that may have presented as secondary or pseudoachalasia.[95] The overall prevalence of esophageal cancer in achalasia is approximately 3%, with an incidence of approximately 197 per 100 000 per year.[30] The incidence of cancer increases significantly after 15 years of symptoms referable to achalasia. However, based on the overall low incidence of esophageal cancer, routine endoscopic screening of patients with achalasia is not generally recommended. It is also possible that successful treatment of achalasia may reduce the risk of cancer, but this has not been proven and several cases have reported carcinoma arising following treatment. Finally, upper airway obstruction has been reported as a complication of achalasia, presumably secondary to extrinsic compression of the posterior aspect of the trachea by the markedly dilated esophageal body.[4,68,78] This particular complication implies dysfunction of upper as well as lower esophageal sphincter function, which is surprising in the light of the skeletal muscle composition of the upper esophageal sphincter.

Other esophageal motor and functional disorders

Diffuse esophageal spasm

Diffuse esophageal spasm is a rare condition, first described by Osgood in 1889. The diagnosis is based upon the finding of the simultaneous, esophageal body contractions (Fig. 9.7). How rapid esophageal contractions need to be in order to be considered simultaneous was examined by Hewson and colleagues, who found that propagation velocities that exceed 6.25 cm/s are associated with esophageal retention.[47] Radiological barium studies demonstrate impaired esophageal emptying and the presence of simultaneous and tertiary contractions that result in the characteristic

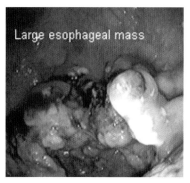
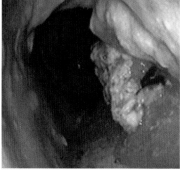

Fig. 9.6 Esophageal squamous cell carcinoma arising in achalasia. These endoscopic photographs demonstrate an exophytic mass in the proximal esophagus of a patient with long-standing achalasia complicated by a chronically dilated esophagus.

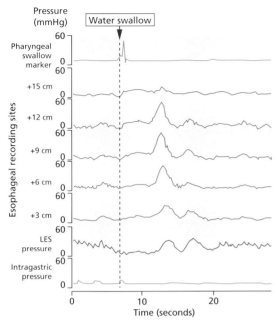

Fig. 9.7 Esophageal manometry in diffuse esophageal spasm. Esophageal motility tracing from a patient with diffuse esophageal spasm, demonstrating simultaneous contractions of the esophageal body with intact lower esophageal sphincter relaxation.

'corkscrew' or 'chain of beads' configuration of the esophagus (Fig. 9.8). High-amplitude, repetitive and long-duration contractions may be present but are not necessary for the diagnosis.[23] Intermittent preservation of esophageal peristalsis should be observed. If every swallow sequence is simultaneous or if failed LES relaxation is noted, the diagnosis of achalasia needs to be entertained. That being said, a number of similarities between the two conditions exist. Both conditions appear to result from a defect in the inhibitory neurotransmission of the esophagus, presumably at the level of the myenteric plexus. Failed deglutitive inhibition

was demonstrated in patients with esophageal spasm using paired swallows and with an artificially created high-pressure zone in the esophageal body.[5,99] Because of the rarity of cases of diffuse esophageal spasm and the even less common need for surgical intervention, histopathological data are few. Limited studies have demonstrated degeneration of vagal fibers, inflammatory infiltration of myenteric plexus and hypertrophy of smooth muscle. Furthermore, several cases have been reported in which transformation from diffuse esophageal spasm into achalasia has been observed. Simultaneous esophageal contractions are not entirely specific for diffuse esophageal spasm and have been reported in patients with diabetes, connective tissue disorders, alcoholism and gastro-esophageal reflux disease.

The management of diffuse esophageal spasm consists primarily of pharmacological therapy and following patients for progression to achalasia. Both calcium channel antagonists and nitrates have demonstrated benefit in uncontrolled trials.[77,109] No data exist on the use of oral anticholinergic agents, although recent studies have found some efficacy in the use of botulinum toxin injections in the LES or distal esophageal body. In patients with dysfunction of the LES, pneumatic dilation therapy has been effective in relieving dysphagia. In severe cases, surgical therapy consisting of a longitudinal myotomy of the distal esophagus may be considered.

Functional chest pain of presumed esophageal origin

The term 'functional chest pain of presumed esophageal origin' has been recommended by the Rome II committee to encompass patients with chest pain that is not caused by cardiac disease or gastro-esophageal reflux disease.[18] Studies from the 1980s postulated

---

Esophageal spasm

1 Rare cause of dysphagia and esophageal pain.
2 Differential diagnosis includes early or atypical presentations of achalasia.
3 Associated with degenerative changes in myenteric plexus in some cases.

4 Data on treatment are scarce.
5 Treatment includes oral or sublingual smooth muscle relaxants. Botulinum toxin injection, pneumatic dilatation and extended myotomy are therapeutic considerations for severe cases.

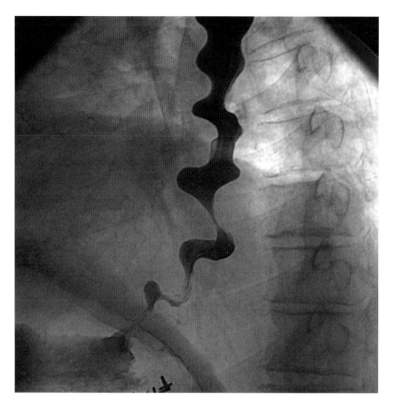

Fig. 9.8 Radiographic examination of diffuse esophageal spasm. Barium swallow illustrating the spiral or 'corkscrew' deformity of the tubular esophagus caused by simultaneous, lumen-obliterated contractions of the circular muscle of the esophageal body.

that esophageal dysmotility, in particular nutcracker esophagus, was an important cause of unexplained chest pain. Nutcracker esophagus is defined by the presence of esophageal contractile amplitudes exceeding 180 mmHg (Fig. 9.9). In one series, esophageal dysmotility was found in 28% of patients with non-cardiac chest pain, of whom nearly half had a nutcracker pattern.[57] Symptoms that have been reported in patients with nutcracker esophagus include chest pain and dysphagia. However, studies have demonstrated poor correlation between the symptoms of nutcracker esophagus and the manometric abnormalities. Furthermore, treatments, such as calcium channel antagonists, that effectively improve the motility abnormalities do not significantly improve symptoms.[91] Additionally, therapies using low-dose antidepressants have improved symptoms while having no effect on the manometric disturbances.[11,17] Thus, it appears at present that nutcracker esophagus is not an important primary cause of chest pain and the use of medications directed at the motility abnormalities for the purpose of relieving chest pain is not supported by the available data. It fol-

lows that the routine use of esophageal manometry in the initial evaluation of patients with non-cardiac chest pain is not recommended.[56] It is important to exclude other treatable conditions, such as gastro-esophageal reflux disease, in patients presenting with non-cardiac chest pain.[1]

As has occurred with the understanding of irritable bowel syndrome, investigations into the mechanism responsible for functional chest pain have shifted away from motility disorders to dysfunction of the brain–gut axis.[18,44,70] Visceral hypersensitivity has been demonstrated using balloon distension studies that have detected significantly lower sensory thresholds in most patients with non-cardiac chest pain compared with controls.[86,87,90] Altered autonomic function has been demonstrated in patients with non-cardiac chest pain in response to mechanical, chemical or electrical stimulation.[51,113] Hyperexcitability within central visceral nociceptive pathways has been demonstrated using the technique of cerebral evoked potentials.[96,97] Finally, as in other functional gastrointestinal disorders, psychological factors, including anxiety, panic and affective

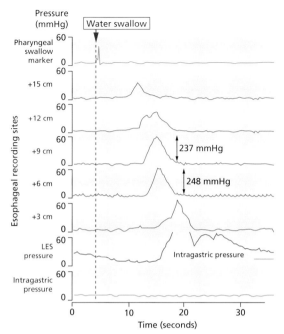

Fig. 9.9 Esophageal manometry in nutcracker esophagus. Esophageal motility tracing from a patient with nutcracker esophagus demonstrating high-amplitude peristaltic contractions of the esophageal body with intact lower esophageal sphincter relaxation.

disorders, have been demonstrated in many patients with non-cardiac chest pain.[37,103] It remains unclear whether such psychological factors are a primary cause of chest pain, serve as triggers to underlying visceral hypersensitivity or act to lower the threshold by which functional chest pain patients choose to seek medical attention.

The management of functional chest pain incorporates reassurance of the benign nature of the patient's condition. The high prevalence of reflux disease among patients with non-cardiac chest pain provides the rationale for anti-reflux therapy as an initial therapeutic trial, even in patients without obvious clinical symptoms or endoscopic signs of gastro-esophageal reflux. As mentioned above, the available evidence does not support the routine use of smooth muscle relaxants. The best evidence for pharmacological treatment of functional chest pain is for pain modulators. In a randomized controlled trial, trazodone was significantly more effective than placebo in relieving symptoms.[17] Similarly, sertraline, a serotonin reuptake inhibitor,

has shown efficacy over placebo in a recent randomized trial.[120] Psychological comorbidities should be addressed in the light of their potential roles as triggers or causes of chest pain. Finally, the role of alternative medicine approaches needs to be defined, given their reported effectiveness in irritable bowel syndrome.

References

1 Achem SR, Kolts BE, Wears R, Burton L, Richter JE. Chest pain associated with nutcracker esophagus: a preliminary study of the role of gastroesophageal reflux [see comments]. *Am J Gastroenterol* 1993; **88**: 187–92.

2 Aggestrup S, Uddman R, Sundler F *et al.* Lack of vasoactive intestinal polypeptide nerves in esophageal achalasia. *Gastroenterology* 1983; **84**: 924–7.

3 Atkinson M, Ogilvie AL, Robertson CS, Smart HL. Vagal function in achalasia of the cardia. *Q J Med* 1987; **63**: 297–303.

4 Becker DJ, Castell DO. Acute airway obstruction in achalasia. Possible role of defective belch reflex. *Gastroenterology* 1989; **97**: 1323–6.

5 Behar J, Biancani P. Pathogenesis of simultaneous esophageal contractions in patients with motility disorders. *Gastroenterology* 1993; **105**: 111–18.

6 Biancani P, Hillemeier C, Bitar KN, Makhlouf GM. Contraction mediated by Ca2+ influx in esophageal muscle and by Ca2+ release in the LES. *Am J Physiol* 1987; **253**: G760–6.

7 Binder HJ, Bloom DL, Stern H, Solitare GB, Thayer WR, Spiro HM. The effect of cervical vagectomy on esophageal function in the monkey. *Surgery* 1968; **64**: 1075–83.

8 Birgisson S, Galinski MS, Goldblum JR, Rice TW, Richter JE. Achalasia is not associated with measles or known herpes and human papilloma viruses. *Dig Dis Sci* 1997; **42**: 300–6.

9 Bortolotti M, Mari C, Lopilato C, Porrazzo G, Miglioli M. Effects of sildenafil on esophageal motility of patients with idiopathic achalasia. *Gastroenterology* 2000; **118**: 253–7.

10 Brackbill S, Shi G, Hirano I. Diminished mechanosensitivity and chemosensitivity in patients with achalasia. *Am J Physiol Gastrointest Liver Physiol* 2003; **285**: G1198–203.

11 Cannon RO 3rd, Quyyumi AA, Mincemoyer R *et al.* Imipramine in patients with chest pain despite normal coronary angiograms. *N Engl J Med* 1994; **330**: 1411–17.

12 Cassella RR, Brown AL Jr, Sayre GP, Ellis FH Jr. Achalasia of the esophagus: pathologic and etiologic considerations. *Ann Surg* 1964; **160**: 474–85.

13 Castagliuolo I, Brun P, Costantini M *et al.* Esophageal achalasia: is the herpes simplex virus really innocent? *J Gastroin-*

test Surg 2004; **8**: 24–30.

14 Chapman J, Joehl RJ, Murayama KM et al. Achalasia treatment: improved outcome of laparoscopic myotomy with operative manometry. *Arch Surg* 2004; **139**: 508–13.

15 Chinn JS, Schuffler MD. Paraneoplastic visceral neuropathy as a cause of severe gastrointestinal motor dysfunction. *Gastroenterology* 1988; **95**: 1279–86.

16 Clark SB, Rice TW, Tubbs RR, Richter JE, Goldblum JR. The nature of the myenteric infiltrate in achalasia: an immunohistochemical analysis. *Am J Surg Pathol* 2000; **24**: 1153–8.

17 Clouse RE, Lustman PJ, Eckert TC, Ferney DM, Griffith LS. Low-dose trazodone for symptomatic patients with esophageal contraction abnormalities. A double-blind, placebo-controlled trial. *Gastroenterology* 1987; **92**: 1027–36.

18 Clouse RE, Richter JE, Heading RC, Janssens J, Wilson JA. Functional esophageal disorders. *Gut* 1999; **45** (Suppl. 2): II31–6.

19 Cohen S, Fisher R, Tuch A. The site of denervation in achalasia. *Gut* 1972; **13**: 556–8.

20 Conklin JL, Du CA, Schulze-Delrieu K, Shirazi S. Hypertrophic smooth muscle in the partially obstructed opossum esophagus. Excitability and electrophysiological properties. *Gastroenterology* 1991; **101**: 657–63.

21 Csendes A, Smok G, Braghetto I, Ramirez C, Velasco N, Henriquez A. Gastroesophageal sphincter pressure and histological changes in distal esophagus in patients with achalasia of the esophagus. *Dig Dis Sci* 1985; **30**: 941–5.

22 Cuilliere C, Ducrotte P, Zerbib F et al. Achalasia: outcome of patients treated with intrasphincteric injection of botulinum toxin [see comments]. *Gut* 1997; **41**: 87–92.

23 Dalton CB, Castell DO, Hewson EG, Wu WC, Richter JE. Diffuse esophageal spasm. A rare motility disorder not characterized by high-amplitude contractions. *Dig Dis Sci* 1991; **36**: 1025–8.

24 Dantas RO, Godoy RA, Oliveira RB, Meneghelli UG, Troncon LE. Cholinergic innervation of the lower esophageal sphincter in Chagas' disease. *Braz J Med Biol Res* 1987; **20**: 527–32.

25 Darnell RB, Posner JB. Paraneoplastic syndromes involving the nervous system. *N Engl J Med* 2003; **349**: 1543–54.

26 de la Concha EG, Fernandez-Arquero M, Conejero L et al. Presence of a protective allele for achalasia on the central region of the major histocompatibility complex. *Tissue Antigens* 2000; **56**: 149–53.

27 de Oliveira JM, Birgisson S, Doinoff C et al. Timed barium swallow: a simple technique for evaluating esophageal emptying in patients with achalasia. *AJR Am J Roentgenol* 1997; **169**: 473–9.

28 Dempsey DT, Kalan MM, Gerson RS, Parkman HP, Maier WP. Comparison of outcomes following open and laparoscopic esophagomyotomy for achalasia. *Surgical Endoscopy* 1999; **13**: 747–50.

29 Dodds WJ, Dent J, Hogan WJ, Patel GK, Toouli J, Arndorfer RC. Paradoxical lower esophageal sphincter contraction induced by cholecystokinin-octapeptide in patients with achalasia. *Gastroenterology* 1981; **80**: 327–33.

30 Dunaway PM, Wong RK. Risk and surveillance intervals for squamous cell carcinoma in achalasia. *Gastrointest Endosc Clin N Am* 2001; **11**: 425–34, ix.

31 Eckardt VF, Krause J, Bolle D. Gastrointestinal transit and gastric acid secretion in patients with achalasia. [Erratum appears in Dig Dis Sci 1989; 34: 1324]. *Dig Dis Sci* 1989; **34**: 665–71.

32 Eckardt VF, Stauf B, Bernhard G. Chest pain in achalasia: patient characteristics and clinical course. *Gastroenterology* 1999; **116**: 1300–4.

33 Eckardt VF, Gockel I, Bernhard G. Pneumatic dilation for achalasia: late results of a prospective follow up investigation. *Gut* 2004; **53**: 629–33.

34 Ejima FH, Dantas RO, Simoes MV, Marin Neto JA, Meneghelli UG. Intraesophageal balloon distension test in Chagas' disease patients with noncardiac chest pain. *Dig Dis Sci* 1998; **43**: 2567–71.

35 Eng C. Seminars in medicine of the Beth Israel Hospital, Boston. The RET proto-oncogene in multiple endocrine neoplasia type 2 and Hirschsprung's disease. *N Engl J Med* 1996; **335**: 943–51.

36 Fass R, Naliboff B, Higa L et al. Differential effect of long-term esophageal acid exposure on mechanosensitivity and chemosensitivity in humans. *Gastroenterology* 1998; **115**: 1363–73.

37 Fleet RP, Dupuis G, Marchand A, Burelle D, Arsenault A, Beitman BD. Panic disorder in emergency department chest pain patients: prevalence, comorbidity, suicidal ideation, physician recognition. *A J Med* 1996; **101**: 371–80.

38 Foster PN, Stewart M, Lowe JS, Atkinson M. Achalasia like disorder of the oesophagus in von Recklinghausen's neurofibromatosis. *Gut* 1987; **28**: 1522–6.

39 Gaumnitz EA, Bass P, Osinski MA, Sweet MA, Singaram C. Electrophysiological and pharmacological responses of chronically denervated lower esophageal sphincter of the opossum. *Gastroenterology* 1995; **109**: 789–99.

40 Gebhart GF. Pathobiology of visceral pain: molecular mechanisms and therapeutic implications IV. Visceral afferent contributions to the pathobiology of visceral pain. *Am J Physiol Gastrointest Liver Physiol* 2000; **278**: G834–8.

41 Ghosh P, Linder J, Gallagher TF, Quigley EM. Achalasia of the cardia and multiple endocrine neoplasia 2B. *Am J Gastroenterol* 1994; **89**: 1880–3.

42 Goin JC, Sterin-Borda L, Bilder CR et al. Functional implications of circulating muscarinic cholinergic receptor autoantibodies in chagasic patients with achalasia. *Gastro-*

enterology 1999; **117**: 798–805.

43 Goldblum JR, Rice TW, Richter JE. Histopathologic features in esophagomyotomy specimens from patients with achalasia. *Gastroenterology* 1996; **111**: 648–54.

44 Goyal RK, Crist JR. Chest pain of esophageal etiology. *Hosp Pract (Off Ed)* 1988; **23**: 15–20.

45 Goyal RK, Hirano I. Mechanisms of disease: the enteric nervous system. *N Engl J Med* 1996; **334**: 1106–15.

46 Guelrud M, Zambrano-Rincones V, Simon C *et al.* Dysphagia and lower esophageal sphincter abnormalities after proximal gastric vagotomy. *Am J Surg* 1985; **149**: 232–5.

47 Hewson EG, Ott DJ, Dalton CB, Chen YM, Wu WC, Richter JE. Manometry and radiology. Complementary studies in the assessment of esophageal motility disorders. *Gastroenterology* 1990; **98**: 626–32.

48 Higgs B, Ellis FH Jr. The effect of bilateral supranodosal vagotomy on canine esophageal function. *Surgery* 1965; **58**: 828–34.

49 Higgs B, Kerr FW, Ellis FH Jr. The experimental production of esophageal achalasia by electrolytic lesions in the medulla. *J Thorac Cardiovasc Surg* 1965; **50**: 613–25.

50 Hirano I, Tatum RP, Shi G, Sang Q, Joehl RJ, Kahrilas PJ. Manometric heterogeneity in patients with idiopathic achalasia. *Gastroenterology* 2001; **120**: 789–98.

51 Hollerbach S, Bulat R, May A *et al.* Abnormal cerebral processing of oesophageal stimuli in patients with noncardiac chest pain (NCCP). *Neurogastroenterol Motil* 2000; **12**: 555–65.

52 Holloway RH, Dodds WJ, Helm JF, Hogan WJ, Dent J, Arndorfer RC. Integrity of cholinergic innervation to the lower esophageal sphincter in achalasia. *Gastroenterology* 1986; **90**: 924–9.

53 Howard PJ, Maher L, Pryde A, Cameron EW, Heading RC. Five year prospective study of the incidence, clinical features, diagnosis of achalasia in Edinburgh. *Gut* 1992; **33**: 1011–15.

54 Hunter JG, Trus TL, Branum GD, Waring JP. Laparoscopic Heller myotomy and fundoplication for achalasia. *Ann Surg* 1997; **225**: 655–64 [discussion 664–5].

55 Jones DB, Mayberry JF, Rhodes J, Munro J. Preliminary report of an association between measles virus and achalasia. *J Clin Pathol* 1983; **36**: 655–7.

56 Kahrilas PJ, Clouse RE, Hogan WJ. American Gastroenterological Association technical review on the clinical use of esophageal manometry [see comments]. *Gastroenterology* 1994; **107**: 1865–84.

57 Katz PO, Dalton CB, Richter JE, Wu WC, Castell DO. Esophageal testing of patients with noncardiac chest pain or dysphagia. Results of three years' experience with 1161 patients. *Ann Intern Med* 1987; **106**: 593–7.

58 Katz PO, Richter JE, Cowan R, Castell DO. Apparent complete lower esophageal sphincter relaxation in achalasia. *Gastroenterology* 1986; **90**: 978–83.

59 Kelly JL, Mulcahy TM, O'Riordan DS *et al.* Coexistent Hirschsprung's disease and esophageal achalasia in male siblings. *J Pediatr Surg* 1997; **32**: 1809–11.

60 Khajanchee YS, VanAndel R, Jobe BA, Barra MJ, Hansen PD, Swanstrom LL. Electrical stimulation of the vagus nerve restores motility in an animal model of achalasia. *J Gastrointest Surg* 2003; **7**: 843–9 [discussion 849].

61 Kimura K. The nature of idiopathic esophagus dilation. *Jpn J Gastroenterol* 1929; **1**: 199–207.

62 Kolbasnik J, Waterfall WE, Fachnie B, Chen Y, Tougas G. Long-term efficacy of botulinum toxin in classical achalasia: a prospective study. *Am J Gastroenterol* 1999; **94**: 3434–9.

63 Konturek JW, Thor P, Lukaszyk A, Gabryelewicz A, Konturek SJ, Domschke W. Endogenous nitric oxide in the control of esophageal motility in humans. *J Physiol Pharmacol* 1997; **48**: 201–9.

64 Kravitz JJ, Snape WJ Jr, Cohen S. Effect of thoracic vagotomy and vagal stimulation on esophageal function. *A J Physiol* 1978; **234**: E359–64.

65 Lee HR, Lennon VA, Camilleri M, Prather CM. Paraneoplastic gastrointestinal motor dysfunction: clinical and laboratory characteristics. *Am J Gastroenterol* 2001; **96**: 373–9.

66 Little AG, Correnti FS, Calleja IJ *et al.* Effect of incomplete obstruction on feline esophageal function with a clinical correlation. *Surgery* 1986; **100**: 430–6.

67 Lucchinetti CF, Kimmel DW, Lennon VA. Paraneoplastic and oncologic profiles of patients seropositive for type 1 antineuronal nuclear autoantibodies. *Neurology* 1998; **50**: 652–7.

68 Massey BT, Hogan WJ, Dodds WJ, Dantas RO. Alteration of the upper esophageal sphincter belch reflex in patients with achalasia [see comments]. *Gastroenterology* 1992; **103**: 1574–9.

69 Mayberry JF. Epidemiology and demographics of achalasia. *Gastrointest Endosc Clin N Am* 2001; **11**: 235–48.

70 Mayer EA, Collins SM. Evolving pathophysiologic models of functional gastrointestinal disorders. *Gastroenterology* 2002; **122**: 2032–48.

71 Mearin F, Mourelle M, Guarner F *et al.* Patients with achalasia lack nitric oxide synthase in the gastro-oesophageal junction. *Eur J Clin Invest* 1993; **23**: 724–8.

72 Mittal RK, Ren J, McCallum RW, Shaffer HA Jr, Sluss J. Modulation of feline esophageal contractions by bolus volume and outflow obstruction. *Am J Physiol* 1990; **258**: G208–15.

73 Moses PL, Ellis LM, Anees MR *et al.* Antineuronal antibodies in idiopathic achalasia and gastro-oesophageal reflux disease. *Gut* 2003; **52**: 629–36.

74 Murray J, Du C, Ledlow A, Bates JN, Conklin JL. Nitric oxide: mediator of nonadrenergic noncholinergic responses of opossum esophageal muscle. *Am J Physiol* 1991; **261**: G401–6.

75 Murray JA, Ledlow A, Launspach J, Evans D, Loveday M, Conklin JL. The effects of recombinant human hemoglobin on esophageal motor functions in humans. *Gastroenterology* 1995; **109**: 1241–8.

76 Niwamoto H, Okamoto E, Fujimoto J, Takeuchi M, Furuyama J, Yamamoto Y. Are human herpes viruses or measles virus associated with esophageal achalasia? *Dig Dis Sci* 1995; **40**: 859–64.

77 Orlando RC, Bozymski EM. Clinical and manometric effects of nitroglycerin in diffuse esophageal spasm. *N Engl J Med* 1973; **289**: 23–5.

78 Panzini L, Traube M. Stridor from tracheal obstruction in a patient with achalasia. *Am J Gastroenterol* 1993; **88**: 1097–100.

79 Pasricha PJ, Rai R, Ravich WJ, Hendrix TR, Kalloo AN. Botulinum toxin for achalasia: long-term outcome and predictors of response [see comments]. *Gastroenterology* 1996; **110**: 1410–15.

80 Pasricha PJ, Ravich WJ, Hendrix TR, Sostre S, Jones B, Kalloo AN. Intrasphincteric botulinum toxin for the treatment of achalasia [see comments]. *N Engl J Med* 1995; **332**: 774–8.

81 Paterson WG. Esophageal and lower esophageal sphincter response to balloon distention in patients with achalasia. *Dig Dis Sci* 1997; **42**: 106–12.

82 Paterson WG, Rattan S, Goyal RK. Experimental induction of isolated lower esophageal sphincter relaxation in anesthetized opossums. *J Clin Invest* 1986; **77**: 1187–93.

83 Patti MG, Pellegrini CA, Horgan S *et al*. Minimally invasive surgery for achalasia: an 8-year experience with 168 patients. *Ann Surg* 1999; **230**: 587–93 [discussion 593–4].

84 Perretta S, Fisichella PM, Galvani C, Gorodner MV, Way LW, Patti MG. Achalasia and chest pain: effect of laparoscopic Heller myotomy. *J Gastrointest Surg* 2003; **7**: 595–8.

85 Qualman SJ, Haupt HM, Yang P, Hamilton SR. Esophageal Lewy bodies associated with ganglion cell loss in achalasia. Similarity to Parkinson's disease. *Gastroenterology* 1984; **87**: 848–56.

86 Rao SS, Hayek B, Summers RW. Functional chest pain of esophageal origin: hyperalgesia or motor dysfunction. *Am J Gastroenterol* 2001; **96**: 2584–9.

87 Rao SS, Hayek B, Summers RW. Impedance planimetry: an integrated approach for assessing sensory, active, passive biomechanical properties of the human esophagus. *Am J Gastroenterol* 1995; **90**: 431–8.

88 Rate AJ, Hobson AR, Barlow J, Bancewicz J. Abnormal neurophysiology in patients with oesophageal motility disorders. *Br J Surg* 1999; **86**: 1202–6.

89 Rice TW, Richter JE, Goldblum JR. Achalasia. A morphologic study of 42 resected specimens. *Gastroenterology* 1996; **111**: 648–54.

90 Richter JE, Barish CF, Castell DO. Abnormal sensory perception in patients with esophageal chest pain. *Gastroenterology* 1986; **91**: 845–52.

91 Richter JE, Dalton CB, Bradley LA, Castell DO. Oral nifedipine in the treatment of noncardiac chest pain in patients with the nutcracker esophagus. *Gastroenterology* 1987; **93**: 21–8.

92 Robertson CS, Martin BA, Atkinson M. Varicella-zoster virus DNA in the oesophageal myenteric plexus in achalasia. *Gut* 1993; **34**: 299–302.

93 Rosati R, Fumagalli U, Bonavina L *et al*. Laparoscopic approach to esophageal achalasia. *Am J Surg* 1995; **169**: 424–7.

94 Ruiz-de-Leon A, Mendoza J, Sevilla-Mantilla C *et al*. Myenteric antiplexus antibodies and class II HLA in achalasia. *Dig Dis Sci* 2002; **47**: 15–19.

95 Sandler RS, Nyren O, Ekbom A, Eisen GM, Yuen J, Josefsson S. The risk of esophageal cancer in patients with achalasia. A population-based study. *JAMA* 1995; **274**: 1359–62.

96 Sarkar S, Aziz Q, Woolf CJ, Hobson AR, Thompson DG. Contribution of central sensitisation to the development of non-cardiac chest pain. *Lancet* 2000; **356**: 1154–9.

97 Sarkar S, Hobson AR. Furlong PL. Woolf CJ. Thompson DG, Aziz Q. Central neural mechanisms mediating human visceral hypersensitivity. *Am J Physiol Gastrointest Liver Physiol* 2001; **281**: G1196–202.

98 Shoenut JP, Micflikier AB, Yaffe CS, Den Boer B, Teskey JM. Reflux in untreated achalasia patients. *J Clin Gastroenterol* 1995; **20**: 6–11.

99 Sifrim D, Janssens J, Vantrappen G. Failing deglutitive inhibition in primary esophageal motility disorders. *Gastroenterology* 1994; **106**: 875–82.

100 Sivarao DV, Mashimo HL, Thatte HS, Goyal RK. Lower esophageal sphincter is achalasic in nNOS(–/–) and hypotensive in W/W(v) mutant mice. *Gastroenterology* 2001; **121**: 34–42.

101 Smith B. The neurological lesion in achalasia of the cardia. *Gut* 1970; **11**: 388–91.

102 Smith VV, Gregson N, Foggensteiner L, Neale G, Milla PJ. Acquired intestinal aganglionosis and circulating autoantibodies without neoplasia or other neural involvement [see comments]. *Gastroenterology* 1997; **112**: 1366–71.

103 Song CW, Lee SJ, Jeen YT *et al*. Inconsistent association of esophageal symptoms, psychometric abnormalities and dysmotility. *Am J Gastroenterol* 2001; **96**: 2312–16.

104 Spiess AE, Kahrilas PJ. Treating achalasia: from whalebone to laparoscope. *JAMA* 1998; **280**: 638–42.

105 Staiano A, Alrakawi A, Clouse RE. Development of a topographic analysis system for manometric studies in the gastrointestinal tract. *Gastroenterology* 2000; **118**: 469–76.

106 Stewart KC, Finley RJ, Clifton JC, Graham AJ, Storseth C, Inculet R. Thoracoscopic versus laparoscopic modified Heller myotomy for achalasia: efficacy and safety in 87 patients. *J Am Coll Surg* 1999; **189**: 164–9 [discussion 169–70].

107 Storch WB, Eckardt VF, Junginger T. Complement components and terminal complement complex in oesophageal smooth muscle of patients with achalasia. *Cell Mol Biol* 2002; **48**: 247–52.

108 Storch WB, Eckardt VF, Wienbeck M *et al.* Autoantibodies to Auerbach's plexus in achalasia. *Cell Mol Biol* 1995; **41**: 1033–8.

109 Swamy N. Esophageal spasm: clinical and manometric response to nitroglycerine and long acting nitrites. *Gastroenterology* 1977; **72**: 23–7.

110 Szymanski PT, Chacko TK, Rovner AS, Goyal RK. Differences in contractile protein content and isoforms in phasic and tonic smooth muscles. *Am J Physiol* 1998; **275**: C684–92.

111 Tottrup A, Forman A, Funch-Jensen P, Raundahl U, Andersson KE. Effects of postganglionic nerve stimulation in oesophageal achalasia: an *in vitro* study. *Gut* 1990; **31**: 17–20.

112 Tottrup A, Fredens K, Funch-Jensen P, Aggestrup S, Dahl R. Eosinophil infiltration in primary esophageal achalasia. A possible pathogenic role. *Dig Dis Sci* 1989; **34**: 1894–9.

113 Tougas G, Spaziani R, Hollerbach S *et al.* Cardiac autonomic function and oesophageal acid sensitivity in patients with non-cardiac chest pain. *Gut* 2001; **49**: 706–12.

114 Trounce JR, Deuchar DC, Kauntze R, Thomas GA. Studies in achalasia of the cardia. *Q J Med* 1957; **36**: 433–43.

115 Tullio-Pelet A, Salomon R, Hadj-Rabia S *et al.* Mutant WD-repeat protein in triple-A syndrome. *Nat Genet* 2000; **26**: 332–5.

116 Tung HN, Schulze-Delrieu K, Shirazi S, Noel S, Xia Q, Cue K. Hypertrophic smooth muscle in the partially obstructed opossum esophagus. The model: histological and ultrastructural observations. *Gastroenterology* 1991; **100**: 853–64.

117 Tung HN, Shirazi S, Schulze-Delrieu K, Brown K. Morphological changes of myenteric neurons in the partially obstructed opossum esophagus. *J Submicrosc Cytol Pathol* 1993; **25**: 357–63.

118 Vaezi MF, Baker ME, Richter JE. Assessment of esophageal emptying post-pneumatic dilation: use of the timed barium esophagram. *Am J Gastroenterol* 1999; **94**: 1802–7.

119 Vaezi MF, Richter JE, Wilcox CM *et al.* Botulinum toxin versus pneumatic dilatation in the treatment of achalasia: a randomised trial. *Gut* 1999; **44**: 231–9.

120 Varia I, Logue E, O'Connor C. Randomized trial of sertraline in patients with unexplained chest pain of noncardiac origin. *Am Heart J* 2000; **140**: 367–72.

121 Verne GN, Hahn AB, Pineau BC, Hoffman BJ, Wojciechowski BW, Wu WC. Association of HLA-DR and -DQ alleles with idiopathic achalasia. *Gastroenterology* 1999; **117**: 26–31.

122 Verne GN, Sallustio JE, Eaker EY. Anti-myenteric neuronal antibodies in patients with achalasia. A prospective study. *Dig Dis Sci* 1997; **42**: 307–13.

123 Wattchow DA, Costa M. Distribution of peptide-containing nerve fibres in achalasia of the oesophagus. *J Gastroenterol Hepatol* 1996; **11**: 478–85.

124 Weber A, Wienker TF, Jung M *et al.* Linkage of the gene for the triple A syndrome to chromosome 12q13 near the type II keratin gene cluster. *Hum Mol Genet* 1996; **5**: 2061–6.

125 Wehrmann T, Kokabpick H, Jacobi V, Seifert H, Lembcke B, Caspary WF. Long-term results of endoscopic injection of botulinum toxin in elderly achalasic patients with tortuous megaesophagus or epiphrenic diverticulum. *Endoscopy* 1999; **31**: 352–8.

126 Wong RK, Maydonovitch CL, Metz SJ, Baker JR Jr. Significant DQw1 association in achalasia. *Dig Dis Sci* 1989; **34**: 349–52.

127 Wychulis AR, Woolam GL, Andersen HA, Ellis FH Jr. Achalasia and carcinoma of the esophagus. *JAMA* 1971; **215**: 1638–41.

128 Yamamura MS, Gilster JC, Myers BS, Deveney CW, Sheppard BC. Laparoscopic Heller myotomy and anterior fundoplication for achalasia results in a high degree of patient satisfaction. *Arch Surg* 2000; **135**: 902–6.

129 Yamato S, Saha JK, Goyal RK. Role of nitric oxide in lower esophageal sphincter relaxation to swallowing. *Life Sci* 1992; **50**: 1263–72.

130 Yamato S, Spechler SJ, Goyal RK. Role of nitric oxide in esophageal peristalsis in the opossum. *Gastroenterology* 1992; **103**: 197–204.

CHAPTER 10

Gastric Disorders

Fernando Azpiroz and Jan Tack

Neuromuscular anatomy and electrophysiology

Functionally, the stomach consists of a proximal part and a distal part, with a sphincter muscle at both ends. The proximal stomach consists of the fundus and part of the gastric corpus. In the proximal stomach, smooth muscle cells do not display electrical oscillations, but they do exert a tonic contractile activity. In the distal part of the stomach, smooth muscle cells display slow waves, which are oscillations of the membrane potential at the rate of three per minute, triggered from an area in the mid-corpus near the greater curvature, the pacemaker region of the stomach. It is now clear that the interstitial cells of Cajal, a specialized type of neural crest-derived cell, located near the myenteric plexus, are the generators of these membrane potential oscillations.[1] Slow waves are not sufficient to generate contractile activity. Phasic contractions are produced by action potential, triggered by neurotransmitter release, at the crest of a slow wave. Thus, the slow waves determine the timing of contractions, while the number of spikes determines the strength of the contractions. Recent observations also support the involvement of interstitial cells of Cajal in nerve-to-muscle neurotransmission.

Like other parts of the gastrointestinal tract, the myenteric plexus is found between the circular and longitudinal muscle layers in the stomach. Cell bodies of intrinsic neurons are grouped in ganglia, whose number increases towards the distal antrum. Although these neurons have numerous connections with vagal (parasympathetic) and splanchnic (sympathetic) extrinsic nerves, the gastric myenteric plexus is also capable of major functional autonomy.

Vago-vagal reflexes play a crucial role in the control of gastric motor activity. The splanchnic or sympathet-ic innervation of the stomach originates from spinal segments T6 to T9. They exert mainly an inhibitory function through the presynaptic inhibition of acetylcholine release from the myenteric plexus and via sympathetic reflexes relaying at prevertebral ganglia or the spinal cord. Perception afferents from the stomach are driven by splanchnic–sympathetic–spinal pathways, while vagal fibers may play only a modulatory role.[2]

Physiology

Interdigestive motility

During fasting, the stomach participates in the cyclic interdigestive motor pattern, alternating periods of quiescence and periods of activity. During the periods of activity the proximal stomach generates a high level tonic contraction with superimposed prolonged phasic contractions with a 1-minute rhythm, whereas the antrum produces shorter phasic contractions at three per minute. The net effect of gastric interdigestive activity is the evacuation of indigestible particles from the stomach to the small bowel. Hence, the absence of gastric phase III activity may promote gastric bezoar formation.

Postprandial activity

Ingestion of food suppresses interdigestive motility, and the gut switches to a fed pattern. The stomach accommodates a rapidly ingested, heterogeneous meal, and delivers into the small bowel a homogenized chyme at the rate adapted to the intestinal processing capability (Fig. 10.1). In response to ingestion, the proximal stomach partially relaxes to accommodate the meal (Fig. 10.2). During the postprandial period the proximal stomach progressively recontracts, and this tonic contraction gently forces intragastric chyme distally. Solid particles are retained and ground in the

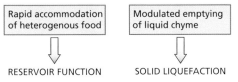

Fig. 10.1 Motor function of the stomach.

antrum by phasic contractions, while liquid chyme is squeezed through the pyloric gate, which determines the final gastric outflow.

The tonic contraction of the proximal stomach during the postprandial period is modulated by several mechanisms. Swallowing produces a transient and brief receptive relaxation that probably has little effect on the accommodation process. Antral filling releases antrofundal relaxatory reflexes, which may play a major role in the early accommodation phase.[3] Nutrients entering the intestine induce a variety of reflexes depending on the type of nutrient and the region of the intestine stimulated. This probably constitutes a fine feedback control to adapt the rate of nutrient delivery to the intestinal processing capability. Other chyme parameters, such as pH and osmolarity, also play a role. Gastric accommodation is modulated by vago-vagal reflexes involving the release of 5-HT, probably at the level of the enteric nervous system, and subsequent activation of nitrergic motor neurons.[4]

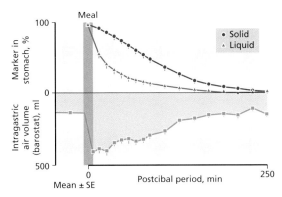

Fig. 10.2. Gastric tone during gastric emptying of a meal. Gastric emptying of solids and liquids was measured by scintigraphy and gastric tone was measured as changes in air volume within an intragastric bag maintained at constant pressure by a barostat. Note gastric relaxation (air volume increases) after meal ingestion, and subsequent tone recovery paralleling gastric emptying. From Moragas *et al.*, *Am J Physiol* 1993; **264**: G112–17, with permission.

Tests of gastric motor function

Measurement of gastric emptying
Radionuclide gastric emptying test
This technique is still considered the standard method for the assessment of gastric emptying rate. Solid and liquid emptying can be assessed separately or simultaneously (Fig. 10.2). The solid and/or liquid meal components are labeled with a (different) radioisotope, usually ^{99}Tc or ^{111}In.[5,6] The number of counts in a given region of interest (proximal, distal or total stomach, small intestine) is measured at regular intervals after ingestion of a meal, using a gamma-camera. The disadvantage is the use of radioactive labels, its high cost and its poor level of standardization of meal composition and measuring times over different laboratories.

^{13}C breath test
The solid or liquid phase of a meal is labeled with a ^{13}C-containing substrate (octanoic acid, acetic acid, glycine or spirulina). As soon as the labeled substrate leaves the stomach, it is rapidly absorbed and metabolized in the liver to generate ^{13}CO$_2$, which appears in the breath. Breath sampling at regular intervals and mathematical processing of its ^{13}CO$_2$ content over time makes it possible to calculate a gastric emptying curve. The advantages of this test are its non-radioactive nature and the ability to perform the test outside a hospital setting. Disadvantages are the absence of standardization of meal and substrate.

Ultrasound
Ultrasound makes it possible to measure the diameter of the gastric antrum as a marker of the emptying rate of a liquid meal. Complex technologies that allow proximal and distal gastric volumes to be calculated have been described. However, the ultrasound technique is operator-dependent, time-consuming and not suitable for solid meals. It is therefore mainly an experimental tool.

Antro-intestinal manometry
Antro-intestinal manometry makes it possible to investigate mechanisms that are involved in the regulation of normal and abnormal gastric emptying.[7] Its clinical application is restricted to referral centers and it is indi-

cated only in cases of suspected intestinal dysmotility, especially in patients with gastroparesis.

The barostat

The gastric barostat consists of a computer-driven air pump connected to an oversized balloon, which can be positioned in the proximal or distal stomach. The barostat maintains a fixed pressure level within the stomach by adapting the intraballoon volume.[5] Measurement of volume changes at a constant low pressure allows changes in gastric tone to be quantified (Fig. 10.2), and measurement of perception at various pressure levels of distension makes it possible to quantify sensitivity to gastric distension. The use of barostat measurement is restricted to research.

Electrogastrography

Cutaneous electrodes can be used to measure the electrical activity of the stomach, which provides information on the frequency and regularity of gastric pacemaker activity, and on changes in the power of the signal after meal ingestion. This technique is an experimental tool.

Gastroparesis

Delayed gastric emptying in the absence of mechanical obstruction is called gastroparesis. In fact, the clinical diagnosis of gastroparesis is established by techniques that evidence a significant delay in gastric emptying.[5,8] Chronic idiopathic gastroparesis is a relatively uncommon but important entity. The diagnosis of gastroparesis should be restricted to patients with objective demonstration of grossly abnormal gastric emptying of both solids and liquids (Fig. 10.3). The perception of pain or nausea may delay gastric emptying secondarily. Hence, special attention has to be paid to patients (for example, those with functional dyspepsia) who experience symptoms during the gastric emptying test.

Pathophysiology

The most important causes of gastroparesis are diabetes mellitus (24%) and postsurgical (19%), but in some patients (33%) no underlying cause is apparent, so their disorder is considered idiopathic. In some of these, an acute onset and the presence of antibodies against neurotropic viruses suggest the involvement of

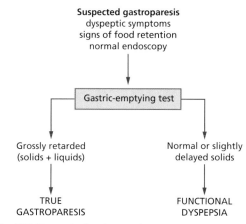

Fig. 10.3 Diagnosis of gastroparesis.

(viral) infections in the pathogenesis of gastroparesis. Gastric emptying may be secondarily delayed by drugs, such as anticholinergics, opioids, L-dopa, tricyclic antidepressants and phenothiazines.

Clinical features

The onset of chronic gastroparesis is usually insidious. The symptoms vary from mild dyspepsia-like complaints (early satiety, epigastric fullness, vague nausea) to severe manifestation of gastric stasis with retention-type emesis (that is, vomiting of food ingested many hours or even days earlier) and nutritional compromise. Nausea and vomiting may occur in some patients during fasting rather than postprandially. Associated complaints, such as dysphagia, diarrhea, constipation and rectal incontinence, may be present, and these suggest a more widespread dysfunction of gut motility. Likewise, extraintestinal manifestations of autonomic neuropathy (bladder dysfunction, orthostatic hypotension), peripheral neuropathy or an extrapyramidal disorder suggest a neuropathic condition. The course of the disease is variable. In some patients the disorder is unremitting, with fluctuations or progressive severity that may lead to inability to eat and incapacitation. In severe cases, even endogenous fasting secretions cannot be emptied, requiring gastric evacuation via a tube. In other patients the disorder may remit spontaneously after a few months with complete recovery.

Management

The diagnostic approach to the patient with gastropa-

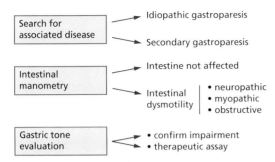

Fig. 10.4 Characterization of gastroparesis.

resis can be undertaken in four stages (Figs 10.3 and 10.4). First, in a patient with dyspeptic-type symptoms and signs of food retention, an endoscopy should be performed. In the absence of organic lesion, gastroparesis is suspected. The diagnosis can be ascertained in a second stage by a gastric emptying test, as detailed above. At this stage it may also be important to search for associated diseases and define whether the gastroparesis is idiopathic or secondary. A third diagnostic stage addresses whether the intestine is also affected. A manometric study of the small intestine will determine whether the motility patterns are normal or whether some type of intestinal dysmotility is present. Finally, confirmation of impairment of the proximal stomach can be sought in a fourth stage by means of the barostat.[5] This procedure, still experimental, can demonstrate a flaccid stomach, characterized by low resting tone and impaired distensibility, and may also allow a therapeutic assay. In each case, the indications to proceed from stage one to four depend on the severity of the symptoms, the nutritional balance of the patient and the availability of the techniques.

Diet should be adapted to the patient's tolerance. In general, large meals should be avoided and if necessary a liquid diet should be given – either homogenized meals or formula diets. Pharmacological treatment of gastroparesis includes gastroprokinetic drugs, such as domperidone and metoclopramide. The former seems preferable, because metoclopramide crosses the blood–brain barrier and may induce extrapyramidal symptoms. Several studies have reported the successful use of cisapride in gastroparesis. However, because of an enhanced risk of QT prolongation with cardiac arrhythmias, the availability of cisapride has been suspended. Short-term studies in diabetic and postsurgi-

cal gastroparesis have reported beneficial effects of treatment with erythromycin (3×250–500 mg).[8] This macrolide antibiotic has prokinetic properties in that it acts as a motilin receptor agonist. In patients with severe gastric stasis, a trial of intravenous administration should be prescribed initially, to normalize gastric emptying before oral administration can be effective. Attempts to develop macrolide prokinetics without antibiotic properties have been disappointing. Some patients require home parenteral nutrition. However, the course of gastroparesis usually exhibits fluctuations and the treatment should be adjusted accordingly (Fig. 10.5). Intensive treatment during the phases of relapse usually lead to symptom remission.

The indications for surgical treatment are exceptional and should be restricted to refractory cases. Gastroenteric anastomosis is ineffective and should not be performed. A surgically implanted jejunal catheter may allow enteral feeding. If the stomach retains endogenous secretions, a drainage gastrostomy may be also used. The effect on gastric emptying of electrical stimulation via implanted electrodes is limited. Subtotal gastric resection with Roux-en-Y enteric anastomosis may be helpful in extreme cases, provided intestinal motility is not affected.

Functional dyspepsia

Functional dyspepsia is defined as persisting or recurrent pain or discomfort centered in the upper abdomen, in the absence of organic disease that readily explains the symptoms.[9] According to recent estimates,

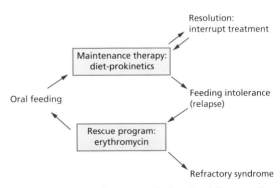

Fig. 10.5 Treatment of gastroparesis. Associated disease and intestinal dysmotility should be treated if pertinent.

functional dyspepsia has a prevalence of 26–29% in the adult population below 65 years old. Functional dyspepsia is probably a heterogeneous disorder, and in the absence of known pathophysiology its diagnosis is based solely on clinical criteria.

Symptoms in functional dyspepsia include pain, early satiety, fullness, bloating, nausea and retching. Heartburn, if present, is strongly indicative of gastro-esophageal reflux disease. A considerable proportion of dyspeptic patients also have irritable bowel symptoms. Based on the clinical presentation, dyspepsia has been classified as ulcer-like when the predominant symptom is pain and dysmotility-like when other uncomfortable, but not painful sensations are present. The value of this classification has been questioned. The relation of symptoms to meals has not been studied in large populations, but some recent data indicate that most patients with ulcer-like dyspepsia experience symptoms during fasting or more than 2 hours after meal ingestion, whereas patients with dysmotility-like dyspepsia report symptoms during the postprandial period.[3]

In the past, there was widespread belief that an underlying gastrointestinal motility disturbance was the cause of dyspepsia. Indeed, a considerable proportion of dyspeptic patients (between 20 and 40% depending on the population studied) exhibit postprandial antral hypomotility associated with a certain delay in solid emptying.[6] The distinction between functional dyspepsia with delayed gastric emptying and idiopathic gastroparesis has not been clearly defined. It may be a matter of degree, and it is perhaps better to reserve the term 'idiopathic gastroparesis' for patients with a well-defined and prominent gastric emptying disorder. Very infrequently, dyspeptic-type symptoms may be due to a neuropathy of the gut, but in the presence of an underlying cause these patients should not be labeled as having functional dyspepsia.

Pathophysiology

A large proportion of patients with functional dyspepsia have increased perception of gastric distension (Fig. 10.6).[2] The same degree of hypersensitivity has been evidenced in patients with ulcer-like and dysmotility-like dyspepsia, but the underlying mechanism is not established.[3] This sensory dysfunction is restrict-

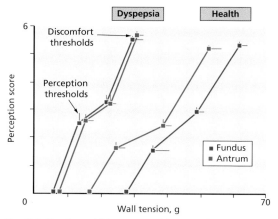

Fig. 10.6 Gastric sensitivity compared between dyspepsia and in healthy subjects. Patients with functional dyspepsia perceived and tolerated significantly lower distension levels in the fundus and antrum. Standardized distensions at fixed tension levels were applied by means of a computerized tensostat. From Caldarella *et al.*, *Gastroenterology* 2003; **124**: 1220–9, with permission.

ed to the gut, because somatic sensitivity is normal in these patients.[7,10]

Some data indicate that altered perception in dyspepsia is associated with impaired enterogastric and antrofundic reflexes that normally modulate the gastric accommodation/emptying process. Gastric hyporeactivity to relaxatory reflexes would predictably result in defective accommodation of the proximal stomach and antral overload. Studies using a gastric barostat have shown reduced proximal gastric relaxation in response to a meal in up to 40% of patients with functional dyspepsia,[11,12] and this may be associated with more prevalent early satiety and weight loss. In at least a subset of patients, this occurs as a consequence of an acute (possibly viral) gastroenteritis, which leads to impaired nitrergic nerve function in the proximal stomach.[13] Scintigraphic and ultrasonographic studies have demonstrated an abnormal intragastric distribution of food in patients with functional dyspepsia, with preferential accumulation in the distal stomach. If the stomach does not relax properly, meal ingestion will result in increased gastric wall tension and symptom perception, particularly in patients with gastric hypersensitivity. Antral overload may also explain the impression of postprandial antral hypomotility, because only occlusive contractions are recorded by manometry. A distended antrum may produce slower grinding of solids, and thus account for the prolonged gastric retention and delayed emptying of solids observed in these patients.

The role of *Helicobacter pylori* in the pathogenesis of functional dyspepsia has been the subject of several studies that have shown variable results, but most studies failed to demonstrate a beneficial effect of *H. pylori* eradication on dyspeptic symptoms.[14]

Recent studies suggest a complex interaction between psychopathological and physiopathological factors in the dyspeptic symptom complex,[15] but their precise role in functional dyspepsia is not clear.

Management

The first decision in a patient with dyspepsia is whether and when to perform upper endoscopy. This will depend on the presence of alarm symptoms, the degree of certainty required by the physician, and the patient's demands. Nevertheless, once the endoscopy is performed, it should not be repeated in the absence of objective indications. Other tests are indicated only in extreme cases, when gastroparesis or intestinal neuropathy is suspected. The barostat, although experimental, may be helpful in some patients by demonstrating gastric hypersensitivity and impaired accommodation. Formal psychological or psychiatric evaluation is indicated if these types of disorders are suspected.

An essential part of the treatment is reassurance and explanation. Depending on the putative pathophysiological mechanisms involved, possible therapeutic options would include antral prokinetics, fundal relaxants and visceral analgesia (Table 10.1). Prokinetics have been used widely in the treatment of functional dyspepsia, but due to a risk of arrhythmias the use of cisapride can be recommended only exceptionally, and the other prokinetics are less efficacious. Tegaserod, a new prokinetic 5-HT4 agonist, is currently under evaluation for the treatment of functional dyspepsia.

Table 10.1 Putative therapeutic options in dyspepsia

Antral prokinetics
Fundic relaxants
Visceral antinociception
Antisecretory drugs

Proton pump inhibitors, frequently used as initial therapy, are often probably more effective in patients with underlying gastro-esophageal reflux disease rather than in those with true dyspepsia.[9] Several drugs aimed at decreasing visceral sensitivity or at enhancing gastric accommodation are currently under investigation, but their efficacy needs to be established in future studies. Some patients may respond to low-dose antidepressants, possibly related to their antinociceptive effects or to psychotherapy.[16]

Dumping syndrome

Dumping syndrome is characterized by rapid gastric emptying accompanied by vasomotor and gastrointestinal symptoms. Dumping syndrome occurs mainly after partial or complete gastrectomy, but may also be observed after vagotomy (intentional or unintentional) at the time of surgery at the gastro-esophageal junction.

Symptoms typically occur after ingestion of a meal. Symptoms are subdivided into early and late dumping (Table 10.2). Early dumping occurs in the first hour after meal ingestion and is associated with both abdominal and systemic symptoms. Late dumping symptoms occur 1–2 hours after a meal and are the expression of reactive hypoglycemia. Most patients suffer from early dumping or a combination of early and late dumping; a minority suffer from late dumping only. Symptoms usually occur within the first weeks after surgery, when patients resume their normal diet. Liquids and meals rich in carbohydrates are poorly tolerated. Severe dumping may lead to weight loss because of fear of food ingestion, and in extreme cases malnutrition may even occur. Quality of life may be severely impaired.[17]

Pathophysiology

Symptoms of early dumping are explained in part by the rapid passage of hyperosmolar contents into the small bowel, accompanied by a shift of fluids from the intravascular compartment to the gut lumen. This induces intestinal distension and gastrointestinal symptoms such as bloating, abdominal pain and diarrhea. The vasomotor symptoms were previously attributed to relative hypovolemia, but the shift of fluid is usually only 300–700 ml, which should not cause such acute

Table 10.2 Dumping symptoms

Early dumping 30–60 min postcibal		Late dumping 90–240 min postcibal
Gastrointestinal	**Vasomotor**	**Hypoglycemia**
Abdominal pain	Flushing	Transpiration
Diarrhea	Palpitations	Palpitations
Borborygmi	Transpiration	Hunger
Bloating	Dizziness	Weakness
Nausea	Tachycardia	Confusion
	Syncope	Tremor
	Orthostatic hypotension	Syncope

symptoms. Enhanced release of several gastrointestinal hormones, including enteroglucagon, vasoactive intestinal polypeptide, peptide YY, pancreatic polypeptide and neurotensin, is thought to cause systemic and splanchnic vasodilation, which is the cause of the vasomotor symptoms.

Late dumping is characterized by symptoms of hypoglycemia. Rapid gastric emptying induces a high glucose concentration in the intestinal lumen. Glucose is rapidly absorbed, which leads to a peak in insulin secretion. Because of the long half-life of insulin and the often very transient character of the initial rise in glycemia, reactive hypoglycemia occurs when all sugars have been absorbed. Enhanced release of glucagon-like peptide-1 is thought to contribute to the extreme changes in glycemia levels after gastrectomy.

Management

Dietary measures are the first step in treating dumping syndrome. Patients are instructed to divide their daily calorie intake over at least six meals, and to avoid drinking during the 2 hours after a meal. Rapidly absorbed carbohydrates should be avoided, and intake of fat and proteins is increased accordingly. Certain food additives, such as pectin, guar gum and glucomannan, can be used. They form a gel with carbohydrates, thereby slowing absorption and delaying transit time.

Acarbose is a powerful inhibitor of intestinal α-glucosidase. Its ingestion slows carbohydrate digestion and blunts postprandial rises in glycemia; hence its application in late dumping. However, acarbose often induces diarrhea, which limits its use. Octreotide is a long-acting synthetic somatostatin analog. It is administered subcutaneously three times daily or intramuscularly once every 2–4 weeks as a slow-release formulation. Octreotide inhibits gastric emptying of liquids, although conflicting data have been reported, and inhibits small bowel transit. It inhibits the release of enteral hormones, thus favorably influencing postprandial vasomotor dumping symptoms. Octreotide inhibits the release of insulin and slows monosaccharide absorption, and thereby prevents late dumping caused by reactive hypoglycemia. Because of its mode of administration and the potential side-effect of gallstone formation, octreotide should be reserved for severe cases that do not respond to more conservative measures. In difficult-to-manage patients, surgery to create a proximal short anti-peristaltic intestinal loop can be considered.

References

1 Huizinga JD, Thuneberg L, Kluppel M, Malysz J, Mikkelsen HB, Bernstein A. W/kit gene required for interstitial cells of Cajal and for intestinal pacemaker activity. *Nature* 1995; **373**: 347–9.

2 Azpiroz F. Gastrointestinal perception: pathophysiological implications. *Neurogastroenterol Motil* 2002; **14**: 1–11.

3 Caldarella P, Azpiroz, F, Malagelada J-R. Antro-fundic dysfunctions in functional dyspepsia. *Gastroenterology* 2003; **124**: 1220–9.

4 Tack J, Demedts I, Meulemans A, Schuurkes J, Janssens J. Role of nitric oxide in the accommodation reflex and in meal-induced satiety in man. *Gut* 2002; **51**: 219–24.

5 Azpiroz F, Malagelada J-R. Gastric tone measured by an electronic barostat in health and postsurgical gastroparesis. *Gastroenterology* 1987; **92**: 934–43.

6 Stanghellini V, Tosetti C, Paternico A *et al.* Risk indicators of delayed gastric emptying of solids in patients with functional dyspepsia. *Gastroenterology* 1996; **110**: 1036–42.

7 Mearin F, Cucala M, Azpiroz F, Malagelada J-R. The origin of symptoms on the brain–gut axis in functional dyspepsia. *Gastroenterology* 1991; **101**: 999–1006.

8 Janssens J, Peeters TL, Vantrappen G *et al*. Improvement of gastric emptying in diabetic gastroparesis by erythromycin. Preliminary studies. *N Engl J Med* 1990; **322**: 1028–31.

9 Talley NJ, Stanghellini V, Heading RC, Koch KL, Malagelada JR, Tytgat GNJ. Functional gastroduodenal disorders. In: Drossman DA, Corazziari E, Talley NJ, Thompson WG, Whitehead WE, eds. *The Functional Gastrointestinal Disorders*, 2nd edn. McLean, Virginia: Degnon, 2000: 299–350.

10 Coffin B, Azpiroz F, Guarner F, Malagelada J-R. Selective gastric hypersensitivity and reflex hyporeactivity in functional dyspepsia. *Gastroenterology* 1994; **107**: 1345–51.

11 Tack J, Caenepeel P, Fischler B, Piessevaux H, Janssens J. Symptoms associated with hypersensitivity to gastric distension in functional dyspepsia. *Gastroenterology* 2001; **121**: 526–35.

12 Salet GAM, Samsom M, Roelofs JMM, van Berge Henegouwen GP, Smout AJPM, Akkermans LMA. Responses to gastric distension in functional dyspepsia. *Gut* 1998; **42**: 823–9.

13 Tack J, Demedts I, Dehondt G *et al*. Clinical and pathophysiological characteristics of acute-onset functional dyspepsia. *Gastroenterology* 2002; **122**: 1738–47.

14 Talley NJ, Vakil N, Ballard ED 2nd, Fennerty MB. Absence of benefit of eradicating *Helicobacter pylori* in patients with nonulcer dyspepsia. *N Engl J Med* 1999; **341**: 1106–11.

15 Fischler B, Vandenberghe J, Persoons P *et al*. Evidence-based subtypes in functional dyspepsia with confirmatory factor analysis: psychosocial and physiopathological correlates. *Gastroenterology* 2001; **120**: 268–76.

16 Calvert EL, Houghton LA, Cooper P, Whorwell P. Long-term improvement in functional dyspepsia using hypnotherapy. *Gastroenterology* 2002; **123**: 1778–85.

17 Vecht J, Masclee AA, Lamers CB. The dumping syndrome. Current insights into pathophysiology, diagnosis and treatment. *Scand J Gastroenterol* 1997; **223** (Suppl.): 21–7.

CHAPTER 11

Small Bowel Disorders

John Kellow

Perhaps more than disorders of any other region of the gut, disorders of small bowel motility serve as a template for the investigation of potential aberrations of the enteric nervous system (ENS) in the functional gastrointestinal disorders. This is because (i) the motor patterns of the healthy small bowel are well characterized and stereotypic, and (ii) distinct histological lesions have been identified in the myenteric plexus, the interstitial cells of Cajal and the enteric smooth muscle. In this chapter, the focus will be on motor and sensory dysfunction of the small bowel, as it is likely that these aspects, more than disordered water and electrolyte transport, are most relevant to the functional gastrointestinal disorders.

Normal small bowel motor and sensory function

Motor activity of the small bowel

The healthy small bowel can generate a number of specific motor patterns to suit its particular functions (Table 11.1). The most striking of these motor events is the migrating motor complex (MMC).[1] This remarkable phenomenon, which traverses most of the human small bowel in the fasting state, clearing digestive residue, has by convention three main components or phases (Fig. 11.1). Phase 3 of the MMC, the most distinctive phase, is a powerful propulsive sequence which commences in the gastric antrum or in the proximal small bowel. The phasic contractions during phase 3 are largely peristaltic, because although they propagate over relatively short distances, their velocity of propagation is considerably greater than the migration velocity of the overall phase 3 sequence itself. During the subsequent motor quiescence of phase 1, the intestine appears relatively refractory to

contractile stimulation. The phase 2 component of irregular contractile activity, which follows phase 1, is also important for propulsion, although the actual proportion of phase 2 contractions that are propagative remains poorly understood. A particular phase 2 contractile pattern, discrete clusters of phasic contractions, can occur in some individuals and is most prevalent in the elderly. With further technological developments for recording patterns of flow, the functional significance of the various components of the MMC will be defined more clearly. Phases 1 and 3 of the MMC biorhythm are generated within the ENS, with modulation by the central nervous system (CNS). Gastrointestinal regulatory peptides, such as motilin, and neurotransmitters, such as serotonin, modulate these phases by both endocrine and paracrine modes. The normal intestinal microflora also appears to provide a stimulatory drive for the initiation and propagation of the phase 3 activity front,[2] while the characteristics of the front are influenced by a variety of other factors, such as the hormonal fluctuations of the menstrual cycle. Phase 2 motor activity, in contrast, depends more on central input, as it is largely abolished during sleep and after vagotomy.

Following ingestion of a meal, or any form of nutrients, there is an immediate change in the contractile pattern of the small bowel to what is conventionally termed the 'postprandial' or 'fed' pattern. This pattern appears to be initiated by a vagal reflex and is maintained by endocrine and paracrine influences. These phasic contractions – of variable frequency, amplitude and propagation – enable the mixing and absorption of luminal contents and their subsequent aboral transport. The duration of this pattern relates, to some extent, to the time taken for digestible solids and liquids to empty from the stomach, but also to

Table 11.1 Normal small bowel phasic contractile activity

Parameter	Description
Fasting motor pattern: migrating motor complex (MMC)	
Phase 3 component (activity front)	A contractile pattern with at least 2 min duration of uninterrupted regular phasic contractions at the maximum frequency for that particular locus of bowel, usually followed by motor quiescence
Phase 3 periodicity	The time interval between the commencement of consecutive activity fronts
Phase 3 propagation velocity	The distance between proximal and distal recording sensors divided by the time interval between the onset of phase 3 at these two sensors
Phase 2 component	A contractile pattern of irregular and intermittent contractions with three or more contractions within 10 min
Phase 1 component	A period of motor quiescence following the phase 3 pattern, which is of variable duration and which is followed by the phase 2 pattern
Postprandial motor pattern	The period from the time of an evident increase in amplitude and/or frequency of contractions after commencement of a meal to the onset of the next phase 3
Discrete clustered contractions	A contractile pattern longer than 5 min with groups of clustered contractions, with or without propagation, and with at least 30 s of quiescence before and after each cluster
Giant migrating contraction	A highly propulsive, prolonged duration (15–20 s) and large amplitude (>30 mmHg) contraction normally confined to the *distal ileum* that clears refluxed cecal contents

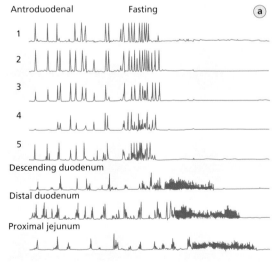
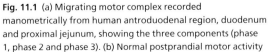
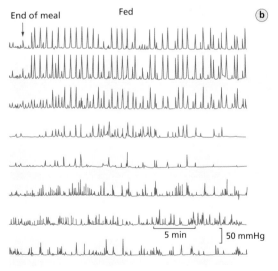

Fig. 11.1 (a) Migrating motor complex recorded manometrically from human antroduodenal region, duodenum and proximal jejunum, showing the three components (phase 1, phase 2 and phase 3). (b) Normal postprandial motor activity in same regions. See text for further details. Reproduced with permission from Malagelada J-R, Camilleri M, Stanghellini V. *Manometric Diagnosis of Gastrointestinal Motility Disorders.* New York: Thieme, 1986: 45.

the caloric content and macronutrient distribution of the meal and the viscosity of the chyme. Thus, a fed pattern duration of about 180 minutes occurs after a mixed meal of 630 kJ, and fat produces a fed pattern of longer duration than carbohydrate or protein. The meal composition also influences the number of isolated pressure waves and short-span pressure wave sequences, but not the number of longer-span sequences. The timing of the meal (for example, breakfast, lunch or dinner) does not appear to affect the contractile response of the intestine to the same nutrient load. Usually, in a person consuming three meals a day, at least one jejunal phase 3 will occur between meals. If snacks are consumed between meals, there may be no MMCs present during the day or even during the entire waking period. The significance of these variations in MMC occurrence during the waking hours, if any, has not been established.

The ileum displays patterns similar to those of the jejunum, but with important differences.[3] The MMC occurs less frequently, and the distinction between fasting and postprandial motor activity is less clear. This may be because remnants of a meal are often retained in the ileum for some hours after return of the MMC in the upper gut. Highly propulsive contractions, termed 'giant migrating contractions' or 'prolonged propagated contractions', are triggered by substances such as short-chain fatty acids, and appear to clear refluxed cecal contents. There is a negative feedback loop that inhibits duodenal and jejunal motility when nutrients are infused into the ileum and colon.[4]

Unlike the phasic contractile activity, the tonic contractile activity of the small bowel remains poorly understood, largely because of technical limitations of recording. It is known, however, that distension of the distal jejunum triggers retrograde reflexes that induce a small and inconstant relaxation (reduction in tone) in the proximal jejunum at a short distance (5 cm), in contrast to a prominent relaxation at a larger distance (40 cm). Also, the distal jejunum does not respond to distension of the proximal jejunum, whereas the proximal jejunum responds similarly to both antegrade and retrograde distension.

Sensitivity of the small bowel
Sensation and sensory processing within the ENS of the human small bowel *in vivo* remain relatively uninves-

tigated. Most studies to date have evaluated the effects of mechanical distension. The conscious perception of such distension has been postulated to be dissociated from the reflex tonic responses described above. In fact, the two processes may be mediated by different mechanisms. It has been shown that perception of two simultaneous small bowel distensions appears to be additive (spatial summation). Sympathetic activation can lead to enhanced perception of proximal duodenal distension without a concomitant increase in the perception of somatic stimuli. Somatic stimuli, for example, TENS (transcutaneous electrical nerve stimulation) can also modify the perception of duodenal distension without interfering with basal gut tone, compliance or reflex responses. The sensitivity of the small bowel appears to be enhanced in the fed state,[5] but further studies are required.

Disordered small bowel motor activity and sensitivity

Important principles and caveats
As is evident from the foregoing discussion, the presence and characteristics of the MMC, and its response to nutrient ingestion, can be used as a marker of the integrity of enteric neuromuscular function. Other measurements, such as small bowel transit assessed scintigraphically, are not helpful in this regard.[6] Indeed, the MMC is the only validated index of small bowel ENS integrated activity that can be monitored *in vivo*. However, because the description of normal small bowel motor patterns continues to evolve, and the available clinico-pathophysiological correlations are limited, the sensitivity and specificity of alterations in small bowel motor patterns are not established. At this time, therefore, a potentially useful clinical role of small bowel manometry is to document seemingly normal small bowel motility in cases where a significant enteric neuromuscular disorder requires exclusion. Moreover, some small bowel disorders which do not primarily affect neuromuscular function, for example Crohn's disease, as well as other systemic disorders, such as chronic renal failure and hepatic cirrhosis, can affect the patterns of small bowel motility. Thus, even prolonged recordings of small bowel motility cannot reliably identify the disease or etiological process responsible for altered motor patterns.

Abnormal motor patterns

Manometric nomenclature is at present largely based on the recognition of specific patterns, such as the characteristic phases of the MMC during fasting and the postprandial pattern. Criteria which can help define the presence of abnormal (proximal) jejunal motor activity, based on prolonged periods of recording, are listed in Tables 11.2 and 11.3. Although computer analysis techniques, including various wave-identification algorithms, artifact rejection techniques and algorithms for the detection of propagated activity, are available, there is no internationally accepted standard. Such analyses, however, produce an improved degree of objectivity in the analysis of pressure tracings and can facilitate the quantitative analysis of relevant parameters for comparison with healthy reference ranges.

Based on our current understanding of manometric recordings of small bowel motor activity in patients with chronic or recurrent symptoms, four main clinico-pathophysiological categories of abnormality can be recognized (Table 11.4):

- type I: patterns consistent with enteric 'neuropathy';
- type II: patterns consistent with enteric 'myopathy';
- type III: patterns consistent with a transient or reversible disorder of small bowel motor function due to mechanical obstruction; and
- type IV: patterns distinct from the above alterations, and tentatively ascribed to 'CNS/ENS dysregulation',

including the acute and chronic influences of central stressors and of mucosal inflammation and altered permeability.

In patients with enteric neuropathy (type I), the motor patterns are typically disorganized and/or uncoordinated (Fig. 11.2).[7] The most compelling abnormality is absence of the MMC, indicating severe enteric dysfunction (assuming a sufficient duration of recording, ideally 24 hours). This finding, however, is rare even in patients with well-documented enteric neuromuscular disease. Retrograde phase 3 MMC propagation can occur rarely, but more common is increased phase 3 frequency or duration. Other alterations include the presence of bursts, sustained uncoordinated phasic activity and postprandial phase 3-like activity, considered to represent evidence of enteric neuropathy because of their frequent occurrence in patients with autonomic neuropathy, and possibly due to loss of inhibitory innervation. These abnormalities may be best detected from recordings during sleep, when normal phase 2 activity is absent. The normal fed pattern may also not be established, despite an adequate nutrient load. It is likely that the presence of several of these abnormalities makes the presence of a neuropathic disorder more likely, but this contention is not evidence-based. In patients with enteric myopathy (type II), in contrast, the normal pattern of contractions is usually preserved, but the amplitude and/or frequency

Table 11.2 Criteria for abnormal jejunal phasic contractile activity

Parameter	Abnormality
Migrating motor complex (MMC)	No MMC per 24 hours of recording
	>3 MMC/3 hours in the awake state
	Phase 3 duration >10 min
	Phase 3 retrograde propagation
	Phasic contraction amplitude <20 mmHg (phase 2 and/or phase 3)
	Phase 2 duration > phase 1 duration (during sleep)
Postprandial motor pattern	Not established after a 400 kcal (or greater) meal
	Duration of postprandial activity <2 hours after a 400 kcal (or greater) meal
Presence of other specific contractile patterns*	Bursts; sustained uncoordinated phasic activity; postprandial phase 3-like activity
	Discrete clustered contractions >30 min
	Non-propagated giant contractions

*See Table 11.3 for descriptions.

Table 11.3 Abnormal specific jejunal contractile patterns

Parameter	Description
Burst	A group of irregular uninterrupted contractions (10 contractions/min or more) >2 min, with 50% or more of contractions >20 mmHg, without propagation
Sustained incoordinated phasic activity	Sustained (>30 min) intense phasic pressure activity occurring in one or more segments of intestine while normal or decreased activity is recorded simultaneously elsewhere
Postprandial phase 3-like activity	Regular phasic contractions at the slow-wave frequency lasting >1 min, occurring 5 min or later after the intake of a meal, and if lasting >2 min then not propagating through a number of channels or not obviously terminating the postprandial pattern
Non-propagated giant contractions	Simultaneous phasic contractions of prolonged duration (>20 s) and large amplitude (> 30 mmHg)

of contractions is reduced in the affected segment (Fig. 11.3).[7] In patients with mechanical obstruction (type III), multiple simultaneous giant contractions have been reported,[8] as well as an increase in discrete clustered contractions.[9] In patients with CNS/ENS dysregulation (type IV), typified by the functional gastrointestinal disorders such as irritable bowel syndrome and functional dyspepsia, a variety of more subtle alterations have been described.[10] These include an increase in the prevalence and duration of discrete clustered contractions, subtle alterations in MMC periodicity and phase 3 amplitude, and alterations in postprandial pattern duration. The relevance of these alterations to the pathophysiology of these syndromes, however, remains to be established. In particular, whether some patients with these manometric alterations represent a less severe form of, or an earlier stage of, the histological lesions associated with type I and II dysmotility is not known, although some evidence to support this contention is available.[11]

Table 11.4 Clinico-pathophysiological classification of jejunal contractile abnormalities

Type	Putative pathophysiology	Manometric abnormalities	Main clinical presentation
I	Enteric neuropathy	Absent MMC (over a 24-hour period) Abnormal duration/propagation of phase 3 component Bursts, sustained incoordinated phasic activity, postprandial phase 3-like activity (esp. during sleep) Lack of establishment of postprandial pattern	Chronic intestinal pseudo-obstruction
II	Enteric myopathy	Low contractile amplitude (phase 2 and/or phase 3 component, postprandial pattern)	Chronic intestinal pseudo-obstruction
III	Mechanical obstruction	Multiple non-propagated giant contractions	Recurrent small bowel obstruction: extrinsic intrinsic
IV	CNS – ENS dysregulation	Altered MMC periodicity, especially diurnally Altered phase 3 amplitude Increased proportion of discrete clustered contractions Altered postprandial pattern duration	Functional gastrointestinal disorder, e.g. functional dyspepsia, irritable bowel syndrome

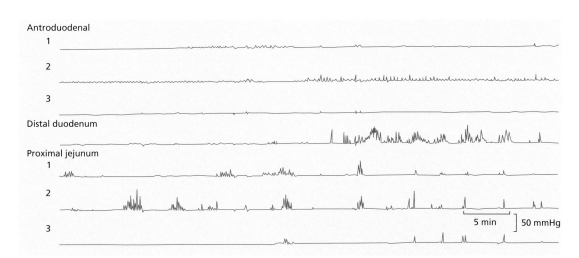

Fig. 11.2 Manometric tracing during fasting from a patient with enteric neuropathy. Note the bursts of contractile activity at several levels of the intestine, with associated tonic change in the duodenum. Reproduced with permission from Malagelada J-R, Camilleri M, Stanghellini V. *Manometric Diagnosis of Gastrointestinal Motility Disorders*. New York: Thieme, 1986: 45.

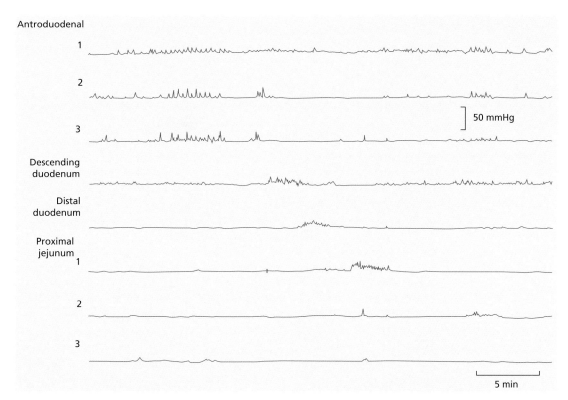

Fig. 11.3 Manometric tracing during fasting from a patient with enteric myopathy. Note the low amplitude but normal propagation of the migrating motor complex and the paucity of other contractile activity in the duodenum and proximal jejunum. Reproduced with permission from Malagelada J-R, Camilleri M, Stanghellini V. *Manometric Diagnosis of Gastrointestinal Motility Disorders*. New York: Thieme, 1986: 45.

Alterations in sensitivity and mucosal permeability

Dysfunction of sensory afferent mechanisms, manifest most commonly as visceral hypersensitivity to mechanical distension, can also be documented in the small bowel.[12] This finding is a feature of patients with irritable bowel syndrome and functional dyspepsia and has been documented using balloon distension or in response to passage of the lumen-occluding contractions of phase 3 of the MMC through the proximal small bowel. It appears that such small bowel hypersensitivity is related to a selective alteration of mechanosensitive pathways. The level of the afferent dysfunction within the brain–gut axis has not been established. However, the abnormal or distorted referral patterns of gut sensation present in these disorders, which are part of the spectrum of visceral hypersensitivity, are believed to reflect secondary sensitization of spinal cord neurons. The complex interactions which arise from different stimuli in different regions of the gut also appear to modify jejunal sensitivity in irritable bowel syndrome to a greater extent than in health.[5] It should be appreciated that studies of visceral hypersensitivity in patients with enteric neuropathy or myopathy have received little attention, so the specificity of visceral hypersensitivity as a marker for functional gastrointestinal disease remains poorly defined. Certainly, for the small bowel, sensitivity testing has not yet entered the clinical area. The intimate relationships between small bowel motor dysfunction and alterations in small bowel sensitivity also require more extensive study.

Both non-immunological and immunological defence mechanisms constitute the small intestinal mucosal barrier to various macromolecules and microorganisms. The recent demonstration of altered small bowel mucosal permeability in some patients with irritable bowel syndrome[13] has refocused attention on the roles of enteric infection and inflammation, food hypersensitivity and intolerance, and chronic stress in provoking alterations in intestinal sensitivity and motility. In animal models, antigenic challenge of sensitized jejunal segments provokes IgE-mediated mucosal and connective tissue mast cell degranulation, serotonin release, prostaglandin synthesis, and direct contractile effects on enteric smooth muscle. Based largely on such studies, it is likely that in acute infective processes affecting the small intestine, multiple giant migrating contractions occur in the jejunum. Further studies in humans are required. There is currently much interest in the neuro-immune regulation of anaphylaxis-induced alterations in enteric motility and secretion, the role of the gut flora, and the contribution of mental stress.[14–16]

Consequences of disturbed small bowel sensorimotor function

The consequences of alterations in normal small bowel sensorimotor function depend not only on the type of abnormality outlined above, but also on whether the alterations are constant (stable or progressive) or intermittent (paroxysmal). The two main consequences are the generation of symptoms and the development of bacterial overgrowth in the small bowel.

Symptoms

The range of symptoms which can emanate from the small bowel is relatively narrow and the symptoms themselves are generally of low specificity (Table 11.5). Moreover, several criteria should in theory be satisfied to define a causal relationship between a symptom and small bowel sensorimotor dysfunction. These are:

- a constant association between the symptom and the motor disorder;
- correlation in time and severity between the symptom and the motor disorder; and
- an improvement in the symptom associated with improvement in the motor disorder.

These criteria are not fulfilled reliably in the case of disorders producing small bowel dysmotility, although for the more severe neuromuscular disorders considered below the first two criteria are often satisfied. Putative mechanisms for the production of symptoms (Table 11.5) include uncoordinated contractile activity, which may lead to pain either directly or indirectly, by affecting the transit of gas or fluid content with subsequent focal gut distension. Rapid transit, with an increase in the volume and rate of ileo-cecal flow, may also produce diarrhea by overwhelming the absorptive capacity of the large bowel. Malabsorption of specific dietary or endogenous compounds, such as fat, carbohydrate and bile acids, can also provoke the secretion or impair the absorption of water and electrolytes. It is probable that normal degrees of local gut distension can, in the presence of visceral hypersensitivity, lead to a range of sensations of variable intensity and

Table 11.5 Gastrointestinal symptoms originating from disturbances in small bowel sensorimotor function

Symptom	Putative mechanism(s)
Pain/discomfort	Visceral hypersensitivity, uncoordinated contractions and/or giant migrating contractions, alterations in intestinal tone
Diarrhea and steatorrhea	Enhanced ileo-cecal volume/flow rates, malabsorption of specific dietary components, small bowel bacterial overgrowth
Abdominal bloating	Impaired gas transit, incomplete small bowel absorption (carbohydrates and sugars), visceral hypersensitivity, delayed ileo-cecal transit of chyme
Abdominal distension	Gas-trapping and/or excessive volumes of intestinal gas with focal gut distension
Nausea/vomiting	Retrograde giant contractions, visceral hypersensitivity

character, such as abdominal discomfort, nausea and abdominal bloating.

Small bowel bacterial overgrowth

Colonization of the small bowel with excess numbers of bacteria, termed 'small bowel bacterial overgrowth' (SBBO), is an almost invariable consequence of small bowel dysmotility that is of sufficient magnitude to affect enteric clearance, such as described earlier in patients with types I and II dysmotility. For example, in patients with small bowel dysmotility due to severe late radiation enteropathy there is a close correlation between impaired MMC activity and colonization with Gram-negative bacteria.[17] In this study, a semiquantitative index of disordered MMC activity, and the presence of bursts, displayed high (>90%) sensitivity and specificity for the detection of significant gram-negative colonization in the proximal small bowel. Other specific conditions associated with small bowel dysmotility and SBBO include diabetic autonomic neuropathy and other causes of extrinsic neural dysfunction, and the syndrome of chronic intestinal pseudo-obstruction considered below. Recently, the presence of SBBO in patients with irritable bowel syndrome has been suggested to be of clinical importance,[18] but further studies are required before investigation and treatment for SBBO in this patient population can be advocated. There is also recent evidence that recurrent spontaneous bacterial peritonitis in patients with hepatic cirrhosis and portal hypertension may be associated with impaired small bowel motility and SBBO.[19] The mechanisms for such dysmotility have not been identified but appear to depend on the severity of the liver disease. In the case of primary biliary cirrhosis, a myogenic component has been suggested. In rodent studies, SBBO has also been demonstrated in acute necrotizing pancreatitis, and in pharmacologically induced delayed small bowel transit.[20,21] Thus, in addition to considering SBBO in conditions which affect the anatomical structure of the small bowel, such as postsurgical syndromes, it is important to consider SBBO in patients with significant small bowel dysmotility of any cause and in whom no structural abnormality is present.

Details of the sequelae of SBBO are beyond the scope of this chapter, but include malabsorption of a variety of micronutrients, such as iron, folate, calcium, vitamin K and vitamin B12, with their attendant clinical features, as well as a number of other symptoms.[22] These include weight loss, chronic diarrhea and steatorrhea, symptoms which can be similar to those of the primary condition. Although the diagnosis of SBBO can be established by a variety of techniques, direct endoscopic aspiration and culture from the upper small bowel is regarded as the gold standard, even though this procedure itself has technical limitations. For the bacterial overgrowth to be regarded as clinically significant, a total concentration of bacteria of more than 10^5 organisms per milliliter is generally taken as the cutoff level. The species likely to be present include bacteroides, anaerobic lactobacilli, coliforms and enterococci. The lactulose hydrogen breath test and the bile acid breath test have relatively high false-negative rates, and results of these investigations need to be interpreted with caution in routine clinical use. The ^{14}C-xylose breath test (with or without a transit marker) appears to have greater sensitivity and specificity, and is the test most widely recommended in children and women of child-bearing age. It may be less useful, however, in SBBO associated with small bowel motility disorders.[23]

Treatment options for SBBO include the use of empirical courses of broad-spectrum antibiotics and/or the use of prokinetic agents in some circumstances. Antimicrobial agents which are regarded as having some efficacy include tetracycline (250 mg q.i.d.), doxycycline (100 mg b.d.), minocycline (100 mg b.d.), amoxycillin–clavulanic acid (850 mg b.d.), cipro-floxacin (500 mg b.d.) and norfloxacin (400 mg b.d.).[22] Some patients respond to a single course of therapy over several weeks, others require cyclical therapy (e.g. one week every month) or even more prolonged courses. The use of prokinetic agents requires further evaluation. One study has shown that treatment with cisapride or antibiotics in patients with liver cirrhosis reversed the documented small bowel dysmotility and SBBO. Probiotic supplements are of theoretical interest, but the limited data available to date do not suggest they have an important role in their currently available forms.

Specific disorders with well-characterized small bowel sensorimotor dysfunction

As discussed earlier, chronic or recurrent small bowel sensorimotor dysfunction occurs as a result of enteric neuropathy, enteric myopathy, local mechanical obstruction or local neuroimmune reactions to luminal antigens, or on the basis of other systemic diseases associated with extrinsic neural denervation or with neurohormonal influences, such as carcinoid syndrome. Extrinsic neural dysfunction can arise from conditions such as diabetes mellitus, spinal cord injury and multiple sclerosis. A number of alterations in small bowel motility have been documented in these disorders, with respect to both the MMC and the postprandial pattern, but these conditions will not be discussed further. Likewise, acute small bowel dysmotility, synonymous with intestinal ileus, is usually secondary to acute self-limited intra-abdominal conditions, such as the immediate postoperative state, acute pancreatitis, or other systemic disease, and will not be discussed further (see review by Delgado-Aros and Camilleri).[24]

Some of the main causes of chronic enteric neuropathy and myopathy affecting the small intestine are shown in Table 11.6. In many of these disorders other regions of the gastrointestinal tract can also be affected, and some evidence suggests that in the neuropathic group more widespread autonomic dysfunction, mostly postganglionic in nature, can occur. All of these disorders can present with the syndrome of chronic intestinal pseudo-obstruction (CIP).

Chronic intestinal pseudo-obstruction

This term refers to a diverse group of disorders characterized by profoundly disturbed intestinal motor function, usually presenting with recurrent or chronic (over months or years) symptoms and signs of intestinal obstruction in the absence of a documented mechanical cause.[25] Obstructive episodes can occur in a highly variable fashion, and between episodes patients may be asymptomatic or suffer milder episodes of abdominal pain, distension and diarrhea. In order for the diagnosis to be considered, it is important to document ileus or gaseous distension, and air-fluid levels, in the small bowel during an attack by plain abdominal X-rays. Mechanical obstruction must be carefully excluded, and barium contrast studies of the entire gastrointestinal tract remain important in defining the distribution and presence of gut dilatation. In patients with myopathy, megaduodenum may occur and the small intestine may appear featureless with a striking lack of haustral markings. In patients with neuropathy, no abnormal dilatation may be evident, but a suggestion of disordered motility may be appreciated on fluoroscopic screening. Scintigraphy using ^{99m}Tc or ^{131}indium-labeled solids in some cases can detect delayed transit through the stomach and small bowel. A new technique using ^{99m}Tc-HIDA, an intravenous tracer excreted in the bile, enables small bowel transit to be determined without the confounding influence of gastric emptying.[26] Small intestinal manometry may reveal disordered contractile patterns, as discussed earlier, and the presumptive diagnosis of a predominantly neuropathic (type I), myopathic (type II) or mixed disorder. If the patient undergoes an operation, or it is undertaken as a primary laparoscopic intervention, a full-thickness biopsy should be obtained and specialized histochemical staining techniques employed to delineate the enteric nerves and ganglia, the intersti-

	Enteric neuropathies	Enteric myopathies
Table 11.6 Disorders associated with chronic enteric neuropathy or myopathy	Familial or sporadic visceral neuropathy	Familial or sporadic visceral myopathy

	Drug-induced, e.g. tricyclic antidepressants, anticholinergics, opiates, vinca alkaloids	Connective tissue disease
		    Scleroderma
		    Mixed connective tissue disease
		    Dermatomyositis
		    Systemic lupus erythematosus

	Infectious/inflammatory
	    Parasitic, e.g. Chagas' disease
	    Viral, e.g. cytomegalovirus, varicella
	    Radiation enteritis
		Primary muscle disease
		    Muscular dystrophies
		    Myotonic dystrophy
		Infiltrative disease, e.g. amyloidosis

	Paraneoplastic	Endocrine diseases
		    Thyroid disease
		    Parathyroid disease

	Systemic neurological disease
	    Parkinson's disease
	    Familial autonomic dysfunction	

tial cells of Cajal (the gut pacemaker cells), and the smooth muscle layers. The role of biopsy is likely to become even more important as newer immunohistochemical techniques for various neural and muscle markers, such as alpha smooth muscle actin, become available in clinical practice. The genetic defects in cell signaling systems, namely the tyrosine kinase receptor RET, its ligand–glial cell line-derived neurotropic factor (GDNF), the endothelin receptor B and its ligand endothelin 3, which have been implicated in the pathogenesis of the aganglionosis of Hirschsprung's disease, have to date not been identified as abnormal in cases of CIP. Characterization of a genetic mutation in a patient with a mitochondrial DNA-related disease with prominent intestinal pseudo-obstruction has, however, been reported.[27] Alteration in the expression of neuronal nitric oxide synthase, associated with disturbed local production of the inhibitory neurotransmitter nitric oxide, has been suggested as a possible contributor to the pathogenesis of the motor dysfunction in CIP.[28]

Primary CIP

In primary CIP (chronic idiopathic intestinal pseudo-obstruction), there is no detectable underlying systemic disease. In this group, disorders of the myenteric plexus are more frequent than that of the smooth muscle, and include the familial visceral neuropathies and myopathies. Screening blood tests, where available, are required to exclude the disorders listed in Table 11.6. Anti-neuronal nuclear antibodies can be documented in some cases. Whether these can be used to diagnose inflammatory enteric neuropathy at an earlier stage remains to be determined. The small bowel is the major site of involvement, but is usually accompanied by colonic involvement – the term 'chronic idiopathic colonic pseudo-obstruction' is used to refer to patients who have isolated colonic pseudo-obstruction. Extra-intestinal manifestations such as urinary dilatation (e.g. megacystis) and other neurological symptoms can be present.[29] In visceral neuropathy, a variety of myenteric plexus abnormalities can be detected, consisting of degeneration and drop-out of neurons with or without inflammation, and neuronal intranuclear inclusions. A number of specific forms have been characterized.[30] Markedly reduced levels of the interstitial cells of Cajal have been documented in some patients.[31] In visceral myopathy there is vacuolar degeneration and fibrosis of one or both layers of the smooth muscle, although the longitudinal muscle is usually more involved than the circular and the involvement may be patchy.

Secondary CIP

Scleroderma is the most common cause of this entity, and varying degrees of pseudo-obstruction occur in up to 40% of patients with this condition, occasionally as an initial presentation.[32] On contrast radiology, there may be a megaduodenum or more widespread intestinal dilatation. Unlike visceral myopathy, the small bowel may show valvular packing and wide-mouthed diverticula or sacculations. At intestinal biopsy, the circular muscle is usually more affected than the longitudinal, and the involvement can be abruptly delineated and focal, and without vacuolar degeneration. It has been suggested that, in patients with mild or early disease, impaired neurotransmitter release may be present prior to the smooth muscle involvement. This hypothesis requires further study, particularly with respect to the small bowel, but small bowel manometric studies have revealed both neuropathic and myopathic forms of dysmotility.[33] A recent study evaluated the active–passive mechanical and sensory properties of the duodenum in scleroderma patients,[34] and provides the most direct evidence to date that visceral hypersensitivity, perhaps due to resetting of the duodenal mechanoreceptors, may contribute to the symptoms experienced by scleroderma patients, and therefore represents a potential therapeutic target.

Treatment options

Therapies for CIP remain limited, and include symptomatic treatment, especially analgesia, nutritional support and treatment of complications. Nutritional strategies include low-fiber, low-lactose or elemental diets with vitamin supplementation. Gastrostomy or jejunostomy feeding may be necessary to maintain weight, and can be given as supplementary nocturnal feeding. Total parenteral nutrition, either intermittently or long-term, may be required if parenteral feeding is not successful.

Drug therapy with prokinetic agents is usually not helpful,[35] especially in visceral myopathy. Tachyphylaxis occurs with metoclopramide and erythromycin, and indeed one study has reported an inhibitory effect of erythromycin on small bowel motility in healthy subjects, especially in the postprandial state.[36] The use of tegaserod in CIP has not been reported. There are case reports of acute exacerbations of CIP responding to intravenous neostigmine. Octreotide induces phase 3 activity fronts in the small intestine, and has been shown to reduce SBBO and to improve symptoms in patients with scleroderma. It may exacerbate gas-

troparesis, however, and may be best administered at night.[37] Treatment of complications includes antibiotic treatment for SBBO and for urinary tract infections. Surgery has a limited role in CIP, in either facilitating enteral nutrition by means of jejunostomy, or improving abdominal distension by venting gastrostomy or enterostomy or by resection of localized disease. A single case report has suggested that hyperbaric oxygenation therapy is effective in the management of myopathic CIP.[38] Small bowel transplantation, alone or with other viscera, is a last resort for patients with intestinal or liver failure, especially children, who have failed all treatment options.[39]

References

1   Vantrappen G, Janssens J, Hellemans J. The interdigestive motor complex of normal subjects and patients with bacterial overgrowth of the small intestine. *J Clin Invest* 1977; **59**: 1158–66.

2   Husebye E, Hellstrom PM, Midvedt T. The intestinal microflora stimulates myoelectric activity of rat small intestine by promoting cyclic initiation and aboral propagation of the migrating myoelectric complex. *Dig Dis Sci* 1994; **39**: 946–56.

3   Kellow JE, Borody TJ, Phillips SF, Tucker RL, Haddad AC. Human interdigestive motility: variations in patterns from oesophagus to colon. *Gastroenterology* 1986; **91**: 386–95.

4   Spiller RC, Trotman IF, Higgins BE. The ileal brake – inhibition of jejunal motility after ileal fat perfusion in man. *Gut* 1984; **25**: 365–74.

5   Evans PR, Kellow JE. Physiological modulation of jejunal sensitivity in health and in the irritable bowel syndrome. *Am J Gastroenterol* 1998; **93**: 2191–6.

6   Argenyi EE, Soffer EE, Madsen MT, Berbaum KS, Walkner WO. Scintigraphic evaluation of small bowel transit in healthy subjects: inter- and intrasubject variability. *Am J Gastroenterol* 1995; **90**: 938–42.

7   Stanghellini V, Camilleri M, Malagelada JR. Chronic idiopathic intestinal pseudo-obstruction: clinical and intestinal manometric findings. *Gut* 1987; **28**: 5–12.

8   Frank JW, Sarr MG, Camilleri M. Use of gastroduodenal manometry to differentiate mechanical and functional intestinal obstruction: an analysis of clinical outcome. *Am J Gastroenterol* 1994; **89**: 339–44.

9   Summers RW, Anuras S, Green J. Jejunal manometry patterns in health, partial intestinal obstruction, and pseudo-obstruction. *Gastroenterology* 1983; **85**: 1290–300.

10 Kellow JE, Phillips SF. Altered small bowel motility in ir-

ritable bowel syndrome is correlated with symptoms. *Gastroenterology* 1987; **92**: 1885–93.

11 Tornblom H, Lindberg G, Nyberg B, Veress B. Full thickness biopsy of the jejunum reveals inflammation and enteric neuropathy in irritable bowel syndrome. *Gastroenterology* 2002; **123**: 1972–9.

12 Evans PR, Bennett EJ, Bak Y-T, Tennant CC, Kellow JE. Jejunal sensorimotor dysfunction in irritable bowel syndrome – clinical and psychosocial features. *Gastroenterology* 1996; **100**: 393–404.

13 Spiller R, Jenkins D, Thornley JP. Increased rectal mucosal enteroendocrine cells, T lymphocytes, and increased gut permeability after acute *Campylobacter* enteritis and post-dysenteric irritable bowel syndrome. *Gut* 2000; **47**: 804–11.

14 Scott RB. Hypersensitivity and food intolerance. In: Phillips SF, Wingate DL, eds. *Functional Disorders of the Gut*. London: Churchill Livingstone, 1998; 121–49.

15 Hart AL, Stagg AJ, Frame M *et al*. The role of the gut flora in health and disease, and its modification as therapy. *Aliment Pharmacol Ther* 2002; **16**: 1383–93.

16 Hart A, Kamm MA. Mechanisms of initiation and perpetuation of gut inflammation by stress. *Aliment Pharmacol Ther* 2002; **16**: 2017–28.

17 Husebye E, Skar V, Hoverstad T, Iversen T, Melby K. Abnormal intestinal motor patterns explain enteric colonization with Gram negative bacilli in late radiation enteropathy. *Gastroenterology* 1995; **109**: 1078–89.

18 Pimentel M, Chow EJ, Lin HC. Normalization of lactulose breath testing correlates with symptom improvement in irritable bowel syndrome: a double-blind, randomized, placebo-controlled study. *Am J Gastroenterol* 2003; **98**: 412–19.

19 Chang CS, Chen GH, Lieu HC, Yen HZ. Small intestinal dysmotility and bacterial overgrowth in cirrhotic patients with spontaneous bacterial peritonitis. *Hepatology* 1998; **28**: 1187–90.

20 Van Felius ID, Akkermans LM, Bosscha K *et al*. Interdigestive small bowel motility and duodenal bacterial overgrowth in experimental acute pancreatitis. *Neurogastroenterol Motil* 2003; **15**: 267–76.

21 Nieuwenhuijs VB, Verheem A, van Duijvenbode-Beumer H *et al*. The role of interdigestive small bowel motility in the regulation of gut microflora, bacterial overgrowth, and bacterial translocation in rats. *Ann Surg* 1998; **228**: 188–93.

22 Toskes PP. Small intestine bacterial overgrowth, including blind loop syndrome. In: Blaser MJ, Smith PD, Ravdin JI, Greenberg HB, Guerrant RL, eds. *Infections of the Gastrointestinal Tract*, 2nd edn. Philadelphia: Lippincott, Williams & Wilkins, 2002: 291–300.

23 Valdovinos MA, Camilleri M, Thomforde GM, Frie C. Reduced accuracy of 14C-D-xylose breath test for detection of

bacterial overgrowth in gastrointestinal motility disorders. *Scand J Gastroenterol* 1993; **28**: 963–8.

24 Delgado-Aros S, Camilleri M. Pseudo-obstruction in the critically ill. *Best Pract Res Clin Gastroenterol* 2003; **17**: 427–44.

25 Mann SD, Debinski HS, Kamm MA. Clinical characteristics of chronic idiopathic intestinal pseudo-obstruction in adults. *Gut* 1997; **41**: 675–81.

26 Gryback P, Jacobsson H, Blonquist L. Scintigraphy of the small intestine: a simplified standard for study of transit with reference to normal values. *Eur J Nucl Med Mod Imaging* 2002; **29**: 39.

27 Garcia-Velasco A, Gomez-Escalonilla C, Guerra-Vales JM, Cabello A, Campos Y, Arenas J. Intestinal pseudo-obstruction and urinary retention: cardinal features of a mitochondrial DNA-related disease. *J Intern Med* 2003; **253**: 381–5.

28 Takahashi T. Pathophysiological significance of neuronal nitric oxide synthase in the gastrointestinal tract. *J Gastroenterol* 2003; **38**: 421–30.

29 Camilleri M, Malagelada JR, Stanghellini V, Fealey RD, Sheps SG. Gastrointestinal motility disturbances in patients with orthostatic hypotension. *Gastroenterology* 1985; **88**: 1852–9.

30 Camilleri M, Carbone LD, Schuffler MD. Familiar enteric neuropathy with pseudo-obstruction. *Dig Dis Sci* 1991; **36**: 1168–71.

31 Streutker CJ, Huizinga JD, Campbell F, Ho J, Riddell RH. Loss of CD117(c-kit)- and CD34-positive ICC and associated CD34-positive fibroblasts defines a subpopulation of chronic intestinal pseudo-obstruction. *Am J Surg Pathol* 2003; **27**: 228–35.

32 Sjogren RW. Gastrointestinal motility disorders in scleroderma. *Arthritis Rheum* 1994; **37**: 1265–82.

33 Greydanus MP, Camilleri M. Abnormal postcibal antral and small bowel motility due to neuropathy or myopathy in systemic sclerosis. *Gastroenterology* 1989; **96**: 110–15.

34 Pedersen J, Chunwen GAO, Egekvist H *et al*. Pain and biomechanical responses to distention of the duodenum in patients with systemic sclerosis. *Gastroenterology* 2003; **124**: 1230–39.

35 Hyman PE, Di Lorenzo C, McAdams L, Flores AF, Tomomasa T, Garvey TQ. Predicting the clinical response to cisapride in children with chronic intestinal pseudo-obstruction. *Am J Gastroenterol* 1993; **88**: 832–6.

36 Medhus AW, Bondi J, Gaustad P, Husebye E. Low-dose intravenous erythromycin: effects on postprandial and fasting motility of the small bowel. *Aliment Pharmacol Ther* 2000; **14**: 233–40.

37 Verne GN, Eaker EY, Hardy E, Sninsky CA. Effect of octreotide and erythromycin on idiopathic and scleroderma-associated intestinal pseudoobstruction. *Dig Dis Sci* 1995; **40**:

1892–901.

38 Yokota T, Suda T, Tsukioka S, Takalashi T. The striking effect of hyperbaric oxygenation therapy in the management of chronic idiopathic intestinal pseudo-obstruction. *Am J*

Gastroenterol 2000; **95**; 285–8.

39 Iyer K, Kaufman S, Sudan D. Long term results of intestinal transplantation for pseudo-obstruction in children. *J Paediatr Surg* 2001; **36**: 174–7.

CHAPTER 12

Colonic Disorders

Charles Murray and Anton Emmanuel

Constipation

Clinical manifestations

Constipation is one of the most common gastroenterological complaints encountered in both secondary and tertiary care, affecting between 2[1] and 27%[2] of the population in Western studies. As a condition it should be considered as a symptom that has multifactorial causes, with a great number of pathophysiological mechanisms involved.

Regardless of the etiology, constipation represents a common symptom in the general population and accounts for approximately £48 million pounds per year spent in the UK on over-the-counter and prescription laxative medication. Most mild cases will respond to dietary manipulation and an increase in dietary fiber, but in those with intractable symptoms treatment remains difficult and may rely on chronic laxative use. Increasingly, behavioural therapy – biofeedback – is being employed in an attempt to avoid this scenario.

For the purpose of this chapter we can broadly classify constipation into three pathophysiological groups: normal transit constipation, slow-transit constipation and evacuatory dysfunction. The last of these encompasses a variety of terms in the literature, including 'pelvic floor dyssynergia', 'anismus' and 'paradoxical pelvic floor contraction'. These will be covered in detail in Chapter 13. An alternative classification is not by physiological abnormality but by potential enteropathic nerve differences. Alternatively, clinical criteria may be used. For the purposes of consensus, the Rome II criteria were formulated for the diagnosis of constipation, and these are listed in Table 12.1.

Normal transit constipation

Normal transit constipation refers to those symptomatic patients in whom colonic transit is normal and there is no evacuatory abnormality to explain their symptoms. It should be noted, however, that there is inevitably some overlap between groups. The condition is sometimes termed 'functional' constipation, and this group of patients have normal or reduced stool frequency and are symptomatic in the presence of objective measurement of normal whole-gut transit. This group may exhibit greater levels of psychosocial distress, occasionally associated with physical or sexual abuse in childhood,[3] which confers a poor prognosis. In physiological terms, investigators argue that the difference between this group and those with constipation-predominant irritable bowel syndrome is that the latter exhibit rectal hypersensitivity.[4] Within this group of patients there is no evidence of an objective bowel pathology, and indeed normal physiological testing (whole-gut transit, barostat studies) supports this.

Table 12.1 Rome II criteria for constipation

Adults

Two or more of the following for at least 12 weeks in the preceding 12 months:

- Straining during >25% of bowel movements
- Lumpy or hard stools for >25% of bowel movements
- Sensation of incomplete evacuation for >25% of bowel movements
- Sensation of anorectal blockage for >25% of bowel movements
- Manual maneuvers to facilitate >25% of bowel movements
- <3 bowel movements per week
- Loose stools not present, and insufficient criteria for irritable bowel syndrome met

Constipation

1 Constipation can be classified as either slow-transit constipation (STC) or rectal evacuatory dysfunction or both.

2 STC is defined by symptoms of constipation with demonstrable slow whole-gut transit.

3 STC represents a heterogeneous group of primarily motor abnormalities.

4 Hypoganglionosis in the enteric nervous system has been demonstrated in some patients with STC.

5 Multiple abnormalities have been demonstrated at a neuroendocrine level in patients with STC and may explain the mixed response to drug therapies.

6 The density of interstitial cells of Cajal is decreased in the colon in some patients with STC.

Slow-transit constipation

Slow-transit constipation (STC) is defined by symptoms of constipation with demonstrable slow whole-gut transit. Consisting predominantly of women, and commonly with onset in childhood, these patients respond poorly to conventional advice to increase fiber and are represented disproportionately in referrals for constipation to secondary and tertiary care. Colonic transit studies, whether scintigraphic or by radio-opaque markers, demonstrate slow transit (Fig. 12.1),

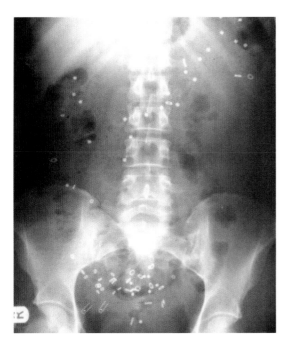

Fig. 12.1 Whole-gut transit study. Three sets of markers are ingested over 3 days and an abdominal film is taken 120 hours after the first markers are ingested.

but invariably no cause for the symptom can be found on further clinical investigation. Idiopathic cases of STC commonly occur in childhood, whereas the onset of STC is also well documented after pelvic surgery and childbirth[5] and has historically been ascribed to damage of the pelvic parasympathetic nerves, although objective evidence of this is lacking.

Physiological disturbances
Motility

A number of motility and sensory physiological disturbances have been demonstrated in patients with STC. This condition has been the focus of much study because it represents a relatively homogeneous patient population with a discrete abnormality. As stated, patients with STC have demonstrable slow colonic transit, but other more specific abnormalities have been shown. A group of STC patients, said to have 'colonic inertia', demonstrate no increase in motor activity after meals or after the intrarectal administration of bisacodyl.[6] Similarly, other patients have demonstrated no response to cholinergic drugs or anticholinesterases such as neostigmine.[7] However, these findings are not consistently seen in all patients with STC. Discrepant findings have been observed when rectosigmoid contractility has been investigated in patients with STC. For example, in contrast to the previously discussed studies, the response to intrarectal bisacodyl has been shown to be both reduced and normal in STC patients,[8,9] and while there is a reduced response to cholinergic stimulation in some studies, it has been normal in others.

In vitro studies using tissue baths have again produced contradictory findings. One study investigating the inhibition by cisapride of the colonic smooth muscle responses induced by carbachol showed that colonic smooth muscle from patients with STC is hypersensitive to cholinergic stimulation.[10] The clinical correlate of this would be increased contractility in response to cholinergic stimulation, which has been shown in some[11] but by no means all studies.[12] What is clear is that these motility effects observed physiologically do not often translate into clinically significant changes.

Some patients appear to have a panenteric abnormality in gut motility, which has been demonstrated throughout the gastrointestinal tract.[13] For this reason it has been suggested that, though representing a heterogeneous group, STC patients should be divided into two groups based on the presence or absence of a panenteric motility disturbance. The argument for this would be that STC patients represent a different pathophysiological group who may have a worse outcome following colonic resection surgery for constipation.[14]

In summary, STC subjects all share the objective abnormality of slow colonic transit, but appear otherwise to represent a heterogeneous group of motor abnormalities.

Sensory abnormalities

The most common reported sensory abnormality in constipation is rectal hyposensitivity, which affects up to 27% of patients with constipation.[15] There is some argument as to whether this is a primary phenomenon or secondary to chronic dysmotility, since it is not found in all patients. However, in a group of patients with idiopathic STC a small-fiber sensory neuropathy has been demonstrated.[16] This study suggested that there is a subgroup of STC patients in whom a more global physiological abnormality is responsible for the development of constipation. Whether this generalized sensory neuropathy is associated with an adverse response to surgery or other therapy remains unknown.

Etiopathogenic theories

The range of abnormalities found in clinical investigations and their often contradictory results suggest there is no one unifying pathophysiological abnormality to explain constipation, and it is therefore no surprise that at an enteric level a variety of abnormalities have been found in patients with STC.

Enteric nervous system abnormalities

Immunohistochemical studies of resected material have suggested that a variety of abnormalities may be present in the enteric nervous system (ENS) in patients with STC, including hypoganglionosis[17] (Fig. 12.2) and a decrease in neuronal structures within the colonic circular muscle.[18] Light microscopy usually fails to reveal any abnormalities in these tissues. Hematoxylin and eosin staining does not identify consistent abnormalities, although some abnormalities, including myenteric plexus degeneration, have been described. On silver staining it is possible to demonstrate a decrease in argyrophilic neurons and intraganglionic filaments,[19] sometimes associated with Schwann cell hyperplasia. Other researchers have failed to show any neuronal reduction in STC. In a study using a control group, no evidence was found of a generalized neuronal reduction when using neuron-specific enolase.[20]

Neuroendocrine system

There is little consistency in the abnormalities detected in these patients at a neuroendocrine level. Studies have shown variously that serotonin cell density may be either increased[21] or decreased.[22] Similarly, expression of peptide YY (Fig. 12.3), substance P and vasoactive intestinal polypeptide in the neurons of the ENS shows marked inconsistency between studies. It has also been reported that there is a more dense innervation of nitric oxide-containing neurons in STC, implying increased inhibitory tone. These contradictory results are perhaps not surprising, given the heterogeneity of the motor and sensory abnormalities described above. This clearly has implications, given the use of serotonergic agonists in the treatment of constipation. The degree of difference in serotonergic expression may in part explain the mixed results seen in clinical trials of these drugs.

Autonomic sensory neuropathy

The presence of a generalized small-fiber autonomic sensory neuropathy has been described in a group of patients with STC who have evidence of both gut and systemic abnormalities.[16] This would suggest a permanent abnormality in these patients. However, behavioral therapy (biofeedback) has been demonstrated to improve both transit and gut-specific autonomic tone in some patients with STC,[23] suggesting

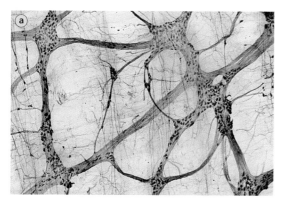 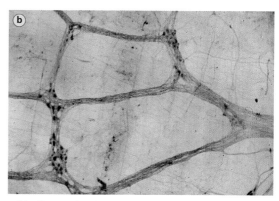

Fig. 12.2 Architecture of the enteric nervous system (myenteric plexus). (a) Normal colon. The nerve network is composed of ganglia and interconnecting nerve fiber strands. Smaller branches ramify from primary and secondary nerve fiber strands and extend into the adjacent muscle layers. Although most neurons are located within the ganglia, some nerve cell bodies are also observed within the nerve fiber strands. (b) Slow-transit constipation. Compared with controls, the meshes of the nerve network are widened and the ganglia are reduced in size, containing a decreased amount of nerve cells. Reprinted with kind permission of Dr Thilo Wedel and Elsevier Publishing (*Gastroenterology* 2002; **123**: 1462).

that a permanent neuropathy cannot be responsible for all cases of idiopathic STC. Similarly, biofeedback has also been shown to improve symptoms and transit in patients with STC following hysterectomy, a condition assumed to be secondary to irreversible pelvic nerve damage.[24]

Decrease in interstitial cells of Cajal

Using c-kit immunoreactivity, two recent studies have demonstrated that there is a decrease in interstitial cells of Cajal (ICC) in patients with STC.[17,18] Since the ICC act as pacemaker cells to the gut, we might intuitively expect a condition in which transit is slow to demonstrate an abnormality at this level. Certainly *W/W*[v] mutant knockout mice, which lack ICC, demonstrate delayed and disordered gut transit. In addition, both of the studies cited[17,18] demonstrated moderate hypoganglionosis in the myenteric plexus.

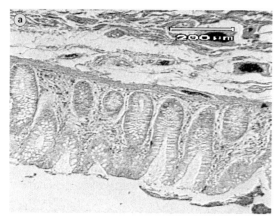 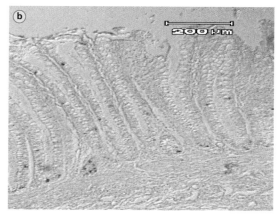

Fig. 12.3 Peptide YY (PYY)-immunoreactive cells in sigmoid colon (a) in a patient with STC and (b) in a control. The control is morphologically normal colon obtained from a patient with colonic carcinoma. Note that the number of PYY cells in the constipated patient is lower than in the control. Reprinted with kind permission of Professor El-Salhy and Blackwell Publishing (*Colorectal Disease* 2003; **5**: 290).

Colonic myopathy

There is no convincing evidence to date that STC is secondary to a colonic myopathy. However, colonic smooth muscle cell inclusion bodies have been found. This suggests that an inclusion body myopathy may arise secondarily to denervation,[25] as similar inclusion bodies are found in the aging gut and also in Chagas' disease, both of which are associated with neuronal degeneration.

Opioid-induced bowel dysfunction

Opiate medication is commonly and effectively used in the treatment of postoperative and chronic pain. Owing to the wide distribution of opioid receptors, in addition to analgesia, a range of side-effects may occur which include drowsiness, respiratory depression and pruritus. The effects of opiate medication on bowel function are well recognized, and these drugs have been used in the control of diarrhea since they slow bowel transit, lead to greater absorption of fluids and decrease luminal propulsive force. In the absence of diarrhea, however, these actions lead to bowel symptoms secondary to opiate use, including gastro-esophageal reflux, nausea, bloating, constipation, and incomplete evacuation. In fact, with chronic treatment these symptoms can be so debilitating that patients may elect to stop opiate medication altogether rather than endure the gastrointestinal side-effects. Over 50% of patients admitted to palliative care units experience opiate-induced bowel dysfunction,[26] and if uncontrolled this can lead to persistent nausea and vomiting, pseudo-obstruction or fecal impaction.

Postoperative ileus

Postoperative ileus refers to the period postoperatively when the recently handled bowel does not have effective peristalsis. It is characterized by distension and accumulation of luminal secretions and can affect the whole gut. It has significant effects both in terms of morbidity and indeed expense, since it prolongs hospital stay and delays recovery. It can occur following any type of surgery, but is most common following abdominal or pelvic procedures. The causes are multifactorial and include an increase in sympathetic autonomic tone to the gut and loss of myoelectric activity, and recently it has been shown that postoperative ileus is maintained by infiltrates activating inhibitory neural pathways.[27] Opioid medication prolongs postoperative ileus at a time when these drugs are needed for analgesia. Other strategies to avoid the use of opioids have therefore been pursued, including the use of non-steroidal anti-inflammatories and epidural local anesthesia. Only the latter has been shown to decrease the duration of postoperative ileus.[28]

Development of new therapies

The analgesic effects of morphine-based drugs are mediated centrally via the μ-opioid receptor. This receptor has been subtyped into $μ_1$, which is central and mediates analgesia, and $μ_2$, which is found in the spinal cord and periphery. Other receptors identified to date are the κ-receptor, δ-receptor and ε-receptor, each class being split further into subtypes. Opioids used in clinical practice are not entirely selective for the μ-receptor, but maintain relative selectivity.

The difficulty with developing drugs to target this opioid-induced bowel dysfunction is that any drug developed would have to be peripherally restricted, since any blockade of the central μ-receptors is likely to block their analgesic effects. Naloxone, a μ-receptor antagonist, has been shown to accelerate whole-gut transit in healthy individuals, and is potentially of use. However, it crosses the blood–brain barrier easily, and at doses required to reverse peripheral effects it will also reverse central analgesia as well.[29]

Two recent μ-receptor antagonists that are peripherally restricted are potential new therapies for opioid-induced bowel dysfunction. Recent studies have demonstrated that both alvimopan[30] and methylnaltrexone[31] reverse opioid-mediated gastrointestinal inhibition without limiting central analgesia in healthy volunteers, and that alvimopan is effective in limiting postoperative ileus.[32]

Diverticular disease

Diverticular disease is a common disorder, affecting 30–50% of the adult population in the developed world. It is much rarer in the developing world and it has been described as a disease of Western civilization. For such a common complaint, data on both the etiology and treatment are limited. This is in part because

---

Diverticular disease

1 Diverticular disease is a common disorder affecting 30–50% of the adult population in the developed world.

2 The condition develops out of a combination of lack of dietary fiber and advancing age, resulting in abnormal colonic pressure distribution.

3 Colonic postprandial motility indices are uniformly elevated, which is not typically observed in subjects without diverticular disease.

4 There may be denervation hypersensitivity in diverticular disease as muscarinic M_3 receptors are upregulated.

5 A decrease in inhibitory neurotransmitters (such as nitric oxide) may have a role in the etiopathogenesis of diverticula.

6 The development of agents modulating metalloproteinase activity or enteric nerve transmission as therapy for diverticular disease is under current investigation.

---

up to 80% of those affected remain asymptomatic and it is therefore difficult to perform representative prospective studies. Most of our epidemiological knowledge is based on barium enema or necropsy studies. Diverticula are out-pouchings of mucosa through the colonic wall. They rarely involve the whole thickness of the wall and therefore are strictly better defined as pseudo-diverticula (Fig. 12.4). In barium enema and necropsy studies, 90% of cases of diverticular disease have left-sided colonic disease and are associated with hypertrophy of the muscle layers. Although there are several theories as to its etiopathogenesis, it is generally agreed that the condition arises out of a combination of lack of dietary fiber and advancing age, resulting in abnormal colonic pressure distribution.

Etiopathophysiology
Fiber hypothesis

Painter and Burkitt, who originally described the condition as a 'deficiency disease of western civilization' in 1971, pointed out that diverticular disease had been on the increase in the Western world since the introduction of milled or refined flour into the diet of most western populations.[33] This in turn led to a

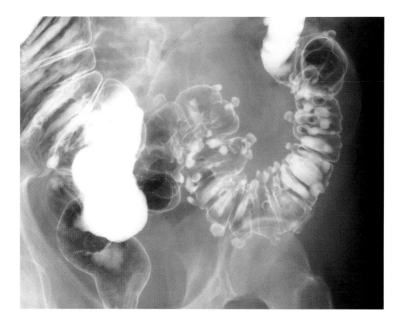

Fig. 12.4 Double-contrast barium enema demonstrating diverticular disease. With kind permission of Dr S Halligan, St Mark's Hospital, Harrow, UK.

decrease in the amount of dietary fiber. This theory was controversial at the time of its initial description, since conventional wisdom for many years held that roughage should be cut down in order to avoid the complications of diverticular disease. The lack of fiber was proposed to lead to harder stools, which spent more time in transit and led to segmentation of the colon with higher intraluminal pressures. The combination of these effects then led to the development of diverticula at points of weakness throughout the bowel wall, which were generally taken to be the sites of the entry of blood vessels.

In support of this theory was the observation that diverticular disease was rare in populations in which the dietary intake of fiber was high, such as African populations. Also, vegetarians, whose intake of fiber is higher, tend to develop fewer diverticula. Interestingly, migration studies have shown that when populations became more westernized and changed their diet the incidence of diverticular disease increased. This has particularly been demonstrated in the black population in South Africa following adoption of a Western diet[34] and also in the Japanese who have settled in Hawaii.[35]

Genetics

In addition to environmental factors (e.g. diet), genetic factors seem also to be important. Unlike Western populations, who develop left-sided disease predominantly, those in the Far East, and in particular Japan, predominantly develop right-sided disease. This is not just a dietary phenomenon, since Japanese people who move to Hawaii do develop more diverticula, but continue to do so on the right side. Additionally, studies have shown that colonic tissue from certain African populations is stronger and more compliant than that of age-matched controls from Western countries.

Extracellular matrix

The presence and structure of collagen within the colonic wall is important for the compliance of the viscus. When there is increased cross-linking of collagen, the wall becomes rigid and non-compliant. In animal studies, when rats are fed on a low-fiber diet they develop increased cross-linking of collagen in the bowel wall.[36] Similarly, this will even occur to a certain extent in rats whose mothers have been fed on a low-fiber diet, suggesting that at least some of the likelihood

of developing diverticula may be conferred *in utero*.[37] Dietary fiber undergoes fermentation in the colon and short-chain fatty acids are produced. Decreased levels of these acids have been demonstrated in animals fed on a low-fiber diet,[38] and it is known that they affect collagen cross-linking. This may involve matrix metalloproteinases, which are known to degrade all classes of extracellular matrix, thereby altering the structure of the colon. Bacterial flora can lead to macrophages, T cells and myofibroblasts secreting these endopeptidases. Hence, alteration of the colonic flora may have some role (secondary to decreased fiber) in the development of diverticula.

Motility abnormalities

The majority of the evidence from manometry studies in diverticular disease suggests that there is an increase in intraluminal pressure within diverticular segments. The literature in human studies is limited, most studies demonstrating that there is baseline elevation of intraluminal pressure within diverticular segments. Additionally, pressure responses to promotility agents such as prostigmine have been found to be exaggerated in diverticular segments, including in the right-sided disease seen most commonly in the Japanese population. This suggests that abnormal distribution of colonic pressure is causally implicated. A more physiological stimulus to motility is eating. There is disagreement between studies as to the degree to which colonic fasting motor activity is altered in diverticular disease. The motility index is a manometrically derived score of colonic motor activity. Motility indices postprandially in diverticular disease are uniformly elevated, which is not always observed in patients without diverticulosis. This supports the potential role of disturbed motility in the generation of diverticula.

Cholinergic denervation

The observation that colonic motility in diverticular segments increased after systemic administration of anticholinesterases led to the hypothesis that this was secondary to hypersensitivity of the cholinergic innervation of colonic smooth muscle. This effect was hypothesized to be specific to affected segments. To assess the level at which this putative cholinergic hypersensitivity was present, electrical field stimulation work demonstrated that diverticular segments demonstrated hypercontractility. It was hypothesized that this was secondary to an increase in cholinergic innervation.[39] Comparing immunohistochemical image analysis between resected diverticular segments and controls, Golder and colleagues, however, have shown that this is not the case.[40] There is in fact a decrease in cholinergic innervation with age, and this is found similarly in patients with or without diverticular disease. However, M_3 muscarinic receptors, which mediate cholinergic neural activity in the colonic smooth muscle are upregulated in the colonic wall of patients with diverticular disease. This suggests that there may be a denervation hypersensitivity in diverticular disease. The role of other receptors, such as the M_2 muscarinic receptors are yet to be elucidated.

Other enteric abnormalities

In contrast to the extensive data with regard to cholinergic transmission, there is little information concerning other non-adrenergic non-cholinergic (NANC) transmitters. Nitric oxide is known from *in vitro* electrical field stimulation experiments to mediate colonic relaxation by NANC neurons. Using nitric oxide synthase inhibitors, Tomita and colleagues demonstrated that nitric oxide also mediated relaxation in diverticular segments, but to a lesser degree.[41] However, it is not clear whether this is a primary etiopathogenic abnormality or whether it is secondary to elevated colonic pressures. It remains possible that a decrease in inhibitory transmitter action has a role to play in the etiopathogenesis of this disease.

Management

The management of complicated diverticular disease remains predominantly surgical. Complications, including abscess formation, perforation, fistulation and diverticular bleeding, often require surgical intervention. In the setting of acute diverticular bleeding there has been some recent literature to support the use of endoscopic injection or clipping to stem the acute bleed, which may avoid unnecessary surgery. Diverticulitis, presenting with abdominal pain and fever, often responds to treatment with intravenous antibiotics unless the complications of perforation, fistulation or abscess occur. Abscesses can be treated initially with radiological drainage with planned definitive resection of the diseased segment at a later date.

The treatment of uncomplicated diverticular disease is more controversial. There is an overlap between the symptoms deemed to be due to diverticular disease and those that are in fact due to irritable bowel syndrome. Hence, surgical resection in this group is not recommended since there may be no effect on symptoms. Medical therapy is limited. Patients are commonly advised to increase their dietary fiber intake, though not all studies show a beneficial effect on symptoms. The use of antispasmodic medications is often recommended, but the evidence for their efficacy is lacking. New therapies are needed for symptomatic treatment in this condition. Pharmacological agents modulating metalloproteinase activity or enteric nerve transmission, leading to an improvement in symptoms or even reversal of early diverticula, are potential therapies of the future.

Megacolon

Classification

The diagnosis of megacolon is based on defined radiological characteristics, with dilatation of the colon to a diameter greater than 6.5 mm at the pelvic brim with no evidence of obstruction (Fig. 12.5).[42] There are physiological and structural features which frequently accompany this structural abnormality. The presentation is with severe constipation and large bowel dilatation. Megacolon can be classified into chronic and acute cases, the latter referring to acute toxic dilatation in the setting of severe inflammation, in which there are no data on enteric nerve function. Chronic cases of megacolon can be further subclassified as congenital, acquired or idiopathic.

Idiopathic megacolon

Idiopathic megacolon refers to cases of large bowel dilatation without organic cause. This and the absence of dilatation of other parts of the gut distinguish it from chronic idiopathic intestinal pseudo-obstruction. Unlike patients with megarectum, who tend to present with incontinence and fecal impaction in childhood and the teenage years, patients with idiopathic megacolon present more in adulthood and commonly complain of constipation, bloating and abdominal pain. Radiological marker studies reveal slow colonic transit, but also a dilated bowel of greater than 6.5 cm above

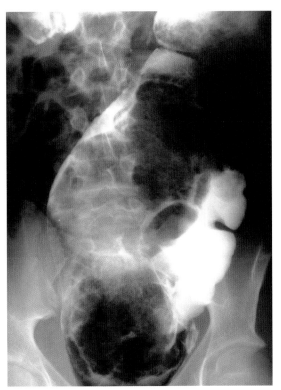

Fig. 12.5 Contrast enema demonstrating a megacolon. The colonic diameter is greater than 6.5 cm at the pelvic rim. With kind permission of Dr S Halligan, St Mark's Hospital, Harrow, UK.

the pelvic rim, which separates these patients from others with STC.[42]

Idiopathic cases of megacolon represent a heterogeneous group, a range of abnormalities having been demonstrated at the ENS level. Abnormalities have been found in some patients in the VIP and nitric oxide inhibitory systems which may contribute to abnormal gut function.[43] Overall, however, the changes are subtle, with some evidence of thickening of the muscularis mucosa and muscularis propria, some muscle fibrosis, and possible decreased innervation of the longitudinal layer.[44] In published studies there are no marked ENS abnormalities in this patient group. There may, however, be significant functional neurotransmitter abnormalities that are as yet undescribed. Drawing a parallel with idiopathic STC, the heterogeneity of this group would suggest multiple etiologies for the phenotype.

Acquired megacolon

Megacolon can occur after acquired insults to the autonomic and enteric nervous systems, such as in the case of Chagas' disease or after spinal cord injury, where the bowel has lost autonomic input. The use of chronic opiate medication can also lead to megacolon.

Chagas' disease

Chagas' disease, caused by the *Trypanosoma cruzi* parasite, is a massive public health problem in South America. Most morbidity comes from its effects on the heart and gastrointestinal tract. In addition to the classically described achalasia-like picture, patients with *T. cruzi* infection can present with involvement of any part of the gastrointestinal tract. Clinically, the effects are seen primarily in the esophagus and colon. Colonic involvement manifests as megacolon. Degeneration and reduction of neuronal density in the myenteric plexus has been demonstrated in affected colonic segments. It has been proposed that the Chagasic megacolon is caused by an autonomic imbalance caused by unopposed inhibitory tone secondary to the destruction of excitatory neural inputs.[45] Recently, circulating antibodies against a colonic muscarinic (M_2) acetylcholine receptor have been identified in these patients, and they may be of pathophysiological importance.[46]

Spinal injury

Bowel symptoms are a significant cause of morbidity and distress in patients with spinal injury. Megacolon is a highly prevalent condition in this patient group. It affects up to 73% of spinal injury patients[47] and is found more often in patients with a longer duration of injury. The causes of this are likely to be multifactorial. There may be loss of parasympathetic tone to the gut, but there is also a large amount of chronic laxative and opiate use in this group. There are no data to support the contention that chronic use of laxative in this group causes functional and ENS changes. Opiates, however, can certainly lead to a structural disturbance (dilatation), though data for ENS changes is lacking.

Congenital megacolon

Hirschsprung's disease

Hirschsprung's disease (HSCR) is a congenital malformation affecting around 1 in 5000 live births, with a

Hirschsprung's disease

1 Hirschsprung's disease is a congenital malformation affecting 1 in 5000 live births with a 3–4:1 male-to-female ratio.

2 Commonly presents in the infant period with failure to pass meconium and bowel obstruction.

3 Full-thickness rectal biopsies are diagnostic and characterized by aganglionosis and overabundance of fibers staining positive for acetylcholinesterase.

4 Diagnosis can be confirmed by the absence of the recto-anal inhibitory reflex.

5 Genetic abnormalities affecting the RET-GDNF-GFRα1 signaling system and the endothelin signaling system are most common.

6 Mutations in genes encoding several transcription factors have been found to be associated with HSCR.

male-to-female ratio of 3–4:1. Although it can present in adulthood, usually with a long history of constipation throughout life, it commonly presents in the infant period with failure to pass meconium, obstruction and occasionally enterocolitis. It is characterized by an aganglionic segment which commonly affects the distal sigmoid and rectum (short segment, approximately 70–80% of cases) (Fig. 12.6). It can, however, affect up to the whole of the large bowel, in which case it is known as 'long segment disease' (approximately

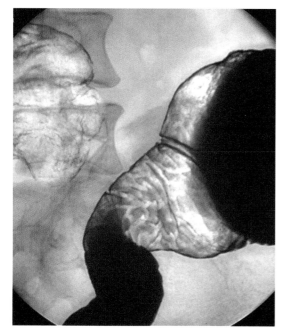

Fig. 12.6 Contrast enema demonstrating Hirschsprung's disease, with a dilated colon above the aganglionic segment. With kind permission of Dr S Halligan, St Mark's Hospital, Harrow, UK.

20%). In addition, an isolated segment of bowel can be involved, and this is known as zonal HSCR. Though commonly an isolated abnormality, HSCR can be associated with other congenital abnormalities, such as part of the Shah–Waardenburg syndrome or with congenital hypoventilation (Onedine's curse).

Embryonic studies of neural crest migration demonstrate that neural crest cells colonize the gut between 6 and 12 weeks and that disruption of this migration leads to the aganglionosis seen in HSCR. Vagal neural crest cells migrate in a rostrocaudal direction to colonize the gut and are not restricted to any particular part of the gut, having the capacity to migrate to and differentiate the distal rectum. However, some enteric neurons migrate from the lumbosacral level and do so in a caudorostral direction. Failure of these neurons to migrate to the whole gut leads to variable degrees of aganglionosis.

Histologically, suction or full-thickness biopsies in HSCR are diagnostic and characterized by aganglionosis and a marked overabundance of extrinsic nerve fibers staining positive for acetylcholinesterase (Fig. 12.7). There is an area adjacent to the aganglionic segment, termed the 'transitional zone', in which there is relative hypoganglionosis. Treatment of HSCR is surgical, by resection of the affected segment with colonic pull-through in a one- or two-stage operation, which can be performed laparoscopically. Problems arise on occasions in which the transitional zone is not fully excised, since these patients tend to develop further motility problems.

Although full-thickness rectal biopsy at least 5 cm above the dentate line is considered the gold standard diagnostic test, the diagnosis can be confirmed in adult cases by demonstrating absence of the recto-anal inhibitory reflex. Normally, the internal anal sphincter

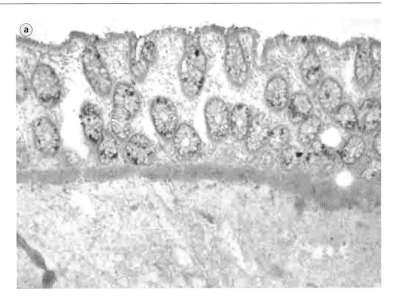

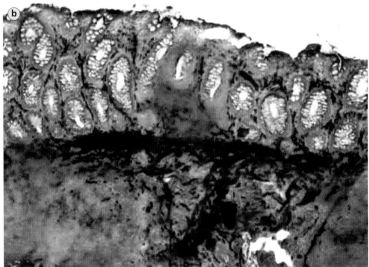

Fig. 12.7 Hirschsprung's disease. (a) Normal colonic biopsy. (b) Acetylcholinesterase staining demonstrating aganglionosis and abundance of extrinsic nerve fibers. With kind permission of Professor Ashley Price, St Mark's Hospital, Harrow, UK.

will relax in response to balloon distension (which mimics the presentation of a stool). However, in HSCR this response is lacking.

Genetics and Hirschsprung's disease

The development of the normal ENS relies on the ability of neural crest cells to differentiate, migrate to the appropriate site, and survive once they are there. In recent years, genetic, and latterly proteomic, studies have begun to unravel the complicated control of ENS development that leads to different phenotypic presentations. The range of genetic abnormalities now characterized in HSCR ranges from single-gene mutations to multiple affected genes with varying modes of inheritance.

Several genes have now been identified which are known to be associated with HSCR. Normal ENS development relies on intact signaling systems and transcription factors. The main signaling systems described to date that are relevant to the development of HSCR are the RET-GDNF-GFRα1 signaling system and the endothelin (ET-3) signaling system.

RET-GDNF-GFRα1 signaling system

The *RET* gene, which maps to chromosome 10q11.2, is the major gene involved in human HSCR, and mutations of this gene account for approximately 50% of familial and sporadic cases of HSCR.[48] As part of the RET-GDNF-GFRα1 signaling system, RET promotes the survival of neurons, mitosis of progenitor cells and differentiation of neurons. *Ret*[-/-] knockout mice have aganglionosis of the small and large intestines and associated renal agenesis. Although *RET* is expressed in human renal tract development, renal agenesis is a rare association with HSCR in humans. The RET receptor tyrosine kinase consists of an intracellular tyrosine kinase, a transmembrane domain and an extracellular domain. Mutations affecting the intracellular domain affect signaling functions, whereas those affecting the extracellular domain affect ligand binding.[49] Multiple mutations have been identified that are associated with HSCR, but can also be associated with the development of other conditions such as familial medullary thyroid carcinoma (FMTC), multiple endocrine neoplasia (MEN) 2A and MEN 2B. Around 5% of patients with HSCR will have an associated MEN 2A or FMTC.[50]

Glial-derived neurotrophic factor (GDNF) is a ligand for the RET receptor and requires the co-receptor GFRα1 for effective signaling.[51] It acts on early ENS precursor cells to stimulate differentiation and in *in vitro* studies can attract migrating ENS cells.[49] Heterozygosity of *GDNF* may contribute to the severity of the HSCR phenotype, but is not responsible for it. Although not described in humans, the *gdnf*[-/-] knockout mouse has a similar phenotype to the *ret*[-/-] mouse. Other members of the GDNF family have now been identified (neuritin, artemin, persephin), but mutations in their genes have not been demonstrated to result in HSCR.

Endothelin (ET-3) signaling system

The endothelin system in the developing embryo may regulate interactions between gut neural crest and mesenchyme cells. The endothelin family consists of ET-1, ET-2, ET-3 and VIP, but it is ET-3 that is important in ENS development via its interaction with the endothelin receptor-B (ET_B). This has been demonstrated in mouse knockout models. The lethal spotted mouse mutant (*ls/ls*) has distal colonic aganglionosis secondary to a mutation in the *Et-3* gene, and colonic aganglionosis is found to a greater extent in the piebald lethal mouse, which lacks the Et_B gene. *ET-3* mutations are associated with approximately 5% of human HSCR cases, with mutations of ET_B accounting for 5–7% of cases. Mutations of the *ET-3* and ET_B genes have been described in presentations of the Shah–Waardenburg syndrome, which is characterized by enteric aganglionosis, skin and hair pigmentation defects and sensorineural hearing loss.[52] As well as ET-3 and ET_B abnormalities, mutations in the endothelin converting enzyme-1 can lead to the presentation of aganglionosis, albeit with associated autonomic, craniofacial and cardiac abnormalities.[53] Mutations of other signaling systems, including the hedgehog signaling system, may have a role in congenital enteric aganglionosis, but, given the widespread role of these systems in embryonic development, it is unlikely that enteric aganglionosis would present without multiple other complex abnormalities.

Nuclear transcription factors

As well as these signaling systems, there are several families of transcription factors which are now known to be important in neuronal differentiation in the ENS. Mutations in the genes producing these factors can lead to a presentation of HSCR. These include *SOX10*, *PHOX2B*,[54] *HASH1*, *HOX11L1*, *PAX3*, *SIP1* and, more recently, *PMX2B*,[55] which have been associated with varying degrees of enteric aganglionosis.

The understanding of the causes of HSCR is thus increasing as our understanding of the genetic control of ENS development evolves.

References

1   Sonnenberg A, Koch TR. Physician visits in the United States for constipation: 1958 to 1986. *Dig Dis Sci* 1989; **34**: 606–11.

2   Pare P, Ferrazzi S, Thompson WG, Irvine EJ, Rance L. An epidemiological survey of constipation in Canada: definitions, rates, demographics, and predictors of health care seeking. *Am J Gastroenterol* 2001; **96**: 3130–7.

3   Leroi AM, Bernier C, Watier A *et al*. Prevalence of sexual abuse among patients with functional disorders of the lower gastrointestinal tract. *Int J Colorectal Dis* 1995; **10**: 200–6.

4   Mertz H, Naliboff B, Munakata J, Niazi N, Mayer EA. Altered rectal perception is a biological marker of patients

with irritable bowel syndrome. *Gastroenterology* 1995; **109**: 40–52.

5   Scott SM, Knowles CH, Newell M, Garvie N, Williams NS, Lunniss PJ. Scintigraphic assessment of colonic transit in women with slow-transit constipation arising *de novo* and following pelvic surgery or childbirth. *Br J Surg* 2001; **88**: 405–11.

6   O'Brien MD, Camilleri M, der Ohe MR *et al.* Motility and tone of the left colon in constipation: a role in clinical practice? *Am J Gastroenterol* 1996; **91**: 2532–8.

7   Bassotti G, Chiarioni G, Imbimbo BP, Betti C, Bonfante F, Vantini I *et al.* Impaired colonic motor response to cholinergic stimulation in patients with severe chronic idiopathic (slow transit type) constipation. *Dig Dis Sci* 1993; **38**: 1040–5.

8   Kamm MA, van der Sijp JR, Lennard-Jones JE. Observations on the characteristics of stimulated defaecation in severe idiopathic constipation. *Int J Colorectal Dis* 1992; **7**: 197–201.

9   Preston DM, Lennard-Jones JE. Pelvic motility and response to intraluminal bisacodyl in slow-transit constipation. *Dig Dis Sci* 1985; **30**: 289–94.

10 Slater BJ, Varma JS, Gillespie JI. Abnormalities in the contractile properties of colonic smooth muscle in idiopathic slow transit constipation. *Br J Surg* 1997; **84**: 181–4.

11 Ferrara A, Pemberton JH, Grotz RL, Hanson RB. Prolonged ambulatory recording of anorectal motility in patients with slow-transit constipation. *Am J Surg* 1994; **167**: 73–9.

12 Waldron D, Bowes KL, Kingma YJ, Cote KR. Colonic and anorectal motility in young women with severe idiopathic constipation. *Gastroenterology* 1988; **95**: 1388–94.

13 Spiller RC. Upper gut dysmotility in slow-transit constipation: is it evidence for a panenteric neurological deficit in severe slow transit constipation? *Eur J Gastroenterol Hepatol* 1999; **11**: 693–6.

14 Glia A, Akerlund JE, Lindberg G. Outcome of colectomy for slow-transit constipation in relation to presence of small-bowel dysmotility. *Dis Colon Rectum* 2004; **47**: 96–102.

15 Gladman MA, Scott SM, Chan CL, Williams NS, Lunniss PJ. Rectal hyposensitivity: prevalence and clinical impact in patients with intractable constipation and fecal incontinence. *Dis Colon Rectum* 2003; **46**: 238–46.

16 Knowles CH, Scott SM, Wellmer A *et al.* Sensory and autonomic neuropathy in patients with idiopathic slow-transit constipation. *Br J Surg* 1999; **86**: 54–60.

17 Wedel T, Spiegler J, Soellner S *et al.* Enteric nerves and interstitial cells of Cajal are altered in patients with slow-transit constipation and megacolon. *Gastroenterology* 2002; **123**: 1459–67.

18 He CL, Burgart L, Wang L *et al.* Decreased interstitial cell of Cajal volume in patients with slow-transit constipation.

Gastroenterology 2000; **118**: 14–21.

19 Krishnamurthy S, Schuffler MD, Rohrmann CA, Pope CE. Severe idiopathic constipation is associated with a distinctive abnormality of the colonic myenteric plexus. *Gastroenterology* 1985; **88**: 26–34.

20 Porter AJ, Wattchow DA, Hunter A, Costa M. Abnormalities of nerve fibers in the circular muscle of patients with slow transit constipation. *Int J Colorectal Dis* 1998; **13**: 208–16.

21 Peracchi M, Basilisco G, Tagliabue R *et al.* Postprandial gut peptide plasma levels in women with idiopathic slow-transit constipation. *Scand J Gastroenterol* 1999; **34**: 25–8.

22 Penning C, Delemarre JB, Bemelman WA, Biemond I, Lamers CB, Masclee AA. Proximal and distal gut hormone secretion in slow transit constipation. *Eur J Clin Invest* 2000; **30**: 709–14.

23 Emmanuel AV, Kamm MA. Response to a behavioural treatment, biofeedback, in constipated patients is associated with improved gut transit and autonomic innervation. *Gut* 2001; **49**: 214–19.

24 Roy AJ, Emmanuel AV, Storrie JB, Bowers J, Kamm MA. Behavioural treatment (biofeedback) for constipation following hysterectomy. *Br J Surg* 2000; **87**: 100–5.

25 Knowles CH, Nickols CD, Scott SM *et al.* Smooth muscle inclusion bodies in slow transit constipation. *J Pathol* 2001; **193**: 390–7.

26 Schug SA, Zech D, Dorr U. Cancer pain management according to WHO analgesic guidelines. *J Pain Symptom Manage* 1990; **5**: 27–32.

27 de Jonge WJ, van den Wijngaard RM, The FO *et al.* Postoperative ileus is maintained by intestinal immune infiltrates that activate inhibitory neural pathways in mice. *Gastroenterology* 2003; **125**: 1137–47.

28 Wattwil M. Postoperative pain relief and gastrointestinal motility. *Acta Chir Scand* 1989; **550** (Suppl.): 140–5.

29 Sykes NP. Oral naloxone in opioid-associated constipation. *Lancet* 1991; **337**: 1475.

30 Schimdt WK. Almivopan (ADL 8–2698) is a novel peripheral opioid antagonist. *Am J Surg* 2001; **182** (5A Suppl.): 27S–38S.

31 Yuan CS, Foss JF, O'Connor M, Toledano A, Roizen MF, Moss J. Methylnaltrexone prevents morphine-induced delay in oral–cecal transit time without affecting analgesia: a double-blind randomized placebo-controlled trial. *Clin Pharmacol Ther* 1996; **59**: 469–75.

32 Taguchi A, Sharma N, Saleem RM *et al.* Selective postoperative inhibition of gastrointestinal opioid receptors. *N Engl J Med* 2001; **345**: 935–40.

33 Painter NS, Burkitt DP. Diverticular disease of the colon: a deficiency disease of Western civilization. *Br Med J* 1971; **2**: 450–4.

34 Segal I, Solomon A, Hunt JA. Emergence of diverticular

disease in the urban South African black. *Gastroenterology* 1977; **72**: 215–19.

35 Stemmermann GN, Yatani R. Diverticulosis and polyps of the large intestine. A necropsy study of Hawaii Japanese. *Cancer* 1973; **31**: 1260–70.

36 Wess L, Eastwood MA, Edwards CA, Busuttil A, Miller A. Collagen alteration in an animal model of colonic diverticulosis. *Gut* 1996; **38**: 701–6.

37 Wess L, Eastwood M, Busuttil A, Edwards C, Miller A. An association between maternal diet and colonic diverticulosis in an animal model. *Gut* 1996; **39**: 423–7.

38 Wess L, Eastwood MA, Edwards CA, Busuttil A, Miller A. Collagen alteration in an animal model of colonic diverticulosis. *Gut* 1996; **38**: 701–6.

39 Tomita R, Tanjoh K, Fujisaki S, Fukuzawa M. Physiological studies on nitric oxide in the right sided colon of patients with diverticular disease. *Hepatogastroenterology* 1999; **46**: 2839–44.

40 Golder M, Burleigh DE, Belai A *et al*. Smooth muscle cholinergic denervation hypersensitivity in diverticular disease. *Lancet* 2003; **361**: 1945–51.

41 Tomita R, Fujisaki S, Tanjoh K, Fukuzawa M. Role of nitric oxide in the left-sided colon of patients with diverticular disease. *Hepatogastroenterology* 2000; **47**: 692–6.

42 Preston DM, Lennard-Jones JE, Thomas BM. Towards a radiologic definition of idiopathic megacolon. *Gastrointest Radiol* 1985; **10**: 167–9.

43 Gattuso JM, Hoyle CH, Milner P, Kamm MA, Burnstock G. Enteric innervation in idiopathic megarectum and megacolon. *Int J Colorectal Dis* 1996; **11**: 264–71.

44 Gattuso JM, Kamm MA, Talbot JC. Pathology of idiopathic megarectum and megacolon. *Gut* 1997; **41**: 252–7.

45 Mathias CJ. Autonomic disorders and their recognition. *N Engl J Med* 1997; **336**: 721–4.

46 Sterin-Borda L, Goin JC, Bilder CR, Iantorno G, Hernando AC, Borda E. Interaction of human Chagasic IgG with human colon muscarinic acetylcholine receptor: molecular and functional evidence. *Gut* 2001; **49**: 699–705.

47 Harari D, Minaker KL. Megacolon in patients with chronic spinal cord injury. *Spinal Cord* 2000; **38**: 331–9.

48 Angrist M, Bolk S, Thiel B *et al*. Mutation analysis of the RET receptor tyrosine kinase in Hirschsprung disease. *Hum Mol Genet* 1995; **4**: 821–30.

49 Newgreen D, Young HM. Enteric nervous system: development and developmental disturbances – Part 1. *Pediatr Dev Pathol* 2002; **5**: 224–47.

50 Mulligan LM, Eng C, Healey CS *et al*. Specific mutations of the RET proto-oncogene are related to disease phenotype in MEN 2A and FMTC. *Nat Genet* 1994; **6**: 70–4.

51 Airaksinen MS, Titievsky A, Saarma M. GDNF family neurotrophic factor signaling: four masters, one servant? *Mol Cell Neurosci* 1999; **13**: 313–25.

52 Edery P, Attie T, Amiel J *et al*. Mutation of the endothelin-3 gene in the Waardenburg–Hirschsprung disease (Shah–Waardenburg syndrome). *Nat Genet* 1996; **12**: 442–4.

53 Hofstra RM, Valdenaire O, Arch E *et al*. A loss-of-function mutation in the endothelin-converting enzyme 1 (ECE-1) associated with Hirschsprung disease, cardiac defects, and autonomic dysfunction. *Am J Hum Genet* 1999; **64**: 304–8.

54 Garcia-Barcelo M, Sham MH, Lui VC, Chen BL, Ott J, Tam PK. Association study of PHOX2B as a candidate gene for Hirschsprung's disease. *Gut* 2003; **52**: 563–7.

55 Benailly HK, Lapierre JM, Laudier B *et al*. PMX2B, a new candidate gene for Hirschsprung's disease. *Clin Genet* 2003; **64**: 204–9.

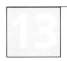

CHAPTER 13

Anorectal Disorders

Adil E Bharucha

Fecal incontinence

Introduction and epidemiology

Fecal incontinence (FI) is the recurrent uncontrolled passage of fecal material, of 1 month or greater duration, in an individual with a developmental age of at least 4 years.[1] Community-based surveys have fostered increasing awareness of the symptom and its detrimental impact on lifestyle and functioning; these consequences are disproportionately severe compared with the medical consequences of FI (Table 13.1).[2] Physicians may under-recognize the prevalence and devastating consequences of FI, perhaps because patients are often embarrassed to discuss the symptom.

Table 13.1 Epidemiology of fecal incontinence

Prevalence of FI in the community ranges from 2% to 15%.

Varying prevalence rates may be attributable to differences in survey techniques, definition of FI and population surveyed.

Prevalence is similar in men and women. Prevalence and severity of FI increased with aging; 47% of nursing home residents in one survey had FI.

Patients with FI are often embarrassed to discuss the symptom with a physician or friends.

FI affects quality of life in >50% of patients. FI may jeopardize employment, and may lead to institutionalization.

Fecal incontinence: key features

1 Distressing symptom attributable to one or more disordered continence mechanisms.
2 Most patients have internal and/or external sphincter weakness. Rectal sensory disturbances (i.e. increased or reduced) and altered bowel habits (i.e. constipation and/or diarrhea) are also important.
3 Common causes include anal sphincter injury resulting from obstetric or iatrogenic trauma and/or pudendal neuropathy caused by obstetric injury or chronic straining.
4 Patients are often embarrassed to discuss the symptom with a physician.
5 Careful characterization of symptoms is useful for gauging severity, understanding pathophysiology and guiding management.

6 Diagnostic testing is guided by clinical features. Anal manometry and ultrasound are used to evaluate sphincter function and structure, respectively. Endoscopy necessary if mucosal disease process is a consideration.
7 Simple measures are often helpful: empathy, patient education, management of altered bowel habits and biofeedback therapy (for sphincter tone and/or rectal sensation).
8 Long-term success rate after surgical repair of anal sphincter defects is poor. More invasive approaches (e.g. graciloplasty) involve considerable morbidity.
9 Colostomy may be the only option for patients with symptoms refractory to other measures.

Table 13.2 Anorectal factors maintaining continence

Factor (method of assessment)*	Physiological functions	Pathophysiology
Internal anal sphincter (anal manometry)	Smooth muscle responsible for maintaining ~70% resting anal tone. Resting tone is maintained by myogenic factors and tonic sympathetic excitation. Relaxes during defecation.	Resting and squeeze pressures are ↓ in most women with FI. Conversely, high sphincter pressures may hinder evacuation, predisposing to FI in some men.
External anal sphincter [anal manometry, *anal EMG* (for neural integrity)]	Tonically-active striated muscle which predominantly contains type I (slow-twitch) fibers in humans. Maintains ~30% of resting anal tone. Voluntary or reflex contraction (i.e. squeeze response) closes the anal canal, preserving continence.	Internal and external sphincter weakness is often caused by sphincter trauma. Obstetric or iatrogenic injuries are common causes of sphincter trauma. Diseases affecting upper or lower motor neuron pathways can also weaken the external sphincter.
Puborectalis (evacuation proctography, *dynamic pelvic MRI*)	Maintains a relatively acute anorectal angle at rest. Contracts further to preserve continence during squeeze.	MRI reveals puborectalis atrophy and/or impaired function in a subset of incontinent patients.
Rectal compliance (*barostat testing*)	By relaxing (i.e. accommodating), the rectum can hold more stool until defecation is convenient.	Rectal compliance is ↓ in ulcerative and ischemic proctitis. Rectal capacity is ↓ in 'idiopathic' FI.
Rectal sensation (perception of latex balloon distension, *barostat testing*)	Rectal distension evokes the desire to defecate and is also critical for initiating the squeeze response when continence is threatened.	↓ rectal sensation occurs in FI, may impair evacuation and continence, and can be ameliorated by biofeedback therapy . Rectal sensation may contribute to the symptom of urgency in FI.
Anal sensation (*electrosensitivity, temperature change*)	The exquisitely sensitive anal mucosa will periodically sample and ascertain whether rectal contents are gas, liquid or stool[38] when the anal sphincters relax.	The extent to which normal or disordered anal sampling reflexes contribute to fecal continence or FI respectively are unclear.

*Italics indicate the test is used in research studies but is not widely available or generally used in clinical practice. ↓ = reduced; ↑ = increased.

Mechanisms of normal and disordered continence

Fecal continence is maintained by anatomical factors, rectal compliance and recto-anal sensation (Table 13.2). Anatomical factors include the anal sphincters and levator ani (i.e. the pelvic floor), rectal curvatures and transverse rectal folds (Fig. 13.1). The rectum is a distensible organ that relaxes, allowing defecation to be postponed until convenient. The perception of rectal distension is indispensable for defecation and for voluntary contraction of the pelvic floor when continence is threatened (Fig. 13.2). Moreover, disturbances of stool consistency, mental facul-ties, and mobility often contribute to FI, particularly in patients who have impaired anorectal continence mechanisms.

Anal sphincter pressures are reduced in most, but not all, incontinent patients.[3] However, anal sphincter pressures do not always distinguish continent from incontinent subjects, underscoring the importance of rectal compliance and sensation in maintaining continence. Impaired rectal sensation allows the stool to enter the anal canal and perhaps leak before the external sphincter contracts.[3,4] On the other hand, exaggerated rectal sensation, perhaps a marker of coexistent irritable bowel syndrome,[5] is associated

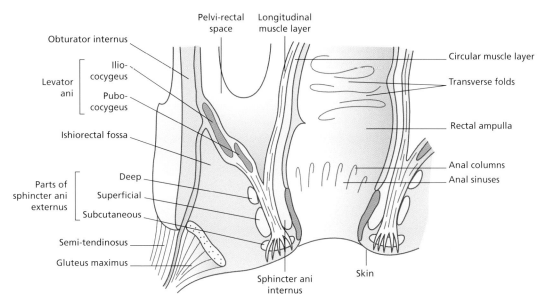

Fig. 13.1 Diagram of a coronal section of the rectum, anal canal and adjacent structures. The pelvic barrier includes the anal sphincters and pelvic floor muscles. Reproduced with permission from Bharucha AE. Fecal incontinence. *Gastroenterology* 2003; **124**: 1672–85.

with reduced rectal compliance, repetitive rectal contractions during rectal distension, external sphincter weakness and exaggerated anal sphincter relaxation during rectal distension.[3] Thus, FI is a heterogeneous disorder, patients often suffering from more than one deficit (Table 13.3).

Etiology

FI is attributable to conditions associated with pelvic floor weakness and/or diarrhea (Table 13.4). Before the advent of endoanal ultrasound, unexplained sphincter weakness was considered 'idiopathic', or attributed to a pudendal neuropathy. Endoanal ultrasound revealed clinically occult internal and external anal sphincter injury in FI and after vaginal delivery in women.[6,7] However, the median age of onset of 'idiopathic' FI is ~ 61 years; that is, several decades after vaginal delivery. This suggests that, in addition to anal sphincter trauma caused by vaginal delivery, other factors – as yet poorly defined, but including aging, menopause, chronic straining, and disordered bowel habits – probably predispose to FI.

The prevalence of FI increases with age and anorectal functions decline with age. Anal pressures are lower in older than in younger, asymptomatic men and women. It is unknown if these effects are attributable to aging alone and/or hormonal changes associated with aging (e.g. menopause) and/or other confounding factors (e.g. obstetric trauma). Previous studies suggested that anal resting and squeeze pressures were lower in older than in younger subjects.[8,9] We recently demonstrated that anal resting pressures did, but squeeze pressures did not decline with age in carefully selected asymptomatic women without other risk factors for pelvic floor trauma.[10] The relative sparing of anal squeeze pressures by aging is consistent with the muscle fiber distribution in the human external anal sphincter. The human external anal sphincter predominantly contains type I (i.e. slow twitch) fibers, which, in contrast to type II fibers, are relatively spared by aging.[11] Rectal compliance also declined with age in asymptomatic women.[10] Taken together, the evidence indicates that reduced anal resting pressure and reduced rectal compliance may predispose to FI.

In men, FI is often attributable to local causes, such as anal fistulae, poorly healed surgical scars or proctitis after radiotherapy for prostate cancer. Idiopathic fecal soiling or leakage in men may also be caused by a long anal sphincter of high pressure that entraps small particles of feces during defecation and subsequently

Table 13.3 Anorectal sensorimotor disturbances in fecal incontinence

Etiology	Anal sphincter pressures	Threshold for internal sphincter relaxation	Threshold for external sphincter contraction	Rectal sensation*	Rectal compliance	Pelvic floor function
Idiopathic	→	→	→	↓ or ↑	↓ or ↑	→
Diabetes mellitus[39]	R ↓; S ↓	↔	NA	↓↓	↔	NA
Multiple sclerosis[39]	R ↔; S ↓↓	→	NA	↓↓	↔	NA
Elderly patients with fecal impaction and incontinence[40]	R ↔; S ↔	→	NA	→	NA	→
Acute radiation proctitis[41]	R ↓; S ↓	NA	NA	↔	→	NA
Chronic radiation injury[42]	NA	NA	NA		→	NA
Ulcerative colitis[43]	S ↓ in FI	↓ (active colitis only)	NA	↑ (active colitis only)	↑ (active colitis only)	NA
Spinal cord injury – high spinal lesion, i.e. T12 or higher[18]	R ↔; S ↓	→	↔	→	→	NA
Low spinal lesion, i.e. below T12	R ↓; S ↓	↔	→	→	↔	NA

Information pertains to patients with underlying disease and FI. ↑ = Increased; ↓ = decreased; ↔ = no change. R = resting; S = squeeze sphincter pressure; NA = not available. *Rectal sensation expressed as volume thresholds for perception; ↑ sensation indicates volume threshold for perception was lower than in normals. Reproduced with permission from Bharucha AE. Fecal incontinence. *Gastroenterology* 2003; **124**: 1672–85.

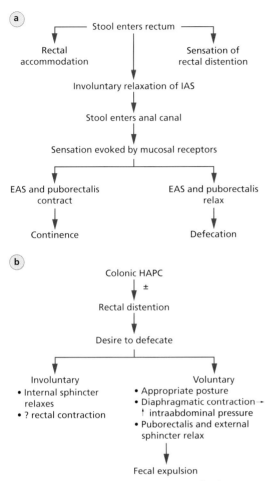

Fig. 13.2 Schematic of events that accompany fecal continence (a) and defecation (b). HAPC, high-amplitude propagated contraction. Panel b is reproduced with permission from Bharucha AE, Camilleri M. Physiology of the colon. In: Pemberton JH, ed. *Shackelford's Surgery of the Alimentary Tract, Vol. IV. The Colon*. 5th edn. Philadelphia: WB Saunders, 2001: 29–39. IAS, internal anal sphincter. EAS, external anal sphincter.

expels them, causing perianal soiling and discomfort.[12] Approximately 5% of patients develop chronic anorectal complications (fistula, stricture and disabling FI) after pelvic radiotherapy.[13] Surgical procedures that may contribute to FI include sphincterotomy and fistulotomy. Postoperative FI affects about 45% of patients after a lateral internal sphincterotomy; 6%, 8% and 1% reported incontinence to flatus, minor fecal soiling and loss of solid stool, respectively, 5 years thereafter.[14]

The risk of FI after a fistulotomy has been reported to range from 18 to 52%, but is perhaps lower with recent modifications.[15]

Several neurological disorders are associated with FI (Table 13.4). Anal sphincter weakness, diminished rectoanal sensation and diarrhea predispose to FI in patients with diabetic neuropathy. Impairment of anorectal function generally parallels the duration of disease.[16] Fifty-one percent of a group of unselected outpatients with multiple sclerosis had FI.[17] Constipation is the predominant symptom after supraconal spinal cord injury; anal resting pressure is relatively preserved and FI is relatively uncommon. In contrast, resting anal sphincter tone is often reduced in patients with spinal cord lesions at or below T_{12}; reduced anal sphincter tone, blunted recto-anal sensation[18] and laxatives predispose to FI in patients with lumbosacral lesions.

Clinical evaluation

A meticulous clinical assessment is necessary to identify the etiology and pathophysiology of FI, establish rapport with the patient, and guide diagnostic testing and treatment. Terms used to reflect the nature and severity of FI include 'staining', 'seepage' (leakage of small amounts of stool) and 'soiling' (of clothes or bedding).

Table 13.4 Etiology of fecal incontinence

Anal sphincter weakness
Injury: obstetric trauma related to surgical procedures, e.g. hemorrhoidectomy, internal sphincterotomy, fistulotomy, anorectal infection
Non-traumatic: scleroderma, internal sphincter thinning of unknown etiology

Neuropathy
Stretch injury, obstetric trauma, diabetes mellitus

Anatomical disturbances of the pelvic floor
Fistula, rectal prolapse, descending perineum syndrome

Inflammatory conditions
Crohn's disease, ulcerative colitis, radiation proctitis

Central nervous system disease
Dementia, stroke, brain tumors, spinal cord lesions, multiple system atrophy (Shy–Drager syndrome), multiple sclerosis

Diarrhea
Irritable bowel syndrome, post-cholecystectomy diarrhea

Reproduced with permission from Bharucha AE. Fecal incontinence. *Gastroenterology* 2003; **124**: 1672–85.

Scales for rating the severity of FI incorporate the nature and frequency of stool loss, number of pads used, severity of urgency, and the impact of FI on coping mechanisms and/or lifestyle–behavioral changes.[19] Quality of life includes not only items connected with coping, behavior, self-perception and embarrassment, but also practical day-to-day limitations, such as the ability to socialize and get out of the house.[20] Patients are affected even by the possibility and unpredictability of incontinence episodes. Thus, the type and frequency of incontinence episodes alone may underestimate the severity of FI in people who are housebound because of FI.

The clinical history provides several insights into the pathophysiology of FI (Table 13.5). The importance of carefully characterizing bowel habits cannot be overemphasized. Stool form and consistency can be described by pictorial stool scales.[21] The terms 'urge FI' and 'passive FI' refer to exaggerated and reduced awareness of the desire to defecate before the incontinence episode, respectively.

A multisystem examination should be guided by the history and by knowledge of underlying diseases. The positive predictive value of digital rectal examination for identifying low resting and squeeze pressures is 67 and 81%, respectively.[22] A digital rectal examination can also evaluate voluntary puborectalis contraction, manifest as normal upward and anterior movement of the puborectalis (i.e. a 'lift') when the subject squeezes. Examination in the seated position on a commode may be more accurate than the left lateral decubitus position for characterizing rectal prolapse, pouch of Douglas hernia or excessive perineal descent.

Diagnostic testing

The extent of diagnostic testing is tailored to the patient's age, probable etiological factors, symptom severity, impact on quality of life and response to conservative medical management. The strengths and limitations of these tests have been detailed elsewhere.[7] Endoscopy to identify mucosal pathology is probably

Table 13.5 The clinical history in fecal incontinence: insights into pathophysiology

Question	Rationale
Onset, natural history and risk factors	Relationship of symptom onset/deterioration to other illnesses may suggest etiology. Natural history may reveal why a patient has sought medical attention.
Bowel habits/ type of leakage	Semiformed or liquid stools, perhaps resulting from laxative use in constipated patients, pose a greater threat to pelvic floor continence mechanisms than formed stools. Incontinence for solid stool suggests more severe sphincter weakness than incontinence for liquid stool only. Management should be tailored to specific bowel disturbance.
Degree of warning before FI	Urge and passive FI are associated with more severe weakness of the external and internal anal sphincter, respectively. These symptoms may also reflect rectal sensory disturbances, potentially amenable to biofeedback therapy.
Diurnal variation in FI	Nocturnal FI occurs uncommonly in idiopathic FI and is most frequently encountered in diabetes and scleroderma.
Urinary incontinence – presence and type	Association between urinary and FI. Same therapy may be effective for both conditions.
Evaluate possible causes of FI	Multisystem diseases causing FI are generally evident on a history and physical examination. The obstetric history must inquire specifically for known risk factors for pelvic trauma, e.g. forceps delivery, episiotomy, and prolonged second stage of labor. Medications (e.g. laxatives, artificial stool softeners) may cause or exacerbate FI.

Modified with permission from Bharucha AE. Fecal incontinence. *Gastroenterology* 2003; **124**: 1672–85.

necessary for FI patients with significant, particularly recent-onset diarrhea or constipation. The extent of examination (sigmoidoscopy or colonoscopy) and consideration of mucosal biopsies are guided by the patient's age, comorbidities and differential diagnosis. The indications for, and extent of, diagnostic testing in FI are evolving. For ambulatory, otherwise healthy patients, anorectal manometry and endoanal ultrasound are useful to document severity of weakness and to identify abnormal sphincter morphology, respectively. Evacuation proctography may be useful to characterize puborectalis contraction, confirm a coexistent evacuation disorder, and/or document the severity of clinically suspected excessive perineal descent or a rectocele. Endoanal MRI is useful for visualizing anal sphincter morphology, particularly external sphincter atrophy (Fig. 13.3), while dynamic MRI can concurrently image the bladder, genital organs and anorectum in real time without radiation exposure (Figs 13.4 and 13.5). However, pelvic MRI is relatively expensive and not widely available. Anal sphincter EMG should be considered for incontinent patients with an underlying disease associated with a neuropathy, such as diabetes mellitus, clinical suspicion of a proximal neurogenic process, or sphincter weakness unexplained by morphology as visualized

by ultrasound. Delayed pudendal nerve terminal motor latencies (PNTML) are widely used as a surrogate marker for pudendal neuropathy. Initial studies suggested that patients with a pudendal neuropathy would not fare as well after surgical repair of sphincter defects compared with patients without a neuropathy. However, the accuracy of delayed PNTML as a marker for pudendal neuropathy has been questioned on several grounds.[23] The test measures only conduction velocity in the fastest conducting nerve fibers, and there are inadequate normative data. Test reproducibility is unknown, and sensitivity and specificity are poor. In fact, in contrast to initial studies, recent studies suggest that the test does not predict improvement, or lack thereof, after surgical repair of anal sphincter defects.

Management

The management must be tailored to clinical manifestations, and includes treatment of underlying diseases, and other approaches detailed in Table 13.6.

Modification of bowel habits

Modification of bowel habits by simple measures is often extremely effective in managing FI. By taking loperamide or diphenoxylate before social occasions

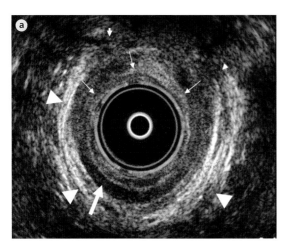

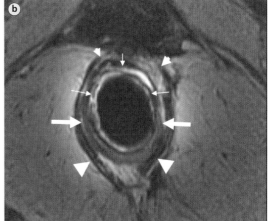

Fig. 13.3 Endoanal ultrasonographic (US; a) and magnetic resonance (MR) images (b) of anal sphincters in a patient with fecal incontinence. The internal anal sphincter is hypoechoic on the US image, while on the MR the internal sphincter is of higher signal intensity than the external sphincter. Thick and thin white arrows indicate normal internal sphincter and tear, respectively (located approximately between 10 and 5 o'clock) on US and MR images. Large and small arrowheads indicate normal-appearing and partially torn external sphincter (between 10 and 2 o'clock), respectively. Reproduced with permission from Bharucha AE. Fecal incontinence. *Gastroenterology* 2003; **124**: 1672–85.

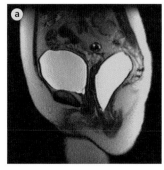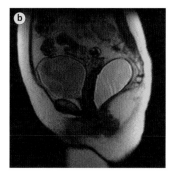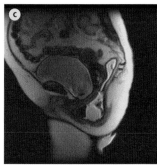

Fig. 13.4 Magnetic resonance fluoroscopic images of the pelvis at rest (a), during squeeze (b), and simulated defecation (c) in a 52-year-old asymptomatic subject after filling the rectum with ultrasound gel. At rest, the pelvic floor was well supported and the anorectal angle measured 126°. Pelvic floor contraction during the squeeze maneuver was accompanied by normal upward and anterior motion of the anorectal junction; the angle declined to 95°. Rectal evacuation was associated with relaxation of the puborectalis, as evidenced by opening of the anorectal junction, widening of the anorectal angle and perineal descent. The bladder base dropped by 2.5 cm below the pubococcygeal line; the 2.8 cm anterior rectocele emptied completely, and was probably not clinically significant; perineal descent (5 cm) was outside the normal range for evacuation proctography. Reproduced with permission from Bharucha AE. Fecal incontinence. *Gastroenterology* 2003; **124**: 1672–85.

or meals outside the home, incontinent patients may avoid having an accident outside the home and gain confidence in their ability to participate in social activities. The serotonin (5-HT$_3$) antagonist alosetron (Lotronex™, GlaxoSmithKline), available under a restricted use program in the USA, is an alternative option when functional diarrhea cannot be controlled by other agents. Patients with constipation, fecal impaction and overflow FI may benefit from a regularized evacuation program, incorporating timed evacuation by digital stimulation and/or bisacodyl/glycerol suppositories, fiber supplementation, and selective use of oral laxatives, as detailed in a recent review.[24]

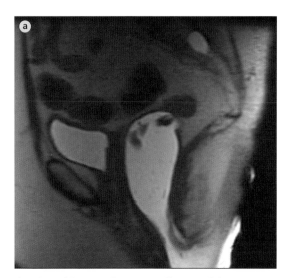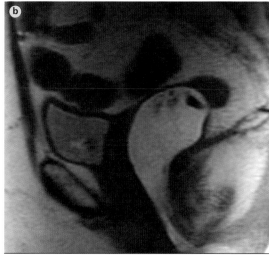

Fig. 13.5 Pelvic magnetic resonance fluoroscopic images at rest (a) and squeeze (b) in a 57-year-old-lady with FI. During squeeze, the puborectalis indentation on the posterior rectal wall was exaggerated compared with rest, and the anorectal angle declined from 143° at rest to 90° during squeeze; however, the anal canal remained patulous. Reproduced with permission from Bharucha AE. Fecal incontinence. *Gastroenterology* 2003; **124**: 1672–85.

Table 13.6 Management of fecal incontinence

Intervention	Side-effects	Comments	Mechanism of action
Incontinence pads*	Skin irritation	Disposable products provide better skin protection than non-disposable products; underpad products were slightly cheaper than body-worn products	Provide skin protection and prevent soiling of linen; polymers conduct moisture away from the skin
Antidiarrheal agents* Loperamide (Imodium) up to 16 mg/day in divided doses Diphenoxylate 5 mg q.i.d.	Constipation	Titrate dose; administer before meals and social events	↑ fecal consistency, ↓ urgency; ↑ anal sphincter tone
Enemas*	Inconvenient; side-effects of specific preparations		Rectal evacuation decreases likelihood of FI
Biofeedback therapy using anal canal pressure or surface EMG sensors;**[28] rectal balloon for modulating sensation		Prerequisites for success include motivation, intact cognition, absence of depression, and some rectal sensation	Improved rectal sensation and coordinated external sphincter contraction ± anal sphincter tone
Sphincteroplasty for sphincter defects**[29]	Wound infection; recurrent FI (delayed)	Restricted to isolated sphincter defects without denervation	Restore sphincter integrity
Sacral nerve stimulation*	Infection	Preliminary uncontrolled trials promising	Unclear; ↑ anal sphincter tone may modulate rectal sensation
Artificial sphincter, gracilis transposition**	Device erosion, failure and infection	Either artificial device or gracilis transposition with/without electrical stimulation	Restore anal barrier

*Grade A, **grade B, ***grade C therapeutic recommendations. Grades A or B are supported by at least one randomized controlled trial, or one high-quality study of non-randomized cohorts. Grade C recommendations are expert opinions generally derived from basic research, applied physiological evidence or first principles, in controlled or randomized trials. ↑ = increased; ↓ = reduced; ± = possible. Adapted from Bharucha AE, Camilleri M. GI dysmotility and sphincter dysfunction. In: Noseworthy JH, ed. *Neurological Therapeutics: Principles and Practice*. London: Martin Dunitz (in press).

Pharmacological approaches

Phenylephrine, an α_1-adrenergic agonist, applied to the anal canal increased anal resting pressure by 33% in healthy subjects and in FI. However, phenylephrine did not significantly improve incontinence scores or resting anal pressure compared with placebo in a randomized, double-blind, placebo-controlled crossover study of 36 patients with FI.[25]

Biofeedback therapy

Biofeedback is based on the principle of operant conditioning. Using a rectal balloon–anal manometry device, patients are taught to contract the external anal sphincter when they perceive balloon distension. Perception may be reinforced by visual tracings of balloon volume and anal pressure, and the procedure is repeated with progressively smaller volumes. In uncontrolled studies, continence improved in about 70% of patients with FI. Though resting and squeeze pressures increased to a variable degree after biofeedback therapy, the magnitude of improvement was relatively small and not correlated to symptom improvement.[26] Perhaps these modest effects are attributable to inadequate biofeedback therapy, lack of reinforcement, and assessment of objective parameters at an early stage after biofeedback therapy. In contrast, sensory assessments, i.e. preserved baseline sensation and improved sensory discrimination after biofeedback therapy, are more likely to be associated with improved continence after biofeedback therapy.[27]

A recent study randomized 171 FI patients to four groups: standard medical/nursing care (i.e. advice only); advice plus verbal instruction on sphincter exercises; hospital-based computer-assisted sphincter pressure biofeedback; and hospital biofeedback plus use of a home EMG biofeedback device.[28] Symptoms improved in approximately 50% of patients in all four groups, and improvement was sustained 1 year after therapy. These results underscore the importance patients attach to understanding the condition, practical advice regarding coping strategies (e.g. diet and skin care), and nurse–patient interaction.

Surgical approaches

Continence improved in up to 85% of patients with sphincter defects after an overlapping anterior sphincteroplasty. For reasons that are unclear, continence deteriorates thereafter. Less than 50% of patients are continent 5 years after the operation.[29] Dynamic graciloplasty and artificial anal sphincter procedures are restricted to a handful of centers worldwide and are

often complicated by infections and device problems which may require reoperation, including removal of the device. A colostomy is the last resort for patients with severe FI.

Minimally invasive approaches

Sacral nerve stimulation is an FDA-approved device that has been implanted in more than 3000 patients with urinary incontinence in the USA. Observations from European studies suggest that sacral nerve stimulation augments squeeze pressure more than resting pressure, may also modulate rectal sensation, and significantly improves continence.[30] Sacral stimulation is conducted as a staged procedure. Patients whose symptoms respond to temporary stimulation over about 2 weeks proceed to permanent subcutaneous implantation of the device. The procedure for device placement is technically straightforward, and device-related complications are less frequent or significant relative to more invasive artificial sphincter devices discussed above.

Rectal evacuation disorders

Pathophysiology

Rectal evacuation disorders are defined by symptoms of difficult defecation caused by a functional disorder

---

Rectal evacuation disorders: key features

1 Normal rectal evacuation involves increased intra-abdominal pressure coordinated with pelvic floor relaxation.

2 Rectal evacuation disorders are defined by symptoms of difficult defecation caused by a functional disorder of the process of rectal evacuation.

3 Most attention has focused on pelvic floor dyssynergia, i.e. impaired relaxation of the puborectalis and/or external anal sphincter during defecation. Other causes include descending perineum syndrome and inadequate propulsive forces.

4 Symptoms: excessive straining and/or anal digitation and/or sense of anorectal blockage

during defecation; sense of incomplete evacuation after defecation; infrequent defecation; hard stools.

5 A careful rectal examination is invaluable.

6 Rectal evacuation disorders cannot be distinguished from normal transit or slow transit constipation by symptoms alone.

7 Diagnostic tests: rectal balloon expulsion test (useful screening test); anal manometry; barium proctography; dynamic pelvic MRI.

8 Colonic transit is often delayed in rectal evacuation disorders.

9 Management: pelvic floor retraining by biofeedback therapy, judicious laxative use/psychological counseling if necessary.

of the process of evacuation. The terms 'anismus', 'pelvic floor dyssynergia', 'puborectalis spasm' and 'descending perineum syndrome' reflect the phenotypic spectrum of rectal evacuation disorders. Anismus reflects increased anal resting tone, while pelvic floor dyssynergia refers to failure of relaxation or paradoxical contraction of the puborectalis and/or external anal sphincter during defecation.[31] The descending perineum syndrome is a sequel of long-standing, excessive straining, which weakens the pelvic floor causing excessive perineal descent.[32] The fourth subgroup within this spectrum of rectal evacuation disorders includes patients who cannot generate the rectal forces necessary to expel stools.

Most attention has focused on pelvic floor dyssynergia or paradoxical sphincter contraction, which can be demonstrated by anal manometry, anal sphincter EMG or defecography (Fig. 13.6).[31] While paradoxical puborectalis contraction is associated with impaired rectal evacuation, the specificity of this finding has been questioned on two grounds. First, some patients with pelvic floor dyssynergia have normal rectal evacuation. Secondly, pelvic floor dyssynergia has been observed in asymptomatic subjects, and in patients with FI or pelvic pain who do not have symptoms of obstructed defecation. Given the inherent limitations of trying to replicate normal defecation in a laboratory, these inconsistencies are not surprising and they underscore the importance of considering symptoms when diagnosing rectal evacuation disorders.[33]

With the exception of Parkinson's disease and multiple sclerosis, rectal evacuation disorders are probably not caused by lesion(s) in the central nervous system. Pelvic floor dyssynergia is associated with anxiety and psychological distress. It is conceivable that psychological distress contributes to pelvic floor dyssynergia by increasing the level of skeletal muscle tension.

Up to 60% of patients with pelvic floor dyssynergia have impaired rectal sensation.[33] Since the desire to defecate is essential for initiating defecation, it is conceivable that diminished rectal sensation, perhaps attributable to a neuropathy, may cause obstructed defecation. Alternatively, reduced rectal sensation may be the result of a change in rectal capacity, or it may be

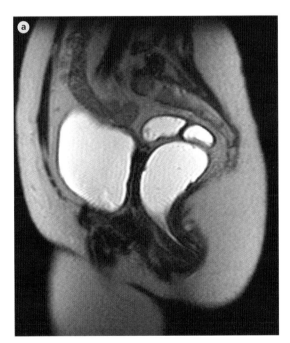
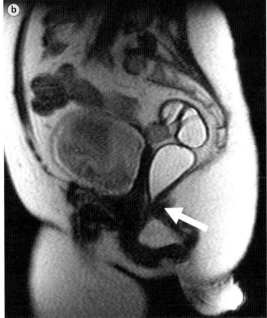

Fig. 13.6 Pelvic MR fluoroscopic images at rest (a) and evacuation (b) in a lady with obstructed defecation. Observe the increased impression of the puborectalis on the posterior rectal wall during evacuation (white arrow) compared with rest.

secondary to retained stool in the rectal vault in obstructed defecation.

Left colonic transit is delayed in up to two-thirds of patients with pelvic floor dyssynergia. It is unclear if delayed left colonic transit is secondary to activation of rectocolonic inhibitory reflexes by stool in the rectum, and/or to physical restriction to passage of stool through the colon, and/or to coexistent colonic motor dysfunction unrelated to obstructed defecation.

Rectal evacuation disorders are primarily attributed to disordered function. However, structural anomalies (e.g. rectoceles and excessive perineal descent) may coexist (Fig. 13.4). Rectoceles are relatively common in older women and infrequently obstruct defecation. On the contrary, clinically significant rectoceles often occur in patients with a primary rectal evacuation disorder and may be secondary to excessive straining.

Perineal descent during defecation is generally reduced in anismus and pelvic floor dyssynergia. However, long-standing, excessive straining can weaken the pelvic floor, causing excessive perineal descent.[32] Excessive perineal descent widens the anorectal angle and impairs the flap valve that normally maintains continence when intra-abdominal pressure increases. Excessive perineal descent has also been implicated as causing stretch-induced pudendal neuropathy. These consequences of excessive perineal descent may explain why patients with the descending perineum syndrome have constipation initially, progressing to FI later.

The mechanisms responsible for inadequate rectal propulsive forces are unclear.[34] Indeed, the relative contributions of abdominal wall motion and rectal contraction to rectal forces during normal defecation are not understood.

Clinical features

Symptoms include infrequent defecation, hard or lumpy stools, excessive straining during defecation, a sense of anal blockage during defecation, use of manual maneuvers to facilitate defecation and a sense of incomplete rectal evacuation after defecation. Anal pain during defecation and a sense of anal blockage are the only symptoms which occur more frequently in rectal evacuation disorders than in functional constipation.[35,36] However, it is not possible to discriminate between obstructed defecation, irritable bowel syndrome and slow-transit constipation based on symptoms alone. The digital anal examination is often extremely useful for confirming a clinical suspicion of obstructed defecation. The examination may reveal prominent external hemorrhoids, an anal fissure, anismus (i.e. increased resistance to passage of the index finger in the anal canal), paradoxical contraction of the puborectalis during simulated defecation, and/or abnormal (i.e. increased or reduced) perineal descent during simulated defecation.

Diagnostic tests

The Rome criteria for pelvic floor dyssynergia include evidence of impaired evacuation, adequate rectal propulsive forces and manometric, EMG or radiological evidence of paradoxical contraction, or failed relaxation of the anal sphincter during attempted defecation. The following considerations are pertinent to these assessments.

- *Increased resting anal pressure.* Though normal ranges are age-, gender- and technique-dependent, an average resting pressure greater than 100 mmHg is probably abnormal and suggestive of anismus.
- *Paradoxical increase in anal pressure during simulated defecation.* Since paradoxical anal sphincter contraction can also occur in asymptomatic subjects, test results must be considered in the overall clinical context.
- *Evacuation proctography* is useful for documenting impaired rectal evacuation, assessing the clinical significance of a rectocele and characterizing anorectal descent during simulated evacuation. Another, perhaps under-recognized, benefit of evacuation proctography is the ability to educate patients about the nature of their disorder by reviewing images with them. More recently, rapid MR imaging sequences have been developed to visualize pelvic floor motion in real time without radiation exposure.[37] The bony landmarks necessary to characterize anorectal motion are more readily visualized by MRI compared with evacuation proctography. Dynamic pelvic MRI can also evaluate urogenital and anorectal prolapse during the same examination.
- *The rectal balloon expulsion test* (Fig. 13.7). When compared with manometry and evacuation proctography, an abnormal balloon expulsion test was 88% sensitive (positive predictive value of 64%) and

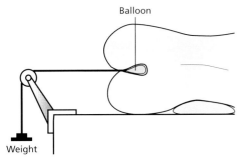

Fig. 13.7 Schematic of rectal balloon expulsion test. The subject is asked to expel a rectal balloon filled with 50 ml of warm water and connected over a pulley to a series of weights. Patients without pelvic floor dysfunction can expel the balloon with no or limited external rectal traction. Patients with pelvic floor dyssynergia require additional external traction to facilitate expulsion of the rectal balloon. Reproduced with permission from Bharucha AE, Klingele CJ. Autonomic and somatic systems to the anorectum and pelvic floor. In: Dyck PJ, Thomas PK, eds. *Peripheral Neuropathy*. 4th edn. Philadelphia: Elsevier, 2004.

89% specific (negative predictive value of 97%) for diagnosing pelvic floor dyssynergia.[36] Thus, a normal rectal balloon expulsion test is extremely useful for excluding pelvic floor dyssynergia in constipated patients.

- *Colonic transit* is often delayed in obstructed defecation. Therefore, it is necessary to exclude obstructed defecation before making a primary diagnosis of slow transit constipation in patients with delayed colonic transit (Fig. 13.6).

Management

Pelvic floor retraining by biofeedback therapy is the cornerstone for managing obstructed defecation. In uncontrolled studies, symptoms improved after pelvic floor retraining in 70% of patients with obstructed defecation; controlled studies are in progress. Pelvic floor retraining facilitates pelvic floor relaxation, and improves coordination between abdominal wall and diaphragmatic contraction and pelvic relaxation during defecation. There is limited objective evidence of improved pelvic floor function after biofeedback therapy. The specific protocols for biofeedback training vary between centers. It is important to concurrently address dietary imbalances (e.g. eating disorders) and psychological disturbances during pelvic floor retraining. Since stool size and consistency influence the ease of defecation, fiber supplements and judiciously used osmotic laxatives are often necessary.

Functional anorectal pain

The Rome diagnostic criteria have maintained the historical characterization of functional anorectal pain as levator ani syndrome and proctalgia fugax.[33] The pathophysiology of these disorders is poorly understood. The often-stated differences in the clinical features of these disorders (Table 13.7) may be blurred in clinical practice.

Acknowledgment

This work was supported in part by USPHS NIH grants RO1 HD 38666 and HD 41129.

References

1 Whitehead WE, Wald A, Norton NJ. Treatment options for fecal incontinence. *Dis Colon Rectum* 2001; **44**: 131–42 [discussion 142–4].

2 Perry S, Shaw C, McGrother C et al. Prevalence of faecal incontinence in adults aged 40 years or more living in the community. *Gut* 2002; **50**: 480–4.

3 Sun WM, Donnelly TC, Read NW. Utility of a combined test of anorectal manometry, electromyography, and sensation in determining the mechanism of 'idiopathic' faecal incontinence. *Gut* 1992; **33**: 807–13.

4 Buser WD, PB Miner Jr. Delayed rectal sensation with fecal incontinence. Successful treatment using anorectal manometry. *Gastroenterology* 1986; **91**: 1186–91.

5 Whitehead WE, Palsson OS. Is rectal pain sensitivity a biological marker for irritable bowel syndrome: psychological influences on pain perception. *Gastroenterology* 1998; **115**: 1263–71.

6 Sultan AH, Kamm MA, Hudson CN, Thomas JM, Bartram CI. Anal-sphincter disruption during vaginal delivery. *N Engl J Med* 1993; **329**: 1905–11.

7 Bharucha A. Fecal incontinence. *Gastroenterology* 2003; **124**: 1672–85.

8 Jameson JS, Chia YW, Kamm MA, Speakman CT, Chye YH, Henry MM. Effect of age, sex and parity on anorectal function. *Br J Surg* 1994; **81**: 1689–92.

9 McHugh SM, Diamant NE. Effect of age, gender, and parity on anal canal pressures. Contribution of impaired anal sphincter function to fecal incontinence. *Dig Dis Sci* 1987; **32**: 726–36.

Table 13.7 Comparison of levator ani syndrome with proctalgia fugax

Clinical feature	Levator ani syndrome	Proctalgia fugax
Prevalence	Relatively common	Extremely rare
Pathophysiology	Unclear. Has been attributed to striated muscle 'tension'	Unclear. Smooth muscle spasm has been implicated. Hereditary form associated with internal anal sphincter hypertrophy
Nature of pain	Relatively chronic, dull, deep-seated rectal pain or urgency, lasting hours	Infrequent episodes (often <5 episodes/year) of relatively sharp, intermittent anal pain lasting seconds to minutes
Tenderness to palpation of puborectalis	Often present	Absent
Diagnostic testing	$\uparrow$ resting anal pressure. Biofeedback therapy may reduce resting anal pressure and reduce pain	Unremarkable
Psychological issues	Elevated score on hypochondriasis, depression, and hysteria scales of MMPI, i.e. the 'neurotic triad' in chronic pain patients	Perfectionistic, anxious, and/or hypochondriacal traits in uncontrolled studies
Management	Uncontrolled studies – electrogalvanic stimulation, biofeedback therapy, digital massage of levator ani, sitz baths and muscle relaxants	Salbutamol inhalation abbreviated episodes in a controlled trial
		Clonidine, amyl nitrate, or nitroglycerin also suggested

$\uparrow$ = increased; $\downarrow$ = decreased; $\leftrightarrow$ = no change. MMPI, Minnesota Multiphasic Personality Inventory.

10 Fox JC, Rath-Harvey D, Helwig PS, Zinsmeister AR, Bharucha AE. Anal sphincter pressures and rectal compliance decline with aging in asymptomatic women. *Gastroenterology* 2002; **122** (Suppl.): A-69.

11 Lexell J, Taylor CC, Sjostrom M. What is the cause of the ageing atrophy? Total number, size and proportion of different fiber types studied in whole vastus lateralis muscle from 15- to 83-year-old men. *J Neurol Sci* 1988; **84**: 275–94.

12 Parellada CM, Miller AS, Williamson ME, Johnston D. Paradoxical high anal resting pressures in men with idiopathic fecal seepage. *Dis Colon Rectum* 1998; **41**: 593–7.

13 Hayne D, Vaizey CJ, Boulos PB. Anorectal injury following pelvic radiotherapy. *Br J Surg* 2001; **88**: 1037–48.

14 Nyam DC, Pemberton JH. Long-term results of lateral internal sphincterotomy for chronic anal fissure with particular reference to incidence of fecal incontinence. *Dis Colon Rectum* 1999; **42**: 1306–10.

15 Del Pino A, Nelson RL, Pearl RK, Abcarian H. Island flap anoplasty for treatment of transsphincteric fistula-in-ano. *Dis Colon Rectum* 1996; **39**: 224–6.

16 Epanomeritakis E, Koutsoumbi P, Tsiaoussis I *et al*. Impairment of anorectal function in diabetes mellitus parallels duration of disease. *Dis Colon Rectum* 1999; **42**: 1394–400.

17 Wiesel PH, Norton C, Glickman S, Kamm MA. Pathophysiology and management of bowel dysfunction in multiple sclerosis. *Eur J Gastroenterol Hepatol* 2001; **13**: 441–8.

18 Sun WM, Read NW, Donnelly TC. Anorectal function in incontinent patients with cerebrospinal disease. *Gastroenterology* 1990; **99**: 1372–9.

19 Vaizey CJ, Carapeti E, Cahill JA, Kamm MA. Prospective comparison of faecal incontinence grading systems. *Gut* 1999; **44**: 77–80.

20 Rockwood TH, Church JM, Fleshman JW *et al*. Fecal incontinence quality of life scale: quality of life instrument for patients with fecal incontinence. *Dis Colon Rectum* 2000; **43**: 9–16 [discussion 16–7].

21 Lewis SJ, Heaton KW. Stool form scale as a useful guide to intestinal transit time. *Scand J Gastroenterol* 1997; **32**: 920–4.

22 Hill J, Corson RJ, Brandon H, Redford J, Faragher EB, Kiff ES. History and examination in the assessment of patients with idiopathic fecal incontinence. *Dis Colon Rectum* 1994; **37**: 473–7.

23 American Gastroenterological Association. American Gastroenterological Association Medical Position Statement on

Anorectal Testing Techniques. *Gastroenterology* 1999; **116**: 732–60.

24 Locke GR 3rd, Pemberton JH, Phillips SF. AGA technical review on constipation. American Gastroenterological Association. *Gastroenterology* 2000; **119**: 1766–78.

25 Carapeti EA, Kamm MA, Phillips RK. Randomized controlled trial of topical phenylephrine in the treatment of faecal incontinence. *Br J Surg* 2000; **87**: 38–42.

26 Bharucha AE. Outcome measures for fecal incontinence: anorectal structure and function. *Gastroenterology* 2004; **126**: S90–8.

27 Wald A, Tunuguntla AK. Anorectal sensorimotor dysfunction in fecal incontinence and diabetes mellitus. Modification with biofeedback therapy. *N Engl J Med* 1984; **310**: 1282–7.

28 Norton C, Hosker G, Brazzelli M. Biofeedback and/or sphincter exercises for the treatment of faecal incontinence in adults. *Cochrane Database Syst Rev* 2000: CD002111.

29 Bachoo P, Brazzelli M, Grant A. Surgery for faecal incontinence in adults. *Cochrane Database of Syst Rev* 2000: CD001757.

30 Rosen HR, Urbarz C, Holzer B, Novi G, Schiessel R. Sacral nerve stimulation as a treatment for fecal incontinence. *Gastroenterology* 2001; **121**: 536–41.

31 Bharucha AE. Obstructed defecation: don't strain in vain! [comment]. *Am J Gastroenterol* 1998; **93**: 1019–20.

32 Bartolo DC, Read NW, Jarratt JA, Read MG, Donnelly TC, Johnson AG. Differences in anal sphincter function and clinical presentation in patients with pelvic floor descent. *Gastroenterology* 1983; **85**: 68–75.

33 Whitehead WE, Wald A, Diamant NE, Enck P, Pemberton JH, Rao SS. Functional disorders of the anus and rectum. *Gut* 1999; **45** (Suppl. 2): II55–9.

34 Rao SS, Welcher KD, Leistikow JS. Obstructive defecation: a failure of rectoanal coordination. *Am J Gastroenterol* 1998; **93**: 1042–50.

35 Grotz RL, Pemberton JH, Talley NJ, Rath DM, Zinsmeister AR. Discriminant value of psychological distress, symptom profiles, and segmental colonic dysfunction in outpatients with severe idiopathic constipation. *Gut* 1994; **35**: 798–802.

36 Minguez M, Herreros B, Sanchiz V *et al.* Predictive value of the balloon expulsion test for excluding the diagnosis of pelvic floor dyssynergia in constipation. *Gastroenterology* 2004; **126**: 57–62.

37 Fletcher JG, Busse RF, Riederer SJ *et al.* Magnetic resonance imaging of anatomic and dynamic defects of the pelvic floor in defecatory disorders. *Am J Gastroenterol* 2003; **98**: 399–411.

38 Miller R, Bartolo DC, Cervero F, Mortensen NJ. Anorectal sampling: a comparison of normal and incontinent patients. *Br J Surg* 1988; **75**: 44–7.

39 Caruana BJ, Wald A, Hinds JP, Eidelman BH. Anorectal sensory and motor function in neurogenic fecal incontinence. Comparison between multiple sclerosis and diabetes mellitus. *Gastroenterology* 1991; **100**: 465–70.

40 Read NW, Abouzekry L. Why do patients with faecal impaction have faecal incontinence. *Gut* 1986; **27**: 283–7.

41 Yeoh EK, Russo A, Botten R *et al.* Acute effects of therapeutic irradiation for prostatic carcinoma on anorectal function. *Gut* 1998; **43**: 123–7.

42 Varma JS, Smith AN, Busuttil A. Correlation of clinical and manometric abnormalities of rectal function following chronic radiation injury. *Br J Surg* 1985; **72**: 875–8.

43 Rao SS, Read NW, Davison PA, Bannister JJ, Holdsworth CD. Anorectal sensitivity and responses to rectal distension in patients with ulcerative colitis. *Gastroenterology* 1987; **93**: 1270–5.

CHAPTER 14

Central Nervous System Injury

Shaheen Hamdy

Introduction

It is now increasingly recognized that the central nervous system (CNS), in particular the brain, plays an important role in modulating gut function. For example, alterations in emotional state can lead to disturbed gastrointestinal symptoms such as diarrhea, dyspepsia and even abdominal pain. Furthermore, alterations in gastrointestinal motility have been described after lesions to the CNS; for instance, symptoms such as dysphagia after stroke, anal incontinence in cerebrovascular disease and multiple sclerosis, and even alterations in small bowel motility following brainstem damage.

In this chapter I will describe current knowledge of the central neural (brain to gut) control of gastrointestinal function in health and after CNS injury, focusing on two specific areas: mechanisms of swallowing and mechanisms of anal continence. In particular, I aim to bring the reader up to date with some newer concepts in relation to the neurophysiology of human cortical swallowing and anal motor function and the associated pathophysiological processes following CNS injury, including dysphagia and anal incontinence. Finally, I will look at future directions; specifically, the potential

therapies that may help in CNS disease states that disrupt the human brain–gut axis.

Mechanisms of swallowing

The physiological events of swallowing

Swallowing is commonly described as having three distinct phases: the oral phase, the pharyngeal phase and the esophageal phase.[1] It was once generally thought that the oral phase is voluntary, whereas the pharyngeal and esophageal phases are involuntary. However, it is now accepted that higher inputs can influence both these latter two phases, probably more in a modulatory capacity. Humans swallow on average once every minute, and this is supplemented by the production of saliva, which, when absent or reduced, inhibits the ability to swallow. Swallowing almost completely tails off during deep (stage 4) sleep but does occur during REM (rapid eye movement) sleep.[2] The oral phase is sometimes described as being preceded by the preparatory phase, particularly when solid or semisolid foods are ingested. Mastication and mixing with saliva occurs at this point, and the bolus is then cupped in the anterior portion of the tongue before being propelled

---

Overview

1 Brain–gut pathways play a key role in executing and modulating many gastrointestinal functions, including swallowing and anal continence.

2 CNS injury can cause profound problems in these functions, resulting in dysphagia and fecal incontinence.

3 Recent functional imaging studies have just begun to shed light on how CNS (brain) injury disrupts gastrointestinal function.

4 Novel therapies, based on these new insights, may improve the rehabilitation of dysphagia and anal incontinence

Swallowing

1 Swallowing is an essential gastrointestinal function that is under strong cerebral control.

2 Swallowing is bilaterally but asymmetrically represented in the human motor cortex.

3 Dysphagia after stroke may be a consequence of damage to the 'dominant' swallowing hemisphere.

4 Recovery of swallowing after dysphagic stroke appears to relate to compensation of function in the undamaged hemisphere.

5 Therapies that can accelerate this compensatory process may in the future help to restore swallowing function in acute stroke.

by an upward and compressing force initiated by the tongue against the hard palate to 'squeeze' the bolus into the pharynx. During this phase, the soft palate rises to seal off the nasopharynx and thus completes the oral phase, which lasts 0.6–1.2 seconds.

The pharyngeal phase typically begins as the bolus reaches the faucial pillars of the hypopharynx. Simultaneously, the larynx and hyoid bone are lifted upwards and forwards by contraction of the strap muscles of the neck. This enlarges the space available for the pharynx to receive the incoming bolus. The bolus is then propelled aborally by sequential contractions of the constrictor muscles of the pharynx, and this is associated with a reflex relaxation of the normally high-toned upper esophageal sphincter to allow passage of the bolus into the esophagus. During transport through the pharynx, respiration is momentarily halted, the swallow usually occurring during expiration. Concurrently, a protective mechanism of aryepiglottic fold closure and approximation of the arytenoid and epiglottic cartilages by contraction of the intrinsic muscles of the larynx then occurs. The whole pharyngeal phase usually takes less than 0.6 seconds.

Thus commences the esophageal phase of swallowing, which comprises a propagated peristaltic wave that propels the bolus at approximately 2–4 cm per second. As the bolus passes through the esophageal body, the lower esophageal sphincter relaxes and the bolus enters the stomach. The esophageal phase lasts between 6 and 10 seconds and the whole process of swallowing usually lasts 12 seconds in total.

The neurophysiology of swallowing

The central neural control of swallowing can be divided into essentially three basic components: an afferent system, an efferent system and a central processor and regulating system (Fig. 14.1).

The afferent system

Afferent input comes from three cranial nerves innervating the muscles of the swallowing tract. These are the trigeminal nerve, the glossopharyngeal nerve and the vagus nerve, the superior laryngeal branch of which appears to have most importance. Stimulation of any of these nerves can initiate or modulate a swallow.[3] These afferent fibers terminate centrally at the level of the brainstem in the tractus solitarius and in the nucleus of the spinal trigeminal system before converging in the nucleus of the tractus solitarius (NTS). There is, however, a second projection, which ascends via a pontine relay to the level of the cortex without transgressing the NTS.[4] The most

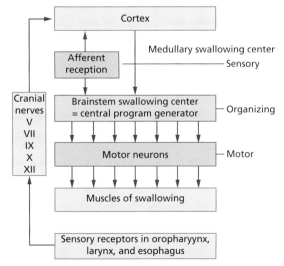

Fig. 14.1 The hierarchical organization of the central regulation of swallowing. Input from the periphery and higher centers converge onto interneurons in the brainstem swallowing center, which generates the sequenced pattern of swallowing via the bulbar motor nuclei. With kind permission from Dr N Diamant.

potent trigger for swallowing is the superior laryngeal nerve, which is matched only by direct stimulation of the nucleus of the tractus solitarius, suggesting that the solitary system is a major contributor of afferent input in swallowing.[3] Importantly, anesthesia of areas innervated by these cranial nerve afferents will disrupt, but will not necessarily completely abolish, the ability to swallow.[5] Sensation from the oral, pharyngeal and laryngeal regions includes a broad range of modalities, including two-point discrimination, vibrotactile detection, somesthetic sensitivity, proprioception, nociception, chemical sensitivity and thermal sensitivity.[6] The oral, pharyngeal and laryngeal mucosae possess an epithelium innervated by both free nerve endings and, within deeper layers, more organized sensory receptors. Of interest, there appear to be chemosensitive receptors that are specifically water-responsive and will not trigger at isotonic levels. There also appear to be different groups of cold-responsive sensory fibers that discharge at around 25–30°C. Mechanical stimuli appear to be the most effective stimuli for exciting NTS neurons within the receptive fields of the oral cavity and epiglottis. Indeed, a moving mechanical stimulus excites more neurons than a static stimulus. When comparing receptive field responsiveness within the oral cavity, it appears that mechanical stimulation is more potent than chemical stimulation, which in turn is more potent than thermal stimulation.[6]

The efferent system

The efferent system comprises motor neuron pools (consisting of the facial motor nucleus, the hypoglossal motor nucleus and the trigeminal motor nucleus) and the vagal motor nuclei (which comprise the nucleus ambiguus and the dorsal motor nucleus of the vagus). Inputs from the brainstem central pattern generator and from suprabulbar regions impinge on these motor nuclei in a manner which synergistically produces the swallow. The cranial motor nuclei mentioned above have subdivisions based on the motor neurons innervating specific muscles. The facial motor nucleus is involved with the labial muscles, for which there are several functions both in swallowing and speech as well as chewing. The hypoglossal nucleus contains the motor neurons innervating the intrinsic and extrinsic muscles of the tongue, which are involved in numerous motor functions, including speech, respiration, licking

and mastication as well as swallowing. The trigeminal motor nucleus contains the motor neuron pools that innervate the mandibular muscles and can be divided into four nuclei that appear to develop at different times during development in the fetus.[6] The nucleus ambiguus is also subdivided into at least four layers: the compact layer, semicompact layer, the loose layer and the external formation. These motor neurons innervate the palatal, pharyngeal, laryngeal and esophageal muscles. Finally, the dorsal motor nucleus of the vagus contains neurons that innervate the esophagus and portions of the proximal gastrointestinal tract. It appears that the earliest motor neuron to develop during swallowing in the fetus is probably the hypoglossal nerve,[6] as tongue activities are present in the fetus at about the same time as the jaw-opening reflex. Indeed, by the eleventh week of development of the human fetus the first pharyngeal motor responses can also be detected.

Whilst lesions to the facial motor nucleus do not implicitly result in dysphagia, lesions to the nucleus ambiguus and, to a lesser extent, the hypoglossal and trigeminal motor nuclei result in more significant dysphagic symptoms.[6] Thus, as a result of input from the NTS and higher centers to the dorsal region of the medulla and the brainstem swallowing center, motoneurons in this region will provide the patterned sequential discharge that activates the oral, pharyngeal and esophageal phases of swallowing.

The central processing and regulatory systems

Brainstem swallowing centre

Much of the research pertaining to the central regulation of human swallowing has focused on the issue of the brainstem swallowing center. This important region is central to the regulation of swallowing in humans and is distributed within the reticular formation just dorsal to the inferior olive, either side of the midline in the medulla.[7] It is believed that this network of neurons and interneurons integrates incoming information from other levels, both central and peripheral, before activating a preprogrammed sequence of responses which then dictate the pattern of swallowing. The concept of a central pattern generator within the brainstem is supported by the fact that, even after disruption of both afferent and efferent fibers to this region, the pattern of swallowing remains essentially unchanged when studied in animals.[7]

It appears that the circuitry of the central pattern generator has different populations of interneurons responsible for the different temporal stages of swallowing. These interneurons have been termed 'early', 'late' and 'very late' neurons, which closely correspond to their muscular counterparts within the oropharynx, lower pharynx and striated muscle portion of the esophagus, and the smooth muscle esophagus, respectively.[8] Functionally, it appears that the brainstem swallowing center can be divided into two divisions: a dorsal medullary region and a ventral medullary region. The dorsal medullary region provides the neurons that initiate the sequential activity of swallowing and can be defined as generating neurons. The ventral medullary region, which includes an area around the nucleus ambiguus, appears to play a switching role in modifying and activating the motor neuron pools controlling swallowing output. Between these two regions there is a short interneuronal network that has both excitatory and inhibitory components and relays information from the dorsal region to the ventral region.

Within both regions of the medulla there are a number of neurotransmitter substances that appear to have relevant roles;[9] for example, the injection of glutamate into the dorsal region of the brainstem evokes pharyngeal swallowing, suggesting that it is excitatory. By comparison, injection of dopamine or norepinephrine appears to inhibit the elicitation of pharyngeal swallowing. It also appears likely that γ-aminobutyric acid, acetylcholine, N-methyl D-aspartate and nitric oxide probably play important roles in the inhibitory and excitatory regulation of swallowing.

In addition to the medullary brainstem swallowing center, there appears to be a separate area within the pontine reticular formation which will also, when stimulated, evoke swallowing. This region, when stimulated at low intensity, will evoke both swallowing and rhythmic jaw movements, but when stimulated at high intensity results in more inhibitory effects. It is likely that pathways from the afferent innervation of swallowing project to this region as well as to the medullary area on their way to the anterolateral cortex. Activation of the pontine region may in fact result in a transcortical reflex to evoke the swallow, rather than the pontine area being directly involved in the initiation of swallowing.

Suprabulbar regions influencing swallowing

There is extensive experimental evidence to support the role of subcortical structures in the control and modulation of swallowing.[10] These regions can be anatomically divided into the hindbrain (comprising the cerebellum), the midbrain (comprising the substantia nigra and the ventral tegmentum) and the basal forebrain (comprising the hypothalamus, amygdala and basal ganglia). In animals, activation of all these sites has been shown to facilitate the swallow response when combined with either superior laryngeal nerve stimulation or cortical stimulation. Evidence from human studies also suggests an important contribution from subcortical areas, for example, dysphagia is a common consequence of Parkinson's disease.[11] This would imply an important role for the basal ganglia in regulating swallowing[11] Indeed, in a recent functional imaging study of human swallowing it was demonstrated that areas including the left amygdala and the left cerebellum, as well as the dorsal brainstem, show increased regional cerebral blood flow during volitional swallowing.[12] The lateralized nature of these activations was of interest and supported the possibility that swallowing displays significant interhemispheric asymmetry in its motor control.

The cerebral cortex has been strongly implicated in the control of swallowing, since numerous investigators have observed that stimulation of the cerebral cortex, both in animals and humans, can elicit the full swallow sequence.[13–14] The areas implicated in these studies seem to be the dorsolateral and anterolateral frontal cortex as well as the premotor cortex, the frontal operculum and also the insula. In fact, much of the information regarding the cerebral localization of human swallowing has relied on inference from studies of swallowing abnormalities following cerebral injury.[15–17] From these reports, a rather diffuse picture has emerged of those areas of the brain considered important; for example, lesions located in the thalamus, pyramidal tracts, frontal operculum and the insula have all been associated with dysphagia. More recently, functional imaging has also established a clear role for the lateral sensorimotor cortex, in particular the right insula, during the process of swallowing.[12,18] More information has come from studies using transcranial magnetic stimulation (TMS) of the human precentral gyrus in understanding the cortical control of swallowing.[19–21] TMS uses a very short, rapidly changing magnetic field to induce electric current in the brain beneath the stimulator. These studies usually employ single shocks given several seconds apart, and after stimulation the cortical evoked motor response can be recorded as electromyographic activity from electrodes housed within an intraluminal catheter inserted into pharynx and esophagus. Following cortical stimulation, the type of response observed is usually a simple electromyographic (EMG) potential which has a latency of about 8–10 milliseconds, compatible with a fairly direct and rapidly conducting pathway from the cortex to the muscle (Fig. 14.2). During these TMS mapping studies the projections to the various swallowing muscles were demonstrated to be somatotopically arranged in the motor strip with the oral muscles most lateral and the pharynx and esophagus more medial. A more interesting finding from a large group of healthy subjects studied was that in most individuals the projection from one hemisphere tended to be larger than

that from the other, suggesting an asymmetrical representation of swallowing between the two hemispheres, independent of handedness. These findings have also been validated with functional imaging techniques such as positron emission tomography (PET) and functional magnetic resonance imaging (fMRI), where cerebral lateralization has been also observed.[12,18,22] These functional imaging studies have, however, identified a number of other cortical areas associated with swallowing, including the anterior cingulate cortex, the premotor cortex (including the supplementary motor cortex), the insular cortex, the frontal opercular cortex and the temporal cortex (Fig. 14.3). Taken together, these observations suggest that swallow-related cortical activity is multidimensional, recruiting brain areas implicated in the processing of motor, sensory and, presumably, attention/affective aspects of the task.

Swallowing dysfunction (dysphagia) after central nervous system injury

Difficulty in swallowing can occur as a consequence of disease of either the anatomical structures involved in

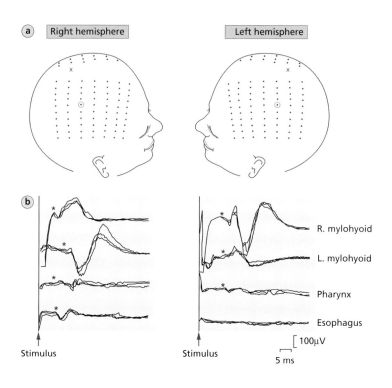

Fig. 14.2 (a) Schematic representations of the sites of stimulation on the scalp grid in relation to the head surface. The cranial vertex is marked by X. (b) Cortically evoked EMG responses recorded in one normal subject from right mylohyoid muscle, left mylohyoid muscle, pharynx and esophagus after transcranial magnetic stimulation of the right and left hemispheres are shown below. The sites of stimulation on the grid from which these responses were obtained are indicated in (a) by the open circles. Responses to three stimuli are superimposed to show reproducibility. The pharyngeal and esophageal responses obtained from the right hemisphere are larger than those from the left hemisphere. *Onset of EMG response. Redrawn with kind permission from *Nature Magazine*.

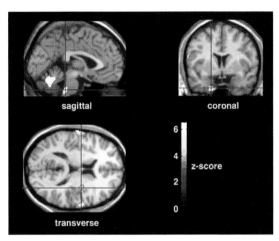

Fig. 14.3 Cerebral representation of human swallowing shown in PET images rendered onto brain MRI sections. Activations can be seen in the bilateral sensorimotor cortex, right insula, left amygdala, cerebellum and brainstem. Reproduced with kind permission from *J Neurophysiol*.

swallowing or, more commonly, of the CNS controlling swallowing (neurogenic dysphagia). The anatomical problems that disrupt swallowing are myriad and include almost any gastrointestinal disease process that affects the oral cavity through to the duodenum. It is therefore important to exclude any intrinsic disease of the gut before making a diagnosis of neurogenic dysphagia in someone presenting with symptoms of swallowing difficulty.

There are many neurological conditions that can disrupt swallowing, including diseases of the muscle or neuromuscular junction or the peripheral nerves, and those affecting the central swallowing centers (Table 14.1).

In addition, it is important to recognize that any pharmacological agent that alters neuromuscular function can produce dysphagia. It is beyond the scope of this chapter to go into detail about the many neurological conditions that can affect swallowing, and for the rest of this section I will discuss the clinical consequences and underlying mechanisms related to dysphagia following cerebrovascular disease, specifically stroke.

Injury to swallowing areas of the motor cortex and/or their connections to the brainstem will usually result in problems with swallowing (dysphagia). The commonest reason for dysphagia in the UK is now stroke. Traditionally, it had been assumed that only strokes producing brainstem or bilateral cortical damage are associated with dysphagia. However, over the last 30 years it has been increasingly recognized that unilateral cerebral lesions can also cause dysphagia.[24–26] Up to half of all stroke patients experience dysphagia, which is associated with life-threatening complications of pulmonary aspiration and malnutrition. Dysphagia leads to increased length of stay in hospital and greater demands on health service resources.

Diagnosing dysphagia after cerebral injury can be difficult and therefore requires a high level of clinical suspicion. The pattern of disordered swallowing after stroke is usually a combination of oral and pharyngeal abnormalities – typically, delayed swallow reflex with pooling or stasis of residue in the hypopharynx associated with reduced pharyngeal peristalsis and weak tongue control, but occasionally esophageal abnormalities may be apparent. This, in combination with a delay in airway closure, can result in significant aspiration of foods and consequent pneumonia.

Mechanism of dysphagia after cerebral injury

While it is relatively easy to appreciate the mechanisms behind dysphagia following bilateral cortical stroke or brainstem disease, the mechanism underlying dysphagia after unilateral cerebral injury, particularly after hemispheric damage, has remained unclear. Possibilities include occult disease in the unaffected

Table 14.1 Causes of swallowing problems after CNS injury

Neuromuscular junction/muscle disease
Polymyositis
Myasthenia gravis
Muscular dystrophies

Peripheral nerve disease
Guillain–Barré syndrome
Polio
Diphtheria

Central swallowing center disease/injury
Stroke and head injuries
Motor neuron disease
Parkinson's disease
Multiple sclerosis

hemisphere, cerebral edema leading to pressure on the adjacent hemisphere or brainstem, and the possibility that swallowing, like speech, may show significant cerebral lateralization. Indeed, in a transcranial magnetic stimulation (TMS) study of the projections from both hemispheres to the swallowing musculature in a large series of pure unilateral hemispheric stroke patients, half of whom had dysphagia, it was observed that while stimulation of the damaged hemisphere produced little or no response in either dysphagic or non-dysphagic patients, stimulation of the undamaged hemisphere evoked much larger responses in the non-dysphagic than in the dysphagic subjects.[26] The conclusion from this study was that the size of the hemispheric projection of the undamaged side to swallowing muscles determined the presence or absence of dysphagia, with the implication that dysphagia would occur if damage had affected the side of the brain with the largest or dominant projection. This observation supported the concept that swallowing is lateralized within the cerebral cortex.

Mechanisms of recovery of swallowing after cerebral injury

Given sufficient time, a large proportion of dysphagic stroke patients eventually recover the ability to swallow.[23] However, the mechanism for this recovery, seen in as many as 90% of the initially dysphagic stroke patients, has remained controversial. In a recent study of stroke using TMS, both dysphagic and non-dysphagic patients were serially mapped over several months while swallowing recovered.[27] The findings of this study showed that the area of pharyngeal representation in the undamaged hemisphere increased markedly in patients who recovered, while there was no change in patients who had persistent dysphagia or in patients who were non-dysphagic (Fig. 14.4). Furthermore, no changes were seen in the damaged hemisphere in any of the groups of patients. These observations imply that, over a period of weeks, the recovery of swallowing after stroke depends on compensatory reorganization in the undamaged hemisphere.

Mechanisms of anal continence

The anal sphincter is a midline muscular structure at the terminus of the gastrointestinal tract that functions to

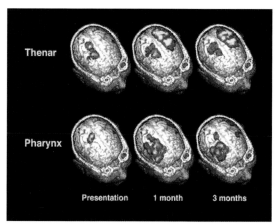

Fig. 14.4 Surface-rendered MRI brain images from a patient after left-sided hemispheric stroke. Topographic data from transcranial magnetic stimulation of the pharyngeal and contralateral thenar muscles are coregistered. The patient was dysphagic at presentation but had recovered swallowing at 1 month. It is evident that, after stroke, the representation of the pharynx in the anterior aspect of the motor cortex and premotor areas expands anterolaterally in the right, unaffected hemisphere at both 1 and 3 months, with little change in the affected left hemisphere. In contrast, the representation of the thenar muscles in the superior motor cortex increases anteriorly and posteriorly in the affected left hemisphere over time, but remains unchanged in the unaffected right hemisphere. Reproduced with kind permission from *Gastroenterology*.

maintain fecal continence. It has two components, the internal sphincter and the external sphincter. Whereas the internal anal sphincter consists of circular smooth muscle and is innervated predominantly by autonomic fibers from the pelvic plexus and sacral spinal cord, the external sphincter is of striated muscle and is innervated by the somatic fibers of the second, third and fourth sacral segments via the pudendal nerve. The neural control of anal continence therefore has sensorimotor contributions from both intrinsic and extrinsic reflexes, the former predominantly via myenteric interaction within the internal anal sphincter and the latter via strong descending volitional interactions with the motor neurons innervating the external anal sphincter.[28]

The neurophysiology of anal continence

Anal continence is an important physiological and socially essential gastrointestinal function, and is regulated by sensorimotor interactions within the anal sphincter and pelvic floor. In particular, contraction of the anal sphincter serves to increase anal canal pressure both voluntarily when the urge to defecate becomes strong and via more involuntary reflexes (for instance, during coughing) when intra-abdominal pressure suddenly rises. In either case, the cerebral cortex is able to modulate this activity via powerful descending inputs to the pelvic plexus and sacral nerves, so that defecation can be resisted until a socially convenient opportunity arises. The importance of cortical influences in the control of the external anal sphincter is well recognized; direct stimulation of the most medial motor cortex adjacent to the interhemispheric fissure will induce anal sphincter contractions.[29] More recent experiments in humans have shown that the corticofugal pathways to the external anal sphincter can be studied non-invasively by recording the electromyographic and manometric responses evoked in response to transcranial electric and magnetic stimulation of the motor cortex.[30,31] These studies have suggested that the motor cortical representation of anal sphincter function is bilateral and, as with swallowing, may display interhemispheric asymmetry (Fig. 14.5).

The peripheral innervation of the external anal sphincter comes from the pudendal nerve. Anatomical and electrophysiological studies of the innervation of the external anal sphincter in animals has shown that most of the pudendal projections to and from the external anal sphincter are centrally organized to spinal segments L6 to S3, the majority with the S1, S2 segments (Fig. 14.6).[32] Furthermore, the motor neurons innervating the external anal sphincter are particularly located in the dorsomedial and ventromedial divisions of Onuf's nucleus in the ventral horn of the spinal cord, while the afferent axonal projections appear to cluster within the marginal zone, intermediate gray and dorsal gray surrounding the gracile nucleus of the dorsal column and lamina 1, around the dorsal horn of the spinal cord. Of interest is the observation that, while there is clear unilateral spinal predominance of these projections during retrograde tracing studies of a single nerve, in both the efferent and afferent pathways there is contralateral axonal connectivity across the midline, suggesting degrees of bilateral convergence. Indeed, in a recent study of pudendal nerve function it was found in a number of healthy volunteers that the evoked muscle potential to pudendal nerve stimu-

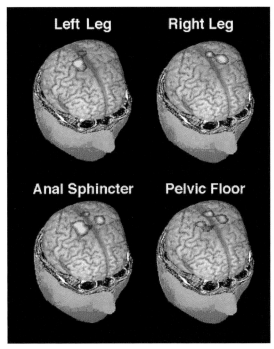

Fig. 14.5 Surface-rendered MRI brain images from a healthy subject. Transcranial magnetic stimulation topographic data of the anorectal and leg muscles are coregistered. It can be seen that the anal sphincter and pelvic floor have representations in the medial motor cortex adjacent to the leg areas. Reproduced with kind permission from *Gastroenterology*.

lation can be quite asymmetrical between the two sides.[33] Furthermore, when pudendal or even lumbar sacral stimulation was used to condition the peripheral pathway, cortical stimulation of the anal region of the motor strip induced much greater responses in the anal sphincter compared with no conditioning.[34] Importantly, stimulation of the pudendal nerve on the side with a larger response induced significantly more facilitation of the cortico-anal pathway than stimulation of the pudendal nerve on the side with the smaller response. This suggests that there may indeed be some functional asymmetry in the pudendal pathways to the anal sphincter, possibly in conjunction with asymmetry at higher levels.

Anal incontinence after CNS Injury

Anal incontinence is a distressing complication of disease of the CNS; for example, injury to the pelvic nerves, as in instrumental delivery at childbirth, will

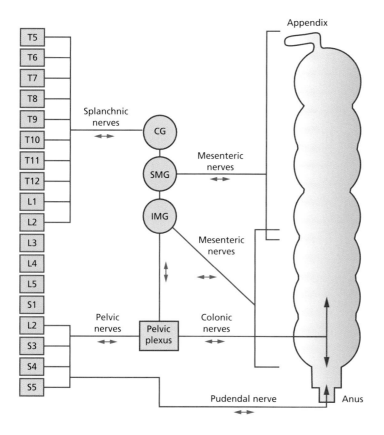

Fig. 14.6 Extrinsic innervation of the colon, rectum and anal sphincter. It can be seen that the anal sphincter is predominantly innervated by the pudendal nerve, which in turn receives its spinal innervation from segments S2–S4. CG, celiac ganglion. SMG, superior mesenteric ganglion. IMG, inferior mesenteric ganglion.

result in significant anal sphincter dysfunction, as well as the disruption of the brain–gut axis from cortex to sphincter seen in conditions such as stroke, multiple sclerosis and spinal injury. In the case of instrumental delivery, anal incontinence has been attributed to pudendal nerve damage. A number of studies have shown clear abnormalities in pudendal nerve function (determined by prolonged nerve conduction terminal latency) in incontinent female patients after vaginal delivery, both with and without instrumental intervention.[35] It is important to mention at this stage that more detailed evaluation of these patients often reveals underlying anatomical defects of the external sphincter as a consequence of the delivery, which also explains the incontinence in many cases.[36] Nonetheless, electrophysiological assessment of pudendal nerve function remains of some importance, as this parameter may be clinically relevant in differentiating patients with fecal leakage from those with solid stool incontinence. There are patients without external anal sphincter defects

who have significant continence problems and whose only demonstrable abnormality is that of pudendal neuropathy.

Fecal incontinence can present in the setting of CNS damage, such as in patients with stroke or frontal lobe damage. For example, it has been demonstrated that fecal incontinence is strongly associated with larger strokes, particularly when the cerebral cortex is involved.[37] Fecal incontinence is also frequently encountered in patients with multiple sclerosis, and one survey of anorectal function in subjects with multiple sclerosis has suggested that there may be central motor mechanisms involved.[38]

Rehabilitation of gastrointestinal dysfunction after CNS injury

The role of sensory stimulation

Modulation of sensory input may also play a central role in sensorimotor cortical plasticity and consequently in neurorehabilitation. Given this effect, Hamdy and colleagues wondered whether modifications of the technique might allow changes in sensory input to drive long-term changes in the motor cortex organization of human swallowing.[39] Evidence for such an effect would have clear relevance for the rehabilitation of dysphagia after CNS injury.

In this study, a 10-minute train of electrical stimuli was applied to the pharynx at a just perceived intensity using a pair of intraluminal electrodes. Motor cortex projections to the pharynx were measured before and after this conditioning input, using TMS. The authors found that, after the pharyngeal input, corticopharyngeal evoked responses were increased for 30 minutes after pharyngeal stimulation, without changes in brainstem reflexes or in responses evoked in response to transcranial electrical stimulation. The implication was that short-term (sensory) stimuli could induce longer-term changes in motor cortical excitability, providing evidence for a driven cross-system effect to increase input. More recent work has suggested that the direction of these changes in the swallowing motor cortex is highly dependent on the frequency, intensity and duration of the stimulus used. Fraser and colleagues showed that, while medium- to low-frequency stimulation ≤ 10 Hz was excitatory, high-frequency pharyngeal stimulation (>10 Hz) resulted in long-lasting cortical inhibition and a reduction in the pharyngeal motor map.[40] In addition, the stronger the stimulation the more pronounced the effect. However, 20 minutes of stimulation appeared no better than 10 minutes.

Sensory-induced plasticity and changes in gastrointestinal function

While evidence from swallowing appears to show a clear effect of sensory stimulation on motor cortex organization, the critical question remains: can sensory-induced plasticity alter gastrointestinal (motor) function? In another study by Fraser and colleagues, fMRI was used to demonstrate that the patterns of pharyngeal input that are associated with enhanced swallowing motor cortical excitability could alter the recruitment pattern of cortical activations associated with the task of swallowing.[40] The group was able to show that pharyngeal stimulation resulted in functionally stronger, bilateral cortical (sensorimotor) activation in areas related to swallowing (Fig. 14.3).

The effects of pharyngeal stimulation have been investigated recently in acute dysphagic stroke patients.[40] The application of 10 minutes of 5 Hz of pharyngeal electrical stimulation at 75% of that maximally tolerated by the patient was used. The stimulation resulted in a long-term (60 minutes) increase in swallowing corticobulbar excitability, predominantly within the undamaged but not the damaged hemisphere. Critically, this was strongly associated with an improvement in swallowing using videofluoroscopy (the standard marker of swallowing performance) during the same time frame.[40] The exciting implication from these results is that that sensory input to the human adult brain can be programmed to promote beneficial changes in plasticity that result in an improvement in gastrointestinal (swallowing) function after cerebral injury. While the more long-term (days to weeks) effects of this approach still need to be established, the observations hold great promise for future treatment strategies.

Repetitive transcranial magnetic stimulation and gastrointestinal function

Repetitive TMS (rTMS) is a non-invasive method capable of producing long-lasting alterations in cortical properties. The accepted maxim is that fast-rate stimulation (5 Hz and above) increases cortical excitability, whereas slow-rate stimulation (1 Hz) reduces cortical excitability.[41]

Following on from the effects of sensory stimulation, the question of whether such changes could be produced by more direct methods of cortical stimulation became intriguing. Thus, to evaluate rTMS as a potential tool for influencing this process, Gow and colleagues examined the effects of limited trains of fast-rate rTMS (5 Hz) on the dominant swallowing motor cortex. In assessing the 'dose' of rTMS to be administered, they chose a frequency of 5 Hz as this had been shown to be optimal for upregulating cortical excitability after afferent stimulation. The effect of active 5 Hz rTMS to the dominant pharyngeal motor cortex was thus compared with a sham procedure, which used an anterior coil tilt. Active stimulation resulted in a significant increase in cortical excitability that lasted more than 1 hour after stimulation.[42] This effect was not noted for the sham procedure. The magnitude of this effect is not as great as that produced by pharyngeal electrical stimulation, which is probably related to the fact that the sensory projection provides a more associative input to M1 than rTMS at the scalp. Although these rTMS data are only available in healthy subjects, there is sufficient promise to proceed to investigate the effect in dysphagic stroke patients.

Neurostimulation may also play a role in anal continence after CNS injury. For example, lumbosacral stimulation, which normally induces sphincter contraction in the external anal sphincter, might be able to condition the anal sphincter muscles in a way that aids anal function in patients with fecal incontinence. Sacral nerve stimulation has been successfully applied to patients with intractable fecal incontinence of multiple etiologies.[43]

Conclusions

Gastrointestinal function is highly dependent on extrinsic neural control. Following CNS injury a number of gastrointestinal functions can be dysregulated, and in many cases they become completely dysfunctional. Human swallowing and anal continence are two highly dependent functions, which, when disrupted by CNS injury, can be devastating for the sufferer. The application of newer neurophysiological methods has just begun to shed light on these important mechanisms, both in health and disease. These observations also provide a window of opportunity for potential therapeutic options, including neurostimulation to rehabilitate dysfunctional swallowing and anal control, with the promise of improved clinical management of these vital functions.

References

1   Kennedy JG, Kent RD. Physiological substrates of normal deglutition. *Dysphagia* 1988; **3**: 24–37.

2   Lichter J, Muir RC. The pattern of swallowing during sleep. *Electroencephalogr Clin Neurophysiol* 1975; **38**: 427–32.

3   Miller AJ. Deglutition. *Physiol Rev* 1982; **52**: 129–84.

4   Car A, Jean A, Roman C. A pontine primary relay for ascending projections of the superior laryngeal nerve. *Exp Brain Res* 1975; **22**: 197–210.

5   Mansson I, Sandberg N. Effects of surface anaesthesia on deglutition in man. *Laryngoscope* 1974; **84**: 427–37.

6   Miller AJ. *The Neuroscientific Principles of Swallowing and Dysphagia*. San Diego: Singular Publishing Group, 1999.

7   Jean A. Brainstem control of swallowing: localisation and organisation of central pattern generator for swallowing. In: Taylor A, ed. *Neurophysiology of the Jaws and Teeth*. London: MacMillan Press, 1990: 294–321.

8   Jean A. Brainstem organisation of the swallowing network. *Brain Behav Evolution* 1984; **25**: 109–16.

9   Bieger D. Central nervous system control mechanisms of swallowing: a neuropharmacological perspective. *Dysphagia* 1993; **8**: 308–10.

10 Bieger D, Hockman CH. Suprabulbar modulation of reflex swallowing. *Exp Neurol* 1976; **52**: 311–24.

11 Bernheimer H, Birkmayer H, Hornykiewicz R. Brain dopamine and the syndromes of Parkinson and Huntington: clinical, morphological and neurochemical correlations. *J Neurol Sci* 1973; **20**: 415–55.

12 Hamdy S, Rothwell JC, Brooks DJ, Bailey DL, Aziz Q, Thompson DG. Identification of the cerebral loci processing human swallowing using H_2O^{15} PET activation. *J Neurophysiol* 1999; **81**: 1917–26.

13 Martin RE, Sessle BJ. The role of the cerebral cortex in swallowing. *Dysphagia* 1993; **8**: 195–202.

14 Penfield W, Boldery E. Somatic motor and sensory representation in the cerebral cortex of man as studied by electrical stimulation. *Brain* 1937; **60**: 389–443.

15 Veis SL, Logemann JA. Swallowing disorders in persons with cerebrovascular accident. *Arch Phys Med Rehabil* 1985; **66**: 372–5.

16 Gordon C, Langton-Hewer R, Wade DT. Dysphagia in acute stroke. *Br Med J* 1987; **295**: 411–14.

17 Horner J, Massey EW. Silent aspiration following stroke. *Neurology* 1988; **38**: 317–19.

18 Hamdy S, Mikulis DJ, Crawley A *et al*. Cortical activation during human volitional swallowing: an event related fMRI study. *Am J Physiol* 1999; **277**: G219–25.

19 Hamdy S, Aziz Q, Rothwell JC *et al*. The cortical topography of human swallowing musculature in health and disease. *Nat Med* 1996; **2**: 1217–24.

20 Hamdy S, Aziz Q, Rothwell JC, Hobson A, Barlow J, Thompson DG. Cranial nerve modulation of human cortical swallowing motor pathways. *Am J Physiol* 1997; **272**: G802–8.

21 Hamdy S, Rothwell JC. Gut feelings about recovery after stroke: the organisation and reorganisation of human swallowing motor cortex. *Trends Neurosci* 1998; **21**: 268–72.

22 Zald DH, Pardo JV. The functional neuroanatomy of voluntary swallowing. *Ann Neurol* 1999; **46**: 281–6.

23 Barer DG. The natural history and functional consequences of dysphagia after hemispheric stroke. *J Neurol Neurosurg Psychiatry* 1989; **52**: 236–41.

24 Meadows J. Dysphagia in unilateral cerebral lesions. *J Neurol Neurosurg Psychiatry* 1973; **36**: 853–60.

25 Daniels SK, Foundas AL. The role of the insular cortex in dysphagia. *Dysphagia* 1997; **12**: 146–56.

26 Hamdy S, Aziz Q, Rothwell JC *et al.* Explaining oropharyngeal dysphagia after unilateral hemispheric stroke. *Lancet* 1997; **350**: 686–92.

27 Hamdy S, Aziz Q, Rothwell JC et al. Recovery of swallowing after dysphagic stroke relates to functional reorganisation in intact motor cortex. *Gastroenterology* 1998; **5**: 1104–12.

28 Christensen J. Motility of the colon. In: Johnson LR, ed. *Physiology of the Gastrointestinal Tract.* New York: Raven, 1983; 445–72.

29 Leyton ASF, Sherrington CS. Observations on the excitable cortex of the chimpanzee, orangutan and gorilla. Q J Exp Physiol 1917; **11**: 135–222.

30 Merton PA, Morton HB, Hill DK, Marsden CD. Scope of a technique for electrical stimulation of the human brain, spinal cord and muscle. *Lancet* 1982; **2**: 597–600.

31 Turnbull GK, Hamdy S, Aziz Q, Singh KD, Thompson DG. The cortical topography of human ano-rectal musculature. *Gastroenterology* 1999; **117**: 32–9.

32 Thor KB, Morgan C, Nadelhaft I, Houston M, De Groat WC. Organization of afferent and efferent pathways in the pudendal nerve of the female cat. *J Comp Neurol* 1989; **288**: 263–79.

33 Hamdy, S, Enck P, Aziz Q, Uengorgil S, Hobson A, Thompson DG. Laterality effects of human pudendal nerve stimulation on cortico-anal pathways: evidence for functional asymmetry. *Gut* 1999; **45**: 58–63.

34 Hamdy S, Enck P, Aziz Q et al. Spinal and pudendal nerve modulation of human cortico-anal motor pathways. *Am J Physiol* 1998; **274**: G419–23.

35 Snooks SJ, Setchell M, Swash M, Henry MM. Injury to innervation of pelvic floor musculature in childbirth. *Lancet* 1984; **2**: 546–50.

36 Sultan AH, Kamm MA, Hudson CN, Thomas JM, Bartram CI. Anal sphincter disruption during vaginal delivery. *N Engl J Med* 1993; **329**: 1905–11.

37 Nakayama H, Jorgensen HS, Pedersen PM, Raaschou HO, Olsen TS. Prevalence and risk factors of incontinence after stroke. *Stroke* 1997; **28**: 58–62.

38 Jameson JS, Rogers J, Chia YW, Misiewicz JJ, Henry MM, Swash M. Pelvic floor function in multiple sclerosis. *Gut* 1994; **35**: 388–90.

39 Hamdy S, Rothwell JC, Aziz Q, Singh KD, Thompson DG. Long-term reorganisation of human motor cortex driven by short-term sensory stimulation. *Nat Neurosci* 1998; **1**: 64–8.

40 Fraser C, Power M, Hamdy S *et al.* Driving plasticity in adult human motor cortex improves functional performance after cerebral injury. *Neuron* 2002; **34**: 831–40.

41 Pascual Leone A, Valls Sole J, Wassermann EM, Hallett M. Responses to rapid-rate transcranial magnetic stimulation of the human motor cortex. *Brain* 1994; **117**: 847–58.

42 Gow D, Rothwell J, Hobson A, Thompson D, Hamdy S. Induction of long-term plasticity in human swallowing motor cortex following repetitive cortical stimulation. *Clin Neurophysiol* 2004; **115**: 1044–51.

43 Rosen HR, Urbarz C, Holzer B, Novi G, Schiessel R. Sacral nerve stimulation as a treatment for fecal incontinence. *Gastroenterology* 2001; **121**: 536–41.

CHAPTER 15

Diarrhea-Predominant Bowel Disorders Following Inflammation and Infection

Robin Spiller

Overview

Diarrhea is a stereotypical response to a wide range of insults characterized by frequent passage of loose or watery stools, often with urgency and colicy abdominal pains. These features reflect increased intestinal fluid secretion, decreased absorption and motor patterns which accelerate transit. As an acute response to infection or inflammation, it has obvious benefit in expelling pathogenic bacteria or toxins. Normally, the process is rapidly self-limiting, ceasing within a few days. However, if the reparative processes fail and the diarrhoeal state persists long after the original insult has passed, then it becomes a disorder requiring treatment. These disorders seen after infection and inflammation will be the subject of this chapter.

Mechanisms of acute infective diarrhea

Infective gastroenteritis is characterized by the rapid onset of abdominal pain, nausea, vomiting and diarrhea, which involve both secretory and motor responses together with inflammation. The relative importance of the secretory and inflammatory responses varies. Cholera is an example of a predominantly secretory diarrhea, while shigellosis and *Campylobacter* enteritis are examples of inflammatory diarrhea. *Vibrio cholerae* induces intestinal secretion by its toxin (CT), which irreversibly switches on en-

---

Key points

Acute diarrhea is a stereotyped response to infection and inflammation.
Mechanisms include increased:
- mucosal secretion
- propulsive motor patterns
- increased visceral sensitivity

Symptoms include:
- abdominal cramps
- frequent loose stools
- urgency

Persistent symptoms may be due to:
- continuing inflammation
- impaired mucosal absorption (Na$^+$, Cl$^-$, water, bile acids)
- persistent enterochromaffin hyperplasia and increased availability of serotonin
- alterations in enteric nerves

Chronic bowel dysfunction can be seen following:
- bacterial gastroenteritis
- acute flare in colitis/ileitis
- acute diverticulitis

terocyte adenyl cyclase (for a review of this and other toxins see Fasano).[1]

Neural amplifier

The effect of CT is amplified markedly by stimulating enteroendocrine cells to release serotonin, which then acts presynaptically to enhance neurotransmitter release and amplify secretomotor reflexes. Similarly, *Rotavirus* toxin and many other pathogens activate mucosal nerves to induce widespread secretion.[2] Neural amplification occurs with all inflammation via the release of sensitizing agents, such as prostaglandins, tachykinins, nerve growth factor and serotonin.[3]

Inflammatory tissue damage

While cholera is associated with only minor inflammation *Campylobacter*, *Salmonella* and *Shigella* infections produce marked mucosal damage, particularly in the terminal ileum and right colon, followed by healing and remodeling. This involves the ingrowth of blood vessels and regenerating nerves together with repopulation of the crypt from the stem cells, with increased production of enteroendocrine cells containing serotonin.[4] Mucosal lymphocytes increase, as does the local production of protective IgA immunoglobulin. The remodeled mucosa has altered function, which will be the focus of this chapter.

Motility patterns associated with acute infectious diarrhea

The general pattern in inflammation is one of inhibition of mixing activity but increased frequency of high-amplitude propagated pressure waves (HAPCs). These have been recorded in infection with enteropathogenic *Escherichia coli*[5] and *V. cholerae*[6] and are likely to cause the abdominal cramps associated with infectious diarrhea. HAPCs can be stimulated by irritants such as sennosides and are blocked by indomethacin,[7] suggesting prostaglandin mediation. Mucosal inflammation causes enterocytes and fibroblasts to secrete prostaglandins. In addition, there is increased serotonin (5-HT) availability, which stimulates peristalsis through 5-HT_3 and 5-HT_4 receptors (see Chapter 18).

Mechanisms of chronic diarrhea

As these acute effects fade, symptoms may remain as some of the changes are very slow to resolve. Abnormal gut permeability and mucosal lymphocytosis is present in the majority of patients 6 months after *Campylobacter* gastroenteritis in spite of the fact that most subjects claim to be asymptomatic.[4] While enterocytes have a half-life of 48 hours, immunocytes and other specialized cells within the mucosa and the lamina propria are much more long-lived. Enteroendocrine cell hyperplasia has been documented to persist for years after infection,[4] and changes in nerve phenotype may also be long-lasting after chronic inflammation.[8] Damage to the terminal ileum may lead to permanent impairment of bile acid reabsorption, which may contribute to postinfective diarrhea reported after *Campylobacter*, *Salmonella* and *Shigella* enteritis.[9] Likewise, the chronic damage induced by recurrent inflammation in poorly controlled ulcerative colitis may lead to colonic shortening and fibrosis. Whether there are changes in mucosal nerves after infection is unknown in man, though it is well described in animal models.[10]

PI-IBS: key points

Develops in approximately 10% of cases of bacterial gastroenteritis. Characterized by:
- frequent urgent stools
- loose stools
- abdominal pain

Associated with:
- accelerated whole-gut transit and increased visceral sensitivity

- increased small bowel permeability
- activation of mucosal immunocytes (ileum, colon and rectum)
- enterochromaffin cell hyperplasia
- increased postprandial serotonin release
- bile acid malabsorption in some patients

Prognosis: 40% recover by 5 years.

Postinfective irritable bowel syndrome (PI-IBS)

Epidemiology

Around 10% of irritable bowel syndrome (IBS) patients claim that infection was the origin of their IBS symptoms. The precise incidence varies widely, being 17% in the UK in primary care but only 6% in the USA in tertiary care.[11] Several prospective studies in Sheffield[12,13] and Nottingham[14,15,16] have shown an incidence of 7–33% (Table 15.1). The higher percentage of new IBS in the studies by Gwee and colleagues[12,13] may reflect the fact that these patients were all hospitalized, whereas the other studies refer to community surveys, in which only approximately 10% were hospitalized. This phenomenon is not unique to the Western world, since the study in China by Wang and colleagues[17] showed a similar picture after an outbreak of salmonellosis (Table 15.1).

Risk factors for developing PI-IBS

These include duration of initial illness, toxigenic *Campylobacter*, female sex, hypochondriasis, neuroticism and adverse life events in the preceding 3 months (Table 15.2). Where multivariate analysis has included psychological factors, it has been shown that female sex is not an independent predictor;[13,18] rather, females appear to be two to three times more likely to develop PI-IBS because they have a higher incidence of psychological disorders. When this is taken into account, sex alone has no predictive value.

Pathology

Serial rectal biopsies from 15 individuals 2, 6 and 12 weeks after *Campylobacter* enteritis showed increased lymphocyte infiltration at 2 weeks and a striking increase in serotonin-containing enteroendocrine cells (also called enterochromaffin or EC cells), though polymorphs and mast cells were not increased (Fig. 15.1). A small group of individuals with long-standing PI-IBS were shown in this study to have similarly increased EC cells and lymphocytes. Gwee and colleagues also showed increased lymphocytes at 3 months in those who developed IBS symptoms. Other cells were not assessed.[13] The relationship between these mucosal changes in the rectum and symptoms were clarified in a subsequent much larger study[16] of the rectal mucosa 3 months after infection, which showed a significant increase in serotonin-containing enteroendocrine (enterochromaffin, EC) cells and T lymphocytes in those who developed PI-IBS. This agrees with several studies which indicate that diarrhea-predominant IBS (D-IBS), both postinfective and without such a history, show signs of immune activation (Table 15.3). The

Table 15.1 Summary of studies reporting increased incidence of IBS following infectious gastroenteritis

Infection	Year	Follow-up (months)	n	Criteria	New IBS (%)	OR (95% CI)	Reference
Prospective studies							
'Gastroenteritis'	1996	3	75	Rome I	31		12
Bacterial	1997	6	390	Rome I	7		14
Bacterial	1999	3	94	Rome I	23		13
Campylobacter	2001	6	188	Rome I	9		15
Campylobacter	2003	3	747	Rome II	13		18
Case–control prospective studies							
Bacterial	1999	12	575, 472	Rome I	4	11.9 (6.7–21)	74
Bacterial	2003	6	500	Rome II	17	10.0 (3–31)	75
Shigella	2004	12–24	295	Rome II	8	10.1	17

'Bacterial' means stool cultures positive, mostly *Campylobacter*, *Salmonella* and *Shigella*.

Table 15.2 Risk factors for developing PI-IBS

Risk factor	Relative risk (95% confidence interval)	Reference
Duration of initial illness		
>21 days	11.4 (2.2–58)	14
>15 days	4.6 (2.1–9.9)	17
Elongating toxin (*Campylobacter*)	10.5 (1.4–76)	15
Female gender	3.4 (1.1–9.5)	14
	2.5*	13
Hypochondriasis	2.0 (1.8–2.5)	13
Adverse life event in previous 3 months	2.0 (1.7–2.4)	13
Age >60 years	0.36 (0.1–0.9)	14

*Not significant after taking psychological factors into account in multivariate analysis.

study of Chadwick and colleagues showed increases in both CD3-positive T lymphocytes and in those carrying the interleukin 2 receptor (CD25), a marker of immune activation.[19] The changes in the rectal mucosa were mirrored throughout the colon. This finding of pancolonic immune activation and the observation of increased small bowel permeability in PI-IBS[4] suggest that these changes are not limited to the rectum. EC hyperplasia is likely to also affect the small bowel since D-IBS patients[20] have increased postprandial serotonin. Interestingly, the most recent study by Wang and colleagues,[17] who obtained terminal ileal biopsies in both PI-IBS and D-IBS without a history of recent infection, showed increased ileal but not colonic mast cells in both groups, supporting earlier studies which also showed ileal mastocytosis in D-IBS patients.[21]

Motility and sensitivity

Whole-gut transit was accelerated 3 months after infection in all infected subjects, but more so in those who developed IBS.[13] Similarly, the threshold for discomfort during balloon distension was also reduced. This would be in keeping with the known sensitizing effects of inflammation on nerve endings.[3]

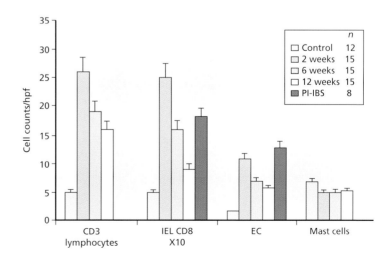

Fig. 15.1 Changes in inflammatory cells in rectal mucosa after *Campylobacter jejuni* infection. Cell counts are per high-power field (x400). Biopsies were taken 2, 5 and 12 weeks after infection. These were compared with those from eight patients with a typical story for PI-IBS following *Salmonella*, *Campylobacter* and unknown infections. Owing to limited material, no data are available for CD3 or mast cells for these patients. IEL CD8, intra-epithelial cytotoxic T cells (scale ×10); EC, enteroendocrine cells (stained positive for synaptophysin). Redrawn from Spiller *et al.*[4]

Site	CD3⁺ T lymphocytes	CD25⁺ lymphocytes	IL-1β mRNA	Mast cells	EC cells	Reference
Rectum	++	ND	+	–	++	13, 76
Rectum	++	ND		–	ND	4
Rectum and colon	++	++		–	ND	19
	++	++			ND	
Rectum	++	+		–	ND	19
Colon and ileum	++	ND	++	–	ND	
	++	ND	++	++	ND	17

ND, not done; + = moderate increase; ++ = marked increased; – = no change.

Evidence of terminal ileal dysfunction in D-IBS

The evidence of terminal ileal inflammation in D-IBS reported by Wang and colleagues[17] is interesting, since inflammatory cytokines such as interleukin-1 (IL-1β) are known to downregulate the apical sodium-dependent bile acid transporter (ASBT) in enterocytes *in vitro*[22] and also in terminal ileal biopsies in patients with Crohn's ileitis.[23] Bile acid malabsorption has been reported in D-IBS[24] and in 16 patients developing D-IBS after gastroenteritis.[9] These patients responded well to cholestyramine, implying that the main cause of diarrhea was bile salt irritation of the colon. A similar conclusion can be drawn from the study by Williams and colleagues, who described a small group with acute onset of severe bile acid malabsorption (less than 5% retention of labelled bile acid at 7 days), who responded very well to cholestyramine.[25] One important clinical clue was that, unlike most D-IBS patients, they described nocturnal diarrhea, something others have also noted.[26]

Clinical features

As many as a quarter of all individuals recovering from bacterial gastroenteritis report that their bowel habit has not returned to normal by 6 months.[14] The characteristic features are abdominal pain and loose or watery stools, which occur on average on two days per week. There was a decrease in hard or lumpy stools but an increase in urgency and repeated defecation. Bloating also increased significantly.[14] Within this larger group of individuals with disturbed bowel habit, there is a smaller subgroup who meet the Rome I criteria for IBS.[27] As would be expected from the definition, these showed more frequent abdominal pain but otherwise had a similar spectrum of symptoms.[14]

Differential diagnosis

Where there is a clear-cut relationship between infection and the onset of IBS symptoms, the probability of another coincidental disease is quite small.

However, when the patient consults some months after the initial illness, the situation may be more confused and a differential diagnosis should be considered (see text box: Differential diagnosis of PI-IBS). If no other diagnosis seems likely after a full history and physical examination and if the Rome I criteria are met in the absence of any alarm features, the diagnosis is unlikely to be incorrect.[28] However, most would advocate simple screening with full blood count, calcium and albumen.[29]

Clinical features of PI-IBS

Experienced by 10% of individuals 6 months after bacterial gastroenteritis. Main features are:
- frequent loose stools
- urgency

- abdominal pain often relieved by defecation
- bloating
- mucus per rectum

Differential diagnosis of PI-IBS

Infection:
- giardiasis
- tropical sprue
- small bowel bacterial overgrowth*

Malabsorption:
- lactose intolerance
- celiac disease

- bile acid malabsorption

Inflammation:
- microscopic colitis*
- Crohn's disease
- ulcerative colitis
- diverticulitis*
- * *More likely over 65 years old.*

Giardiasis should be considered if diarrhea persists. It is a ubiquitous organism found throughout the world and not restricted to those who have traveled to the tropics. Microscopy of stools for cysts is unreliable and only provides a diagnosis in 50%. If symptoms include marked nausea and weight loss, a duodenal biopsy and brush should be performed and will show adherent microorganisms.[30] Tropical sprue is rarely diagnosed other than in those returning from a spell in the tropics. Biopsies show patchy villous atrophy and the condition responds well to broad-spectrum antibiotics. Small bowel contamination may present acutely in the elderly, though they often have obvious predisposing features, such as achlorhydria, previous gastrointestinal surgery with blind loop formation, or small bowel diverticulosis.

Lactose intolerance is well recognized as a transient event after gastroenteritis in infants and probably occurs in adults. However, in adults there is already quite a high incidence of lactose intolerance depending on the racial origin, varying from 10% in northwest Europeans to 40% in West Africa, 60% in Asia and 90% in Chinese.[31] Even with marked hypolactasia, symptoms are rarely experienced unless the individual has a substantial milk intake[32] (more than an equivalent of 240 ml milk per day). Only in such circumstances is a trial of lactose exclusion worthwhile.

Celiac disease is present in 1% of the normal population and 5% of the IBS population,[33] so endomysial antibodies should also be assessed. Onset after infection is well recognized, presumably reflecting enhanced immune activation by the infection exacerbating a pre-existing but clinically covert condition.

Inflammatory bowel disease has a low *a priori* probability (1 per 1000 of the population) but can flare after a bout of gastroenteritis. It should be considered particularly if there are any sinister features, such as anemia, rectal bleeding or weight loss.

Microscopic colitis has been described with an acute onset and should be considered especially in the middle aged and elderly. This is now diagnosed in 10% of patients being colonoscoped for painless diarrhea in Sweden,[34] and 20% of those older than 70 years.

Bile salt malabsorption has already been mentioned as part of the spectrum of PI-IBS. Symptoms of diverticular disease may become acutely worse after a bout of diverticulitis.[35] Here, however, the severity and length of pain associated with abdominal tenderness makes this unlikely to be confused with gastroenteritis.

Rarely, but of great importance, there is the possibility of carcinoma of the colon. Symptom onset is usually insidious, but this condition should be considered when there is a change of bowel habit in a middle-aged or elderly individual. Indeed, because the consequences of missing such a diagnosis are so serious, most guidelines recommend the imaging of the colon to exclude a structural legion of the colon in all patients with new symptoms beginning after the age of 45. Where there is a family history of colon cancer at an early age, this age limit should be lowered.[29]

Investigation and management

If any of the screening tests are positive or if symptoms are severe or atypical, the next stage of investigations would include mucosal biopsies from both the small bowel to diagnose celiac disease and colonic biopsies to exclude microscopic colitis. A lactose breath test may be indicated if the patient consumes more than 240 ml of milk daily and a selenium[75] homocholic acid taurine

(SeHCAT) test if there is nocturnal diarrhea. However, in most cases the screening test will be normal and the clinical course excludes serious organic disease. Management should commence at the very first consultation with a clear statement that it is most likely that the diagnosis will be PI-IBS. The essentially benign nature of the condition should be explained and the patient should be reassured that they do not have colonic cancer, which many fear. Treatments can then be divided into dietary, pharmacological and psychological methods.

Dietary management

A normal individual's stool output is strongly influenced by dietary fiber. Twenty grams of fiber in the form of bran accelerates colonic transit and increases stool weight. Vegetable fiber is somewhat less effective, while readily fermentable fibers have still less effect.[36] A careful dietary history therefore should establish whether there is excessive fiber intake. Where this is the case, a reduction would be appropriate. Since dietary manipulation can be tedious, many have advocated a strict exclusion diet as an initial first step. Those who respond to this with resolution of diarrhea can then reintroduce possible offending items one by one and so identify a modified diet which will minimize symptoms. Items which are typically found to cause symptoms include dairy and wheat products.[37]

Pharmacological treatment

While reduction of dietary fiber may improve symptoms somewhat, urgency and cramps may remain and drug therapy will be required. Only the last drug described in this section has been specifically tested in PI-IBS. Most of the recommendations are therefore extrapolated from studies of D-IBS patients, at least some of whom will be postinfective.

Opiates

Loperamide is an effective anti-diarrheal agent, reducing stool frequency and stool water,[38,39] though it appears less effective as regards abdominal pain.[40] Codeine phosphate is also highly effective, but it does cause nausea and sedation in some individuals, which may limit its use.[41]

5-HT$_3$ antagonists (see also Chapter 18)

As a class, these slow colonic transit[42] and inhibit the colonic activation caused by eating.[43] Alosetron showed efficacy in several large trials in D-IBS, improving stool consistency and decreasing urgency. Overall, IBS symptoms responded in around 60% of patients compared with 45% of those receiving placebo. Meta-analysis (Cremonini and colleagues)[44] gives a number needed to treat of 7.0 (95% CI 5.74–9.43), indicating that 11–17% of D-IBS patients will respond specifically to this treatment. Side-effects included severe constipation and ischemic colitis (1 in 750; for review see Kamm).[45] These side-effects led to its withdrawal, though it has been reintroduced now under strict controls. Cilansetron is a novel 5HT3 antagonist which has been shown to be effective and safe in a 6-month study of D-IBS patients.[46] A dose of 2mg t.i.d resulted in significant relief of IBS symptoms (59%), abdominal pain or discomfort (61%) and abnormal bowel habits including diarrhea and urgency (64%). This study suggested that both males and females responded to treatment with relief of abdominal pain/discomfort in 57%/64% and relief from abnormal bowel habits such as diarrhea and urgency in 60%/67% for males/females respectively.

Cholestyramine

Cholestyramine can be dramatically effective in the subgroup with terminal ileal damage and bile salt malabsorption. When SeHCAT retention at 7 days is less than 5%, nearly all patients respond.[25,9] Unfortunately, cholestyramine tastes unpleasant and patients often discontinue it. Nevertheless, a therapeutic trial of the treatment may be useful in demonstrating the mechanism of diarrhea, even if patients subsequently prefer to use loperamide to manage their condition.

Anti-inflammatory treatment

We recently undertook a proof of principle trial of prednisolone 30 mg daily for 3 weeks, starting 3 months after infection. This was poorly tolerated, and although lymphocyte numbers fell EC counts did not alter, nor did symptoms improve.[74] The treatment may need to be given earlier or for longer. Trials with better-tolerated agents are indicated.

Psychological treatments

Since anxiety, depression and adverse life events are all risk factors for PI-IBS, tackling such issues may be helpful in improving quality of life regardless of bowel symptoms. However, since PI-IBS patients tend to have a lower incidence of psychiatric disease than IBS patients without a history of infection,[47] such treatments have not been tried specifically in PI-IBS.

Prognosis

There is only one prospective study, which indicates that around 40% have recovered by 6 years.[48] Symptoms are therefore likely to be chronic, though they do not appear to be progressive and some patients recover spontaneously. A much earlier study implied that adverse psychological features predicted a poorer outcome,[49] a conclusion supported by Neal and colleagues.[48]

IBS-like symptoms in IBD in remission

Epidemiology

There are two substantial surveys which indicate that IBS symptoms are frequent in patients with inflammatory bowel disease (IBD) who appear by other measures to be in remission.[50,51] This is true for both ulcerative colitis and Crohn's disease, though the symptoms appear more severe in Crohn's disease.[51] The main symptoms are as expected: pain and urgency. The presence of rectal bleeding in active ulcerative colitis makes the clinical definition of relapse and remission easier than it is in Crohn's disease, in which small areas of inflammation could be easily missed.

Pathology

Before the advent of effective treatment, barium enemas were often reported as showing a 'hose-like', rigid, narrowed left colon even in remission. Now there is much better treatment, these appearances are rare; however, more subtle changes may persist, such as loss of crypts and mucus cells.

The mucosal nerves show increased substance P staining in patients with ulcerative colitis who required significant steroid treatment during the previous year[8] and, as described by Holzer in Chapter 17, tachykinin receptors are upregulated in IBD patients. Decreased staining for VIP immunoreactivity has also been noted in IBD,[52] and experimental colitis leads to destruction of nitrergic neurons.[53] There is frequent evidence of distorted and abnormal nerves with altered peptide content in resected Crohn's disease specimens, though the functional significance remains to be determined.[54] Bile salt malabsorption in patients with a damaged terminal ileum remains a possible cause of diarrhea without inflammation, as does small bowel contamination where stricturing has occurred.

Motility and sensitivity

Decreased compliance and increased rectal sensitivity have been documented in acute colitis[55] and in some cases with chronic disease.[56] Studies in quiescent ulcerative colitis suggest that visceral hypersensitivity is paradoxically not a feature.[57] When ulcerative colitis patients are subjected to repetitive sigmoid distension, they do not show the decrease in thresholds for pain perception seen in IBS patients (Fig. 15.2). Studies of brain activation suggest that, under such circumstances, IBS patients fail to show activation of the periaqueductal gray,[58] an area associated in animals with descending antinociceptive pathways.[59] Failure of such antinociceptive mechanisms may be a feature of depression, which is more often associated with IBS than with IBD.

Clinical features

Although mean stool weights and colonic transit times are within the normal range,[60] some IBS-like symptoms, such as abdominal pain, diarrhea and bloating,

---

IBS-like symptoms in IBD in remission: key points

Some IBS-like symptoms are experienced by approximately 50% of IBD patients in remission.

Urgency and abdominal pain are the commonest symptoms.

Abnormalities in physiology include
• reduced rectal compliance

• increased sensitivity to rectal distension

Abnormalities in neuropeptides include
• increased substance P
• decreased VIP

Opiates are the main treatment at present.

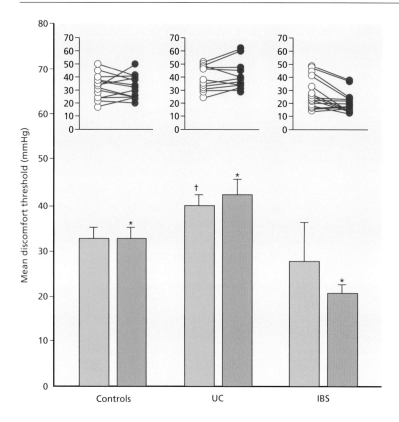

Fig. 15.2 Mean discomfort threshold (green bars) during rectal balloon distension in patients with ulcerative colitis (UC) compared with IBS patients. Blue bars show thresholds after 10 minutes of repetitive distension of the sigmoid colon with a balloon to 60 mmHg pressure. Individual data points are shown above. While IBS patients showed sensitization, no such effect was seen in either colitic patients or controls.[57] Reproduced by permission of BMJ Journals.

are reported in around 50% of patients. They are more likely in those with longer duration of colitis.[51] Importantly, urgency is reported in over 10%.[60] This is a major cause of impairment of quality of life because it leads to fear of going out and severely curtails social activity.

Clinical management

This is similar to PI-IBS, the main measures being dietary modification and drugs. While opiates are generally contraindicated in acute colitis for fear of precipitating toxic megacolon, they are reasonable treatments for urgency and frequency in those in whom inflammation appears quiescent. 5-HT$_3$ antagonists are also likely to be effective by virtue of their antisecretory effects. Cholestyramine could also be tried, particularly in patients with Crohn's disease.

Prognosis

There is no systematic study of prognosis, but given that inflammatory bowel disease has a remitting relapsing course, the prognosis must be guarded.

Symptoms following acute diverticulitis

Epidemiology

Diverticulosis is an extremely common condition of the elderly in industrialized countries. Its incidence is strongly associated with a reduced intake of fruit and vegetables and an increased intake of meat.[61] Radiological evidence of diverticulosis is found in two-thirds of individuals aged 75 and older in the UK. Recent surveys indicate that, while the majority are asymptomatic, a small number suffer from recurrent lower abdominal discomfort. The probability of being symptomatic is doubled by a prior episode of diverticulitis.[35]

Pathology following acute diverticulitis

Fecoliths impacting within diverticula can breach the epithelium, causing acute diverticulitis, following which there is marked smooth muscle hypertrophy and fibrosis.[62] Several morphological studies have indicated abnormalities of the enteric nervous system in diverticular disease,[63] while physiological studies on isolated

---

Symptoms following acute diverticulitis: key points

Uncomplicated diverticulosis is probably asymptomatic.
Acute diverticulitis doubles the risk of symptoms.
Symptoms include:
- recurrent, short-lived abdominal pain
- urgency, diarrhea and incontinence

Abnormalities of circular muscle include:
- thickening
- cholinergic hypersensitivity

Abnormalities in innervation associated with symptoms include:
- impaired nitrergic inhibitory pathways
- increased tachykinins and galanin

Prophylactic antibiotics are the only treatments shown to be of benefit in randomized controlled trials.
Surgical resection may benefit recurrent diverticulitis but not coincidental irritable bowel syndrome.

---

muscle strips suggest overactive excitatory cholinergic[64] and decreased inhibitory nitrergic pathways.[65] More recently, we have shown disorganization of the enteric nervous system with altered phenotype (increased staining of substance P and neurokinin K). This change in the neurochemical coding may reflect damage to nerves followed by regrowth with an altered phenotype. Mucosal biopsies also show that symptomatic patients show increased staining with other markers of neural injury, such as galanin and tachykinins.[66] The significance of these changes is as yet unclear.

Abnormal motility and sensitivity

Narrowing of the lumen and thickening of smooth muscle is associated with increased intraluminal pressures, a feature most marked in patients with symptoms.[67] There is also evidence of hypersensitivity to rectal balloon distension in patients with symptomatic but not asymptomatic diverticular disease, similar to that seen in IBS.[68] Whether this correlates with altered innervation remains to be shown.

Clinical features

While most patients with diverticulosis are asymptomatic, those who have suffered an attack of acute diverticulitis exhibit a high frequency of abnormal bowel symptoms, as shown by Simpson and colleagues.[35] The predominant symptoms were loose stools and urgency, which occurred on a median of 5 and 3 days per week, respectively, with frequent bouts of pain. This was associated with a surprising frequency of incontinence, reported by 16% of patients, and an increased inci-

dence of passage of mucus per rectum and abdominal bloating. Paradoxically, hard stool with straining was also seen, though to a lesser extent.[35]

Differential diagnosis

These are characteristically elderly patients. Depending on the barium enema report, a colonoscopy may also be warranted to exclude a local neoplasm or colitis. Other causes of diarrhea should also be considered (see text box: Differential diagnosis of PI-IBS) and if incontinence is a feature then careful evaluation of the anal sphincter is warranted (see Chapter 13)

Treatment

There are few randomized control trials of treatment. Long-term treatment with the poorly absorbed antibiotic rifaximin appears to reduce the incidence of recurrent pain,[69] possibly by inhibiting episodes of diverticulitis. Fiber supplements reduce the frequency of constipation but do not alter pain and may exacerbate diarrhea.[70] Opiates should be used with caution to avoid aggravating constipation, though they may be useful to allow patients to leave their homes and travel without fear of incontinence.

Where pain is persistent and CT scanning shows the presence of bowel wall thickening,[71] resection of the diseased segment should be considered, though the results are variable.[72,73] Patient selection therefore needs to be careful. In particular, care should be taken to avoid operating on patients with IBS, in whom diverticulosis is an incidental finding. In making this diagnosis, it would be helpful to note a long-standing

---

Summary and conclusions

1 Diarrhea and inflammation are part of normal defenses against infection.
2 Incomplete resolution of inflammation leads to disease.
3 Inflammation-induced structural alterations in

the nerves and enteroendocrine system may be long-lasting.
4 Careful assessment of patients may allow definition of mechanisms that allow specific treatments.

---

history of abdominal pain which predates the age at which diverticulosis is likely.

Conclusions

Much remains to be learnt. Acute inflammation on its own settles rapidly. Genetic polymorphisms in the immune response may predict who will develop postinflammatory syndromes. Likewise, whether EC hyperplasia induces symptoms may depend on polymorphisms of the serotonin transporter. The lack of visceral hypersensitivity in ulcerative colitis suggests that inflammation alone is not enough and emphasizes the importance of central influences on pain perception. We should therefore remember Hippocrates, who in 400 BC stated 'For this is the great error of our day, that the physicians separate the soul from the body'. Although the conditions described show important peripheral changes in the gut, ultimately symptoms are experienced in the brain. We ignore this at our peril.

References

1 Fasano A. Cellular microbiology: can we learn cell physiology from microorganisms? *Am J Physiol* 1999; **276**: C765–76.
2 Lundgren O, Svensson L. Pathogenesis of rotavirus diarrhea. *Microbes Infect* 2001; **3**: 1145–56.
3 Bueno L, Fioramonti J, Delvaux M, Frexinos J. Mediators and pharmacology of visceral sensitivity: from basic to clinical investigations. *Gastroenterology* 1997; **112**: 1714–43.
4 Spiller RC, Jenkins D, Thornley JP *et al.* Increased rectal mucosal enteroendocrine cells, T lymphocytes, and increased gut permeability following acute *Campylobacter* enteritis and in post-dysenteric irritable bowel syndrome. *Gut* 2000; **47**: 804–11.
5 Sjogren RW, Sherman PM, Boedeker EC. Altered intestinal motility precedes diarrhea during *Escherichia coli* enteric infection. *Am J Physiol* 1989; **257**: G725–31.
6 Koch KL, Martin JL, Mathias JR. Migrating action-potential complexes in vitro in cholera-exposed rabbit ileum. *Am J Physiol* 1983; **244**: G291–4.
7 Staumont G, Fioramonti J, Frexinos J, Bueno L. Changes in colonic motility induced by sennosides in dogs: evidence of a prostaglandin mediation. *Gut* 1988; **29**: 1180–7.
8 Watanabe T, Kubota Y, Muto T. Substance P containing nerve fibers in rectal mucosa of ulcerative colitis. *Dis Colon Rectum* 1997; **40**: 718–25.
9 Niaz SK, Sandrasegaran K, Renny FH, Jones BJ. Postinfective diarrhoea and bile acid malabsorption. *J R Coll Physicians Lond* 1997; **31**: 53–6.
10 De Giorgio R, Barbara G, Blennerhassett P *et al.* Intestinal inflammation and activation of sensory nerve pathways: a functional and morphological study in the nematode infected rat. *Gut* 2001; **49**: 822–7.
11 Longstreth GF, Hawkey CJ, Mayer EA *et al.* Characteristics of patients with irritable bowel syndrome recruited from three sources: implications for clinical trials. *Aliment Pharmacol Ther* 2001; **15**: 959–64.
12 Gwee KA, Graham JC, McKendrick MW *et al.* Psychometric scores and persistence of irritable bowel after infectious diarrhoea. *Lancet* 1996; **347**: 150–3.
13 Gwee KA, Leong YL, Graham C *et al.* The role of psychological and biological factors in postinfective gut dysfunction. *Gut* 1999; **44**: 400–6.
14 Neal KR, Hebden J, Spiller R. Prevalence of gastrointestinal symptoms six months after bacterial gastroenteritis and risk factors for development of the irritable bowel syndrome: postal survey of patients. *Br Med J* 1997; **314**: 779–82.
15 Thornley JP, Jenkins D, Neal K, Wright T, Brough J, Spiller RC. Relationship of *Campylobacter* toxigenicity *in vitro* to the development of postinfectious irritable bowel syndrome. *J Infect Dis* 2001; **184**: 606–9.
16 Dunlop SP, Jenkins D, Neal KR, Spiller RC. Relative importance of enterochromaffin cell hyperplasia, anxiety, and depression in postinfectious IBS. *Gastroenterology* 2003; **125**: 1651–9.
17 Wang L-H, Fang X-C, Pan G-Z. Bacillary dysentery as a causative factor of irritable bowel syndrome and its pathogenesis. *Gut* 2004; **53**: 1096–1101.

18 Dunlop SP, Jenkins D, Neal KR, Spiller RC. Clinical and histological features of post-infectious IBS: relative importance of enterochromaffin cell hyperplasia, anxiety and depression. *Gastroenterology* 2003; **125**, 1651–9.

19 Chadwick VS, Chen W, Shu D *et al*. Activation of the mucosal immune system in irritable bowel syndrome. *Gastroenterology* 2002; **122**: 1778–83.

20 Houghton LA, Atkinson W, Whitaker RP, Whorwell PJ, Rimmer MJ. Increased platelet depleted plasma 5-hydroxytryptamine concentration following meal ingestion in symptomatic female subjects with diarrhoea predominant irritable bowel syndrome. *Gut* 2003; **52**: 663–70.

21 Weston AP, Biddle WL, Bhatia PS, Miner PB Jr. Terminal ileal mucosal mast cells in irritable bowel syndrome. *Dig Dis Sci* 1993; **38**: 1590–5.

22 Chen F, Ma L, Sartor RB *et al*. Inflammatory-mediated repression of the rat ileal sodium-dependent bile acid transporter by c-fos nuclear translocation. *Gastroenterology* 2002; **123**: 2005–16.

23 Jung D, Fantin AC, Scheurer U, Fried M, Kullak-Ublick GA. Human ileal bile acid transporter gene ASBT (SLC10A2) is transactivated by the glucocorticoid receptor. *Gut* 2004; **53**: 78–84.

24 Merrick MV, Eastwood MA, Ford MJ. Is bile acid malabsorption underdiagnosed? An evaluation of accuracy of diagnosis by measurement of SeHCAT retention. *Br Med J* 1985; **290**: 665–8.

25 Williams AJK, Merrick MV, Eastwood MA. Idiopathic bile acid malabsorption. A review of clinical presentation, diagnosis, and response to treatment. *Gut* 1991; **32**: 1004–6.

26 Sinha L, Liston R, Testa HJ, Moriarty KJ. Idiopathic bile acid malabsorption: qualitative and quantitative clinical features and response to cholestyramine. *Aliment Pharmacol Ther* 1998; **12**: 839–44.

27 Drossman DA, Thompson WG, Talley NJ, Funch-Jensen P, Janssens J, Whitehead WE. Identification of sub-groups of functional gastrointestinal disorders. *Gastroent Int* 1990; **3**: 159–72.

28 Vanner SJ, Depew WT, Paterson WG *et al*. Predictive value of the Rome criteria for diagnosing the irritable bowel syndrome. *Am J Gastroenterol* 1999; **94**: 2912–17.

29 Jones J, Boorman J, Cann P *et al*. British Society of Gastroenterology guidelines for the management of the irritable bowel syndrome. *Gut* 2000; **47** (Suppl. 2): ii1–19.

30 Vesy CJ, Peterson WL. Review article: the management of giardiasis. *Aliment Pharmacol Ther* 1999; **13**: 843–50.

31 Simoons FJ. The geographic hypothesis and lactose malabsorption: a weighing of the evidence. *Dig Dis Sci* 1978; **23**: 963–79.

32 Suarez FL, Savaiano DA, Levitt MD. A comparison of symptoms after the consumption of milk or lactose-hydrolyzed milk by people with self-reported severe lactose intolerance. *N Engl J Med* 1995; **333**: 1–4.

33 Sanders DS, Carter MJ, Hurlstone DP *et al*. Association of adult coeliac disease with irritable bowel syndrome: a case–control study in patients fulfilling ROME II criteria referred to secondary care. *Lancet* 2001; **358**: 1504–8.

34 Olesen M, Eriksson S, Bohr J, Jarnerot G, Tysk C. Microscopic colitis: a common diarrhoeal disease. An epidemiological study in Orebro, Sweden, 1993–1998. *Gut* 2004; **53**: 346–50.

35 Simpson J, Neal KR, Scholefield JH, Spiller RC. Patterns of pain in diverticular disease and the influence of acute diverticulitis. *Eur J Gastroenterol Hepatol* 2003; **15**: 1005–10.

36 Cummings JH, Branch W, Jenkins DJA, Southgate DAT, Houston H, James WPT. Colonic response to dietary fibre from carrot, cabbage, apple, bran, and guar gum. *Lancet* 1978; **1**: 5–9.

37 Parker TJ, Naylor SJ, Riordan AM, Hunter JO. Management of patients with food intolerance in irritable bowel syndrome: the development and use of an exclusion diet. *J Hum Nutr Dietet* 1995; **8**: 159–66.

38 Cann PA, Read NW, Holdsworth CD, Barends D. Role of loperamide and placebo in management of irritable bowel syndrome (IBS). *Dig Dis Sci* 1984; **29**: 239–47.

39 Efskind PS, Bernklev T, Vatn MH. A double-blind placebo-controlled trial with loperamide in irritable bowel syndrome. *Scand J Gastroenterol* 1996; **31**: 463–8.

40 Jailwala J, Imperiale TF, Kroenke K. Pharmacologic treatment of the irritable bowel syndrome: a systematic review of randomized, controlled trials. *Ann Intern Med* 2000; **133**: 136–47.

41 Palmer KR, Corbett CL, Holdsworth CD. Double-blind cross-over study comparing loperamide, codeine and diphenoxylate in the treatment of chronic diarrhea. *Gastroenterology* 1980; **79**: 1272–5.

42 Gore S, Gilmore IT, Haigh CG, Brownless SM, Stockdale H, Morris AI. Colonic transit in man is slowed by ondansetron (GR38032F), a selective 5-hydroxytryptamine receptor (type 3) antagonist. *Aliment Pharmacol Ther* 1990; **4**: 139–44.

43 Prior A, Read NW. Reduction of rectal sensitivity and post-prandial motility by granisetron, a 5 HT3-receptor antagonist, in patients with irritable bowel syndrome. *Aliment Pharmacol Ther* 1993; **7**: 175–80.

44 Cremonini F, Delgado-Aros S, Camilleri M. Efficacy of alosetron in irritable bowel syndrome: a meta-analysis of randomized controlled trials. *Neurogastroenterol Motil* 2003; **15**: 79–86.

45 Kamm MA. Review article: the complexity of drug development for irritable bowel syndrome. *Aliment Pharmacol Ther* 2002; **16**: 343–51.

46 Bradette M, Moennikes H, Carter F, *et al*. Cilansetron in

irritable bowel syndrome with diarrhea predominance (IBS-D): efficacy and safety in a six month global study. *Gastroenterology*, 2004; **126** (Suppl. 2); A-42.

47   Dunlop SP, Jenkins D, Spiller RC. Distinctive clinical, psychological, and histological features of postinfective irritable bowel syndrome. *Am J Gastroenterol* 2003; **98**: 1578–83.

48   Neal KR, Barker L, Spiller RC. Prognosis in post-infective irritable bowel syndrome: a six year follow up study. *Gut* 2002; **51**: 410–13.

49   Chaudhary NA, Truelove SC. The irritable colon syndrome. *Q J Med* 1962; **123**: 307–22.

50   Isgar B, Harman M, Kaye MD, Whorwell PJ. Symptoms of irritable bowel syndrome in ulcerative colitis in remission. *Gut* 1983; **24**: 190–2.

51   Simren M, Axelsson J, Gillberg R, Abrahamsson H, Svedlund J, Bjornsson ES. Quality of life in inflammatory bowel disease in remission: the impact of IBS-like symptoms and associated psychological factors. *Am J Gastroenterol* 2002; **97**: 389–96.

52   Kubota Y, Petras RE, Ottaway CA, Tubbs RR, Farmer RG, Fiocchi C. Colonic vasoactive intestinal peptide nerves in inflammatory bowel disease. *Gastroenterology* 1992; **102**: 1242–51.

53   Mizuta Y, Isomoto H, Takahashi T. Impaired nitrergic innervation in rat colitis induced by dextran sulfate sodium. *Gastroenterology* 2000; **118**: 714–23.

54   Belai A, Boulos PB, Robson T, Burnstock G. Neurochemical coding in the small intestine of patients with Crohn's disease. *Gut* 1997; **40**: 767–74.

55   Rao SS, Read NW. Gastrointestinal motility in patients with ulcerative colitis. *Scand J Gastroenterol* 1990; **172** (Suppl.): 22–8.

56   Loening-Baucke V, Metcalf AM, Shirazi S. Rectosigmoid motility in patients with quiescent and active ulcerative colitis. *Am J Gastroenterol* 1989; **84**: 34–9.

57   Chang L, Munakata J, Mayer EA, Schmulson MJ, Johnson TD, Bernstein CN *et al*. Perceptual responses in patients with inflammatory and functional bowel disease. *Gut* 2000; **47**: 497–505.

58   Naliboff BD, Derbyshire SW, Munakata J *et al*. Cerebral activation in patients with irritable bowel syndrome and control subjects during rectosigmoid stimulation. *Psychosom Med* 2001; **63**: 365–75.

59   Zhuo M, Gebhart GF. Facilitation and attenuation of a visceral nociceptive reflex from the rostroventral medulla in the rat. *Gastroenterology* 2002; **122**: 1007–19.

60   Rao SS, Holdsworth CD, Read NW. Symptoms and stool patterns in patients with ulcerative colitis. *Gut* 1988; **29**: 342–5.

61   Simpson J, Scholefield JH, Spiller RC. Pathogenesis of colonic diverticula. *Br J Surg* 2002; **89**: 546–54.

62   Simpson J, Scholefield JH, Spiller RC. Origin of symptoms in diverticular disease. *Br J Surg* 2003; **90**: 899–908.

63   Stoss F, Meier-Ruge W. Diagnosis of neuronal colonic dysplasia in primary chronic constipation and sigmoid diverticulosis endoscopic biopsy and enzyme-histochemical examination. *Surg Endosc* 1991; **5**: 146–9.

64   Golder M, Burleigh DE, Belai A *et al*. Smooth muscle cholinergic denervation hypersensitivity in diverticular disease. *Lancet* 2003; **361**: 1945–51.

65   Tomita R, Tanjoh K, Fujisaki S, Fukuzawa M. Physiological studies on nitric oxide in the right sided colon of patients with diverticular disease. *Hepatogastroenterology* 1999; **46**: 2839–44.

66   Simpson J, Sundler F, Jenkins D, Spiller RC. Increased expression of galanin in mucosal nerves of patients with painful diverticular disease. *Gut* 2003; **52**: 318.

67   Cortesini C, Pantalone D. Usefulness of colonic motility study in identifying patients at risk for complicated diverticular disease. *Dis Colon Rectum* 1991; **34**: 339–42.

68   Clemens CHM, Samuel M, Roelofs J, van Berge Henegouwen GP, Smout AJPM. Colorectal visceral perception in diverticular disease. *Gut* 2004; **53**: 717–22.

69   Papi C, Ciaco A, Koch M, Capurso L. Efficacy of rifaximin in the treatment of symptomatic diverticular disease of the colon. A multicentre double-blind placebo-controlled trial. *Aliment Pharmacol Ther* 1995; **9**: 33–9.

70   Ornstein MH, Littlewood ER, Baird IM, Fowler J, North WR, Cox AG. Are fibre supplements really necessary in diverticular disease of the colon? A controlled clinical trial. *Br Med J Clin Res Ed* 1981; **282**: 1353–6.

71   Ambrosetti P, Becker C, Terrier F. Colonic diverticulitis: impact of imaging on surgical management – a prospective study of 542 patients. *Eur Radiol* 2002; **12**: 1145–9.

72   Charnock FM, Rennie JR, Wellwood JM, Todd IP. Results of colectomy for diverticular disease of the colon. *Br J Surg* 1977; **64**: 417–19.

73   Moreaux J, Vons C. Elective resection for diverticular disease of the sigmoid colon. *Br J Surg* 1990; **77**: 1036–8.

74   Dunlop SP, Jenkins D, Neal KR *et al*. Randomized, double-blind, placebo-controlled trial of prednisolone in post-infectious irritable bowel syndrome. *Aliment Pharmacol Ther* 2003; **18**: 77–84.

75   Rodriguez LA, Ruigomez A. Increased risk of irritable bowel syndrome after bacterial gastroenteritis: cohort study. *BMJ* 1999; **318**: 565–6.

76   Parry SD, Stansfield R, Jelley D *et al*. Is irritable bowel syndrome more common in patients presenting with bacterial gastroenteritis? A community-based, case–control study. *Am J Gastroenterol* 2003; **98**: 327–31.

77   Gwee KA, Collins SM, Read NW *et al*. Increased rectal mucosal expression of interleukin 1beta in recently acquired post-infectious irritable bowel syndrome. *Gut* 2003; **52**: 523–6.

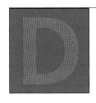

Advances in Pharmacotherapy

CHAPTER 16

Functional Targets for Pharmacotherapy: An Overview

L Ashley Blackshaw

Introduction

The aim of this section is to bring readers up to date with the latest ideas and developments in drug treatment of functional gastrointestinal diseases, with a focus on peripheral targets. This chapter will briefly outline what there is to aim at in terms of cellular targets, and the advantages and disadvantages of targeting

each one (Table 16.1). Subsequent chapters will detail the progress with individual targets, in particular neurokinins and serotonin.

Secretory cells

Because functional gastrointestinal diseases are generally regarded as involving disordered sensation and

Table 16.1 Functional targets along the brain–gut axis and the arguments for and against their relevance as targets for treatment of functional diseases

Target	For	Against
1 Secretory cells	Specific, easy to target historically	Potentially disrupt digestion
2 Smooth muscle	Likely benefit in constipation and diarrhea	General target; effects on vascular smooth muscle, etc. possible
3 Interstitial cells of Cajal	Possibility of targeting pacemaker and neuromuscular roles separately	Possible generalized effects throughout gut
4 Enteroendocrine cells	Strong association with IBS; increased numbers	Mediator release from these cells difficult to target
5 Mast cells	Mucosal mast cells have strong association with IBS	Risk of influencing normal inflammatory responses
6 Intrinsic enteric nerves	Association with motor patterns underlying constipation and diarrhea	Motility effects likely throughout gut
7 Extrinsic spinal afferent nerves	Specific, strong association with pain and discomfort	Possible overlap with effects on somatic sensory pathways
8 Extrinsic vagal afferent nerves	Specific, prominent role in satiety, gastric emptying and reflux	Restricted to non-painful symptoms
9 The central nervous system	Likely to be origin of abnormality in several patient groups	General target; side-effects in other systems likely

Targets 1–8 have the additional advantage over target 9 of being accessible by peripherally restricted drugs.

motility, rather than secretion, the first targets that spring to mind are neural and muscular targets. However, it is worth considering secretory cells as targets in certain circumstances. Exocrine secretions of the gut include acid, pepsin, bicarbonate, proteolytic enzymes, absorptive cofactors and mucus. Their point of addition to and removal from the progressing digesta is crucial to normal function. Furthermore, the major target of gastrointestinal medications over the last 30 years has been the parietal cell, simply because it is the source of hydrochloric acid in the stomach and is involved in damage to the duodenal and esophageal mucosa in ulcer disease and reflux disease, respectively. Although these conditions are distinct from functional gastrointestinal disease as defined earlier in this book, there are large gray areas in which patients who are endoscopy-negative will respond well to acid suppression. Therefore, the prescription of proton pump inhibitors is a good first-line approach to non-cardiac chest pain, particularly because many of these patients have positive esophageal pH monitoring tests,[1] indicating an underlying abnormality in gastroesophageal reflux. Bile secretion may be associated with functional gastrointestinal disease, as a trigger either for motor patterns or for symptoms.[2] Although bile production and release may be quite normal in patients, there is evidence for disordered absorption in diarrhea-predominant disease. The idea that bile may contribute to symptoms was tested by Edwards and colleagues,[3] who showed that perception of rectal distension was exacerbated by a bile enema in normal individuals. The effect on symptoms of chronic exposure of the distal gut to bile has not been evaluated, and remains a major potential source of lowered sensory thresholds in IBS.

Smooth muscle and interstitial cells of Cajal

The topic of whether functional gastrointestinal diseases are predominantly motor or sensory disorders has been debated intensely. Although irritable bowel syndrome (IBS) is classified mainly according to bowel habit, the motor patterns that give rise to diarrhea or constipation are ill-defined. It is probably therefore inappropriate to target smooth muscle function in general. A therapy that reduces the strength of colonic contractions will correspondingly reduce symptoms arising from these contractions – an approach used with some success in a minority of cases.[4] However, because receptors on smooth muscle and contractile mechanisms are broadly similar throughout the non-sphincteric gut, there is also the potential of such a therapy slowing gastric emptying and colonic transit, which may detract substantially from the desired effect. Interstitial cells of Cajal (ICC) represent an attractive target as they may subserve a number of roles relevant to functional diseases. Recent evidence has placed them in the important position of neuromuscular intermediaries. Thus, they are involved in translating the release of excitatory and inhibitory neurotransmitters from enteric nerves into excitation and inhibition (respectively) of the smooth muscle.[5] They are also involved in pacemaker activity, and therefore the control of contractile rhythms in the gut. Distinct populations of ICC are involved in each of these functions, making each one a selective target for either neuromuscular function or contractile rhythms. More recently, ICCs have been proposed to play a role in sensory function, being closely apposed between sensory endings and smooth muscle (see Chapter 1).[6] Whether their interaction with sensory nerves is chemical or structural and whether it is strong enough to constitute a real target is yet to be established. Nonetheless, there is emerging evidence that loss of ICC may be associated with a defect in the function of sensory nerves. The question of how to modify inhibitory motor function, excitatory motor function or sensory function independently in ICC is one that has not been raised in earnest. However, advances in the basic understanding of how this cell type subserves these different functions may quickly provide options for drug targeting in functional diseases.

Enteroendocrine cells

Enteroendocrine cells represent in many cases the first line of gut chemosensitivity. They have long been established as the link between nutrient arrival in the gut and secretory responses. Indeed, such links were the key to our original understanding of the endocrine function of the body. Hormones such as cholecystokinin (CCK), secretin and gastrin are released by subpopulations of enteroendocrine cells, and have direct and indirect effects on the secretory function of the pancreas and stomach. It was many years between these discoveries and those that related enteroendocrine cells with the sensory function of the gut. The most prominent candidates in this regard are CCK and serotonin (5-HT). Both of these are released from the small intestine, and 5-HT is also released from the large intestine. CCK is released from D cells by fatty acids and acts on vagal afferent endings positioned locally to evoke action potentials that are transmitted to the brainstem (see below). A wide range of sensory and reflex responses may ensue, including satiety, nausea, reduced gastric emptying, all of which are symptoms of functional gastrointestinal disease. This link between CCK and symptoms has prompted considerable effort in developing antagonists to the CCK receptors present on vagal afferents (CCK1 receptors). It is not the purpose of this chapter to detail the pharmacotherapy of functional gastrointestinal disease. However, the reduction of symptoms by CCK1 receptor antagonism after a lipid meal serves to demonstrate the fact that intervention with the actions of enteroendocrine cell products may be an effective strategy in functional disease.[7] Of course, CCK has many roles in addition to its contribution to sensory function, and these are the main reason for the lack of specificity (and probably lack of success) of CCK antagonists in the clinic.

Serotonin is released mainly from enterochromaffin cells that line the whole gut. The stimuli for 5-HT release are many and varied, and include distension, pH, nutrients, transmitters and toxins.[8] The release of 5-HT by mechanical forces underlies one of the major theories about the triggering of peristalsis, which holds that many types of mechanical stimulus in the gut trigger peristalsis by distortion of enterochromaffin cells. The 5-HT released then acts on endings of submucous plexus neurons, which in turn activate the ascending and descending pathways involved in the motor program.[9] Although it is certain that 5-HT influences strongly the initiation of peristalsis, whether its role is essential or facilitatory is still debated. In addition to acting on intrinsic enteric neurons, 5-HT also activates extrinsic sensory nerves, both in the vagal[10] and the spinal supply throughout the gastrointestinal tract.[11] This may occur as a paracrine action on mucosal sensory endings or following circulation. Concentrations of plasma 5-HT are sufficient to activate sensory nerves, particularly in

diarrhea-predominant IBS, in which levels are much higher than normal after a meal.[12] Its source is correspondingly increased in the form of larger numbers of enterochromaffin cells.[13] Given its source and its targets in both the extrinsic and intrinsic innervation, there is the potential for 5-HT to have effects on peristalsis and sensory function independently. It is therefore possible that current drug therapies targeted to 5-HT receptors may have dual actions on both these systems. This may not always be desirable, particularly in the constipating action of 5-HT$_3$ receptor antagonists.[4] In Chapter 18, Fabrizio De Ponti outlines the potential for agonists and antagonists of several of the 5-HT receptors as pharmacotherapies in functional gastrointestinal diseases.

As far as enteroendocrine cell mediators that have potential relevance to functional diseases are concerned, 5-HT and CCK represent only the tip of the iceberg. It is beyond the scope of this article to detail all of them, so the reader is referred to reviews by Dockray[14] and Ahlman and Nilsson.[15]

Mast cells

Mast cells are increasingly being implicated in the pathophysiology of functional gastrointestinal diseases, in particular IBS. They constitute both effectors and sensors along neural pathways in addition to their specific roles in inflammation and immune responses. Depending on their origin and species, they may release 5-HT and therefore trigger cascades of sensory activation similar to those described above for enterochromaffin cells. They also contain histamine, tryptases, cytokines and nerve growth factor. These factors may be released by both IgE-dependent (antigen) and non-IgE-dependent (bacterial toxins, neurotransmitters, etc.) stimuli.[16] Mast cells may be one of the final mediators of the effects of stress on gastrointestinal functions, by virtue of their sensitivity to corticotropin releasing factor (see Chapters 8 and 19). Mucosal mast cells are increased in numbers in IBS in a way that correlates closely with symptoms.[17] They are also more frequently degranulated, suggesting ongoing stimulation in disease. There are also abundant mast cells in the muscle, serosa and mesentery that are candidates for activating extrinsic sensory nerves, and the role of these relative to mucosal mast cells is yet to be explored.

Intrinsic enteric nerves

Within the enteric nervous system (ENS), there are at least 18 classes of neuron by recent estimates (see also Chapter 1). These are classified according to their functional role and the transmitters they contain. The approach to understanding enteric nerves as targets for pharmacotherapy has been mainly to find a drug or mechanism (receptor, enzyme, channel), and subsequently investigate which classes of enteric neurons are most likely to be involved in its action on motility. The result is a relatively poor understanding of the detail of drug targets in the ENS. Part of the reason for the current situation is probably the fact that several classes of enteric neuron can be found in the same ganglion; often complex chemical coding is the only way to identify each class. Significant progress has been made by the identification of neuronal classes by retrograde labeling from their destination and by correlation of electrophysiological and morphological features. A class of neuron that has provoked particular interest recently is the Dogiel type II/AH neuron. Due to their projections, morphology and electrophysiological responses, they are proposed to serve a sensory function within the ENS and are known as intrinsic primary afferent neurons (IPANs). Understanding of their adequate physiological and pathophysiological stimuli is developing rapidly. Chemical stimulation of the mucosa may activate IPANs either directly or via release of mediators, including 5-HT, from enteroendocrine cells.[18] Distension of the muscle layers may also activate IPANs,[19] but whether they are sensitive to both types of stimulus is not yet established. This knowledge would be an important step in targeting selectively the mechanosensory or chemosensory reflexes initiated by IPANs. They outnumber extrinsic sensory nerves by severalfold and have the advantage of being confined to their organ of innervation. This means that peripherally restricted drugs may modify aspects of both sensory transduction and onward transmission, which is not possible in extrinsic sensory nerves. Serotonergic drugs are considered to exert many of their effects on both transduction in IPANs and transmission from them. The major transmitters contained within IPANs are acetylcholine and tachykinins. However, these are also the major transmitters in the excitatory motor neurons of the ENS that innervate smooth muscle and ICC,

which limits the potential selectivity of drugs acting on cholinergic and tachykininergic pathways. Peter Holzer in Chapter 17 outlines the potential for tachykinins and their receptors at both of these locations as targets in functional gastrointestinal disease.

Extrinsic vagal and spinal afferent nerves

Sensory information from the gastrointestinal tract reaches the central nervous system (CNS) via the vagal and spinal nerves. These follow the same anatomical paths as the autonomic efferent innervation, so that the vagal innervation extends mainly over the proximal part of the gut and the spinal innervation is provided by the splanchnic nerves throughout most of the gut, and the pelvic nerves in the distal gut.[20] Extrinsic afferent pathways are all relevant to functional gastrointestinal disease as they may all give rise to symptoms directly. This is the reason why there is an intense focus on extrinsic sensory nerves as functional targets for novel pharmacotherapies. This focus has already borne fruit, which may provide clues as to which targets are worth investigating in the future. Although all pathways can be associated with symptoms, this is not normally the case. We are, on the whole, blissfully unaware of events in the gut with the exception of the occasional pang of hunger or pleasant fullness after a meal. The fact that many more events are perceivable in functional gastrointestinal disease, which are generally unpleasant, means that thresholds are lowered at some point along sensory pathways. The way in which primary afferents give rise to perceived sensations and how these may be altered in functional diseases are dealt with by Klaus Bielefeldt and Gerald Gebhart in Chapter 3. The present chapter will focus instead on how the different classes of primary afferents may be separated into classes according to the location of their endings (Fig. 16.1), the pathways they follow, and their potential as targets in functional diseases. Vagal afferents have been classified mainly according to the layer of gut in which they terminate, because the location of endings to a large extent determines their sensitivity. This is supported by anatomical and electrophysiological evidence. Spinal afferents are increasingly becoming classified in a similar way to vagal afferents, particularly with the adoption of similar methods for studying both

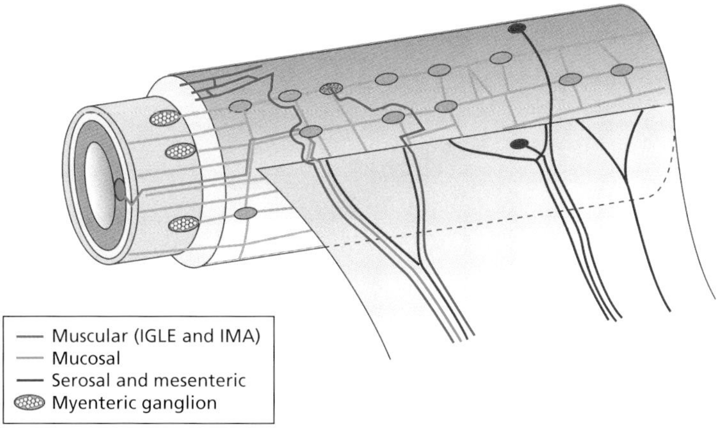

Fig. 16.1 Three classes of extrinsic sensory fibers may be described according to the location of their receptive fields. Some of these may have multiple receptive sites and some may have dual mechanoreceptive function (muscular/mucosal receptors). See also Chapter 1. IGLE, intraganglionic laminar endings. IMA, intramuscular endings.

— Muscular (IGLE and IMA)
— Mucosal
— Serosal and mesenteric
⬭ Myenteric ganglion

pathways. Traditionally, they have been classed according to their thresholds to distension, but this may have led to several classes being overlooked because of their insensitivity to distension.

Mucosal receptors

Mucosal receptors respond briefly to fine tactile stimulation of the mucosal surface but not to distension of the gut wall.[20] Anatomical evidence shows projections of vagal endings into the lamina propria which presumably correspond to this functional class of afferents. They are most likely to function as detectors of particles or texture, and may possibly signal flow when functioning as a population, in a similar way to the sensory innervation of the oral and anal regions. Mucosal tactile information from most of the gut is unlikely to be registered as conscious perception, even in pathophysiological states. It therefore most likely plays a role in the fine tuning of reflexes and transmission along sensory pathways with other modalities. In addition to their mechanosensory role, mucosal receptors have been shown to respond to a number of chemical mediators, including CCK, 5-HT, norepinephrine, opioids, bradykinin, purines and prostaglandins. They also respond to intraluminal changes in osmolarity, acidity and alkalinity and bile concentration. This spectrum of sensitivity has led to a major focus on mucosal receptors in the generation of satiety, nausea and vomiting from the upper gastrointestinal tract, because most evidence is from vagal afferents which are known to be connected with these functions. Mucosal receptors

have, however, been identified in all pathways to the gastrointestinal tract, and similar mechanosensitivity has recently been shown for vagal, splanchnic and pelvic mucosal receptors.[21–24] It remains to be determined whether their chemosensitivity is likewise preserved across pathways, although there are indications that sensitivity to acid, osmolarity, 5-HT and bile is shared between vagal and splanchnic populations.[10,11,21,23] The functional role of splanchnic and pelvic mucosal afferent mechano- and chemosensitivity is not well understood, but may serve to modulate transmission along spinal pathways detecting colorectal distension, as shown by recordings from second-order neurons in the dorsal horn.[25] Until a more precise understanding of the roles of mucosal receptors in separate pathways is reached, their relevance as targets for functional diseases remains speculative. However, it is encouraging that vagal mucosal receptors have already provided targets for anti-emetic therapies (see below, Modulation of extrinsic sensory nerves).

Muscular receptors

Tension receptors (also known as muscular receptors) have resting activity that is often modulated in phase with ongoing contractions. They are mechanosensitive to contractions and distension with a slowly adapting, linear relationship to wall tension. Depending on the pathway, this may be within or beyond the physiological range. Vagal afferents tend to saturate their responses at relatively low levels of distension, whereas splanchnic and pelvic afferents continue to increase their firing well into the noxious range. There is evidence for two populations of spinal distension-sensitive afferents, one with low thresholds, like vagal afferents, and one with high thresholds that respond only slightly at subnoxious levels[26] (see also Chapter 3). Low-threshold tension receptors as a population signal the amplitude, pattern and direction of luminal contractions to the CNS that is important in triggering reflexes controlling gastrointestinal function. Responses of vagal tension receptors to distension are also important in signaling food intake and mediating satiety and fullness. Although there are varying accounts of the chemosensitivity of tension or muscular receptors in different organs, their location within the muscle layers (see Chapter 1) suggests that signaling of contractions and distension is their main function. A population identified so far only in the vagal and pelvic innervation at either end of the gut is known as tension/mucosal (or muscular/mucosal) receptors.[22,24] They show features of both tension receptors and mucosal receptors. Presumably their role is a composite of those described for tension receptors and mucosal receptors. The exquisite responsiveness of muscular receptors to distension coupled with the characteristic hypersensitivity to distension in functional disease patients makes these neurons a prime target for pharmacotherapy. How this may be achieved is discussed below (see Modulation of extrinsic sensory nerves).

Serosal and mesenteric receptors

These have low resting activity and respond only briefly to noxious intensities of organ distension. This is not surprising in view of their lack of penetration of the gut wall. It is possible that these receptors identified *in vitro* correspond to the high threshold/phasic mechanoreceptors described earlier *in vivo*,[27] which were also shown to have receptive fields outside the gut wall, although a direct comparison is not possible. The function of serosal and mesenteric receptors may be as purely nociceptive mechanoreceptors that signal gross distension or distortion of the gut. However, they may instead or additionally signal changes in blood flow, a role that is favored by their close proximity to blood vessels.[28] Further to this role, they are frequently found to be chemosensitive, and respond to low concentrations of 5-HT and other mediators.[11,21,29] This places them in a good position to be systemic detectors of

mediator release from the gut mucosa. It is not yet possible to determine which of these three functions is the more likely to be the major role of serosal and mesenteric receptors, nor is it possible to reconcile their serving all three functions simultaneously. However, it is clear that they form a major part of the pelvic and splanchnic innervation of the colon and rectum. Interestingly, mesenteric receptors are confined to the splanchnic innervation, whereas serosal receptors are evident in all three pathways.[24] This may suggest that there are discrete functions of each type. Their chemosensitivity to chemical mediators makes serosal and mesenteric receptors potential targets in functional diseases.

Silent nociceptors

Based on parallels with somatosensory pathways, another class of primary afferents has been proposed that may be distinct from the three above. They are known as 'silent nociceptors' (or 'mechanically insensitive afferents') as they are normally silent at all times, but develop activity and mechanosensitivity during and after inflammation through the action of inflammatory mediators. These afferents have been identified in the pelvic innervation of the colon *in vivo*,[26] but it is possible that they may turn out to belong to one of the classes described above when investigated *in vitro*. The location of their receptive fields is not yet known, and this may provide important clues as to how they relate to the other classes. As their name suggests, they are considered to be exclusively involved in mediating pain from the gut, and may thus constitute a highly specific target in functional diseases.

Modulation of extrinsic sensory nerves

For many years, the focus on the modulation of function in extrinsic afferents was driven by the concept of their activation by endogenous chemical mediators, and the use of antagonists to block this activation. A good example of this was the involvement of 5-HT in nausea and vomiting, which was shown to depend on vagal innervation. Antagonists for 5-HT$_3$ receptors are successful in reducing nausea and vomiting after radiation, and this effect can be attributed to the blockade of action of 5-HT released from the intestinal mucosa on vagal mucosal receptors.[30] More recently, κ-opioid agonists were shown to inhibit directly the responses of colonic distension-sensitive afferents, thus demonstrating that it was not necessary to identify endogenous mediators for a drug to block. In fact, the lack of endogenous activation of receptors may confer a higher degree of selectivity of agonist drugs acting upon them. This approach is limited only by the fact that the receptor in question must be inhibitory on nerve function and localized on primary afferent endings. The κ-agonists have attracted intense interest in the treatment of functional gastrointestinal disease, several clinical trials showing promise.[31] Our laboratory has focused on other inhibitory G-protein-coupled receptors, including GABA$_B$, metabotropic glutamate and galanin receptors. All these have been shown to inhibit mechanosensitivity in vagal afferents and, to some extent, spinal afferents. GABA$_B$ receptors have been shown in addition to reduce transmission centrally, and thus have a double action. This is attributable for their potent inhibition of the triggering of transient lower esophageal sphincter relaxations following gastric distension,[32] and has important implications for the pharmacotherapy of gastro-esophageal reflux disease. The number of other potentially useful G-protein-coupled receptors is impressive, although many of these are currently 'orphaned', i.e. their natural ligands have yet to be discovered. Any of these receptors that may exist on extrinsic primary afferents are potential candidates for targeting in functional gastrointestinal diseases, particularly if they can be targeted selectively in the periphery, thereby avoiding CNS side-effects. Other drug targets on extrinsic sensory nerves are emerging, including ion channels

(see also Chapter 3) which are summarized in Fig. 16.2 and in other reviews.[20,29]

The central nervous system

Upon reaching the spinal cord, sensory information from the gut is subject to a high degree of convergence with signals from somatic structures. This is the neurophysiological correlate of referred sensation. From the spinal dorsal horn upwards, sensory pathways are therefore shared between the gut and the rest of the body. Pharmacological intervention at these points is therefore unlikely to be specific for gut sensations. Despite this, there are areas of the prefrontal and cingulate cortex that are specifically activated during the processing of sensory input from the gut, in particular affective aspects of the stimulus. These areas of the brain are therefore potentially selective targets for the treatment of functional disease. The therapeutic effect of alosetron is associated with reduced activation in these areas,[33] and suggests that it may be sufficient to alleviate the unpleasantness associated with a sensation without reducing the intensity of the sensation *per se*.

Conclusions

Although sensory pathways from the gastrointestinal tract from the brain are obvious targets for the pharmacotherapy of functional gastrointestinal disease, it is clear from the literature that there are several other cell types that may make equally useful targets. Because of

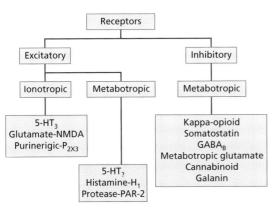

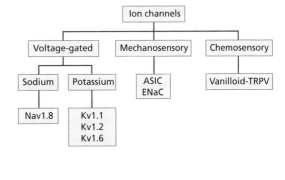

Fig. 16.2 Potential pharmacological targets on extrinsic sensory neurons. Some receptors and ion channels emerging from recent literature and conferences are shown. See also references 20 and 29.

the increasing evidence for specialization within and between pathways, it is also clear that extrinsic primary afferents should not be treated as a homogeneous population. Although details of pharmacological targets are not the subject of this chapter, these are many and varied. They include inhibitory and excitatory neurotransmitter receptors, enzymes, ion channels and intracellular mechanisms.

References

1. Richter JE. Gastroesophageal reflux disease as a cause of chest pain. *Med Clin North Am* 1991; **75**: 1065–80.

2 Spiller RC. Postinfectious irritable bowel syndrome. *Gastroenterology* 2003; **124**: 1662–71.

3 Edwards CA, Brown S, Baxter AJ, Bannister JJ, Read NW. Effect of bile acid on anorectal function in man. *Gut* 1989; **30**: 383–6.

4 Camilleri M. Management of the irritable bowel syndrome. *Gastroenterology* 2001; **120**: 652–68.

5 Sanders KM, Ordog T, Ward SM. Physiology and pathophysiology of the interstitial cells of Cajal: from bench to bedside. IV. Genetic and animal models of GI motility disorders caused by loss of interstitial cells of Cajal. *Am J Physiol Gastrointest Liver Physiol* 2002; **282**: G747–56.

6 Fox EA, Phillips RJ, Byerly MS, Baronowsky EA, Chi MM, Powley TL. Selective loss of vagal intramuscular mechanoreceptors in mice mutant for steel factor, the c-Kit receptor ligand. *Anat Embryol (Berl)* 2002; **205**: 325–42.

7 Feinle C, D'Amato M, Read NW. Cholecystokinin-A receptors modulate gastric sensory and motor responses to gastric distension and duodenal lipid. *Gastroenterology* 1996; **110**: 1379–85.

8 Larsson I. Studies on the extrinsic neural control of serotonin release from the small intestine. *Acta Physiol Scand* 1981; **499** (Suppl.): 1–43.

9 Pan H, Gershon MD. Activation of intrinsic afferent pathways in submucosal ganglia of the guinea pig small intestine. *J Neurosci* 2000; **20**: 3295–309.

10 Blackshaw LA, Grundy D. Effects of 5-hydroxytryptamine on discharge of vagal mucosal afferent fibres from the upper gastrointestinal tract of the ferret. *J Auton Nerv Syst* 1993; **45**: 41–50.

11 Hicks GA, Coldwell JR, Schindler M *et al.* Excitation of rat colonic afferent fibres by 5-HT(3) receptors. *J Physiol* 2002; **544**: 861–9.

12 Houghton LA, Atkinson W, Whitaker RP, Whorwell PJ, Rimmer MJ. Increased platelet depleted plasma 5-hydroxytryptamine concentration following meal ingestion in symptomatic female subjects with diarrhoea predominant irritable bowel syndrome. *Gut* 2003; **52**: 663–70.

13 Spiller RC, Jenkins D, Thornley JP *et al.* Increased rectal mucosal enteroendocrine cells, T lymphocytes, and increased gut permeability following acute *Campylobacter* enteritis and in post-dysenteric irritable bowel syndrome. *Gut* 2000; **47**: 804–11.

14 Dockray GJ. The G. W. Harris Prize Lecture. The gut endocrine system and its control. *Exp Physiol* 1994; **79**: 607–34.

15 Ahlman H, Nilsson. The gut as the largest endocrine organ in the body. *Ann Oncol* 2001; **12** (Suppl. 2): S63–8.

16 Yu LC, Perdue MH. Role of mast cells in intestinal mucosal function: studies in models of hypersensitivity and stress. *Immunol Rev* 2001; **179**: 61–73.

17 Barbara G, Stanghellini V, De Giorgio R *et al.* Activated mast cells in proximity to colonic nerves correlate with abdominal pain in irritable bowel syndrome. *Gastroenterology* 2004; **26**: 693–702.

18 Bertrand PP, Kunze WA, Furness JB, Bornstein JC. The terminals of myenteric intrinsic primary afferent neurons of the guinea-pig ileum are excited by 5-hydroxytryptamine acting at 5-hydroxytryptamine-3 receptors. *Neuroscience* 2000; **101**: 459–69.

19 Kunze WA, Furness JB, Bertrand PP, Bornstein JC. Intracellular recording from myenteric neurons of the guinea-pig ileum that respond to stretch. *J Physiol* 1998; **506**: 827–42.

20 Blackshaw LA, Gebhart GF. The pharmacology of gastrointestinal nociceptive pathways. *Curr Opin Pharmacol* 2002; **2**: 642–69.

21 Lynn PA, Blackshaw LA. *In vitro* recordings of afferent fibres with receptive fields in the serosa, muscle and mucosa of rat colon. *J Physiol* 1999; **518**: 271–82.

22 Page AJ, Blackshaw LA. An *in vitro* study of the properties of vagal afferent fibres innervating the ferret oesophagus and stomach. *J Physiol* 1998; **512**: 907–16.

23 Page AJ, Martin CM, Blackshaw LA. Vagal mechanoreceptors and chemoreceptors in mouse stomach and esophagus. *J Neurophysiol* 2002; **87**: 2095–103.

24 Brierley SM, Jones RCW, Gebhart GF, Blackshaw LA. Splanchnic and pelvic mechanosensory afferents signal different qualities of colonic stimuli in mice. *Gastroenterology* 2004; **127**: 166–78.

25 Andrew LK, Blackshaw LA. Colonic mechanoreceptor inputs to rat lumbo-sacral dorsal horn neurones: distribution, thresholds and chemosensory modulation. *Neurogastroenterol Motil* 2001; **13**: 333–7.

26 Sengupta JN. The sensory innervation of the colon and its modulation. *Curr Opin Gastroenterol* 1997; **13**: 246–60.

27 Haupt P, Janig W, Kohler W. Response pattern of visceral afferent fibres, supplying the colon, upon chemical and mechanical stimulation. *Pflugers Arch* 1983; **398**: 41–7.

28 Brunsden AM, Jacob S, Bardhan KD, Grundy D. Mesenteric

afferent nerves are sensitive to vascular perfusion in a novel preparation of rat ileum *in vitro. Am J Physiol Gastrointest Liver Physiol* 2002; **283**: G656–65.

29 Kirkup AJ, Brunsden AM, Grundy D. Receptors and transmission in the brain–gut axis: potential for novel therapies. I. Receptors on visceral afferents. *Am J Physiol Gastrointest Liver Physiol* 2001; **280**: G787–94.

30 Andrews PLR, Davis CJ, Bingham S, Davidson HIM, Hawthorn J, Maskell L. The abdominal visceral innervation and the emetic reflex: pathways, pharmacology, and plasticity. *Can J Physiol Pharmacol* 1990; **68**: 325–45.

31 Delvaux M. Pharmacology and clinical experience with fedotozine. *Expert Opin Invest Drugs* 2001; **10**: 97–110.

32 Blackshaw LA. Receptors and transmission in the brain–gut axis: potential for novel therapies. IV. GABA(B) receptors in the brain–gastroesophageal axis. *Am J Physiol Gastrointest Liver Physiol* 2001; **281**: G311–15.

33 Berman SM, Chang L, Suyenobu B *et al.* Condition-specific deactivation of brain regions by 5-HT3 receptor antagonist Alosetron. *Gastroenterology* 2002; **123**: 969–77.

CHAPTER 17

Tachykinin Receptor Antagonists: Silencing Neuropeptides with a Role in the Disturbed Gut

Peter Holzer

Tachykinins: mouth-watering yet emetogenic

In 1931, Ulf S von Euler and John H Gaddum reported that both gut and brain contained a substance which caused contraction of intestinal smooth muscle but was different from any of the endogenous compounds known at that time. The effects of the powdery extracts were marked as *P* on the kymograph tracings, so that since 1934 the term 'substance P' (SP) has been used in the literature.[1] In the late 1960s, SP appeared on the stage as a hypothalamic peptide causing copious salivary secretion, a biological activity which greatly helped Susan E Leeman and her laboratory to identify SP as undecapeptide.[2] SP turned out to be the mammalian counterpart of a family of peptides which had been extracted from amphibian and non-vertebrate species and given the name 'tachykinins' by Vittorio Erspamer.[3] Soon, novel members of this peptide family were discovered, and in mammals SP was joined by neurokinin A (NKA) and neurokinin B (NKB).[4] The first two tachykinin genes, now termed *TAC1* and *TAC3* by the Human Genome Organisation Nomenclature Committee (http://www.gene.ucl.ac.uk/nomenclature), were characterized in the late 1980s, and the pharmacological evidence for a heterogeneity of tachykinin receptors was corroborated by the identification of three tachykinin receptor genes[5] called *TACR1*, *TACR2* and *TACR3*. From 1991 onwards, potent non-peptide antagonists selective for the tachykinin NK_1, NK_2 or NK_3 receptor were developed, which made possible the thorough exploration of the pathophysiological implications of tachykinins.[6] In 2003, the first NK_1 receptor antagonist was successfully turned into a drug, and aprepitant was approved for the combination treatment of chemotherapy-induced emesis.[7] Meanwhile, the family of mammalian tachykinins has been expanded by the discovery of hemokinin 1, endokinin A, endokinin B and chromosome 14 tachykinin-like peptide 1 (C14TKL-1).[8]

Molecular characteristics of tachykinins and tachykinin receptors

The common structural feature of tachykinins is their amidated C-terminal amino acid sequence F-*X*-G-L-M-NH_2 (Fig. 17.1), which is fundamentally important for their affinity to tachykinin receptors and biological activity.[3,6,8] Currently, three tachykinin genes have been identified, but the gene encoding C14TKL-1 has not yet been characterized (Table 17.1). SP and NKA are derived from the *TAC1* gene (previously called *PPT-A* for preprotachykinin A), whose primary ribonucleic acid (RNA) transcript is alternatively spliced to produce four different types of mRNA (Table 17.1) which either encode SP or SP plus NKA and some N-terminally extended forms of NKA, such as neuropeptide K and neuropeptide γ (Fig. 17.1). The *TAC3* (*PPT-B*) gene gives rise to NKB, while the human *TAC4* (*PPT-C*) gene is alternatively processed to yield hemokinin 1 and/or endokinin A, B, C or D (Fig. 17.1 and Table 17.1). Endokinin A and endokinin B are N-terminally elongated forms of human hemokinin 1 (Fig. 17.1), whereas endokinin C and D are not tachykinins in the strict sense because their C-terminal sequence is F-X-G-L-*L*-NH_2

The tachykinin system as drug target in gastrointestinal disease

The tachykinin system in the gut
- The tachykinin substance P (SP) and neurokinin A (NKA) are expressed in intrinsic enteric neurons and extrinsic primary afferent neurons.
- Upon release, tachykinins can influence most digestive effector systems by interaction with tachykinin NK_1, NK_2 and NK_3 receptors.

Functional implications of tachykinins in the gut: SP and NKA
- Mediate slow synaptic transmission in the enteric nervous system.
- Participate in enteric motor regulation, especially in the colon.
- Facilitate ion and fluid secretion.
- Exert proinflammatory effects.
- Are transmitters of nociceptive afferent pathways.
- Contribute to emetic reflex transmission in the brainstem.

Physiological versus pathophysiological roles of tachykinins in the gut
- Physiologically, SP and NKA are backup cotransmitters of cholinergic enteric neurons and nociceptive afferent neurons.
- Pathophysiologically, the expression of tachykinins and their receptors is profoundly altered in gastrointestinal disorders of various etiology.
- In inflammatory bowel disease and experimentally induced gastrointestinal inflammation, the enteric nervous system is remodeled such that the tachykininergic innervation becomes more prominent relative to the cholinergic innervation.
- Tachykinin receptor antagonists are little active in the normal gut but can correct functional manifestations of experimental inflammation, such as dysmotility, hypersecretion and hyperalgesia.

Therapeutic perspectives
- Antagonism of tachykinin receptors is a promising option for the treatment of inflammatory bowel disease, irritable bowel syndrome, vomiting and abdominal hyperalgesia.
- Antagonists targeting multiple tachykinin receptors may be more efficacious than selective mono-receptor antagonists.

Fig. 17.1 Amino acid sequence of major mammalian tachykinins.

Substance P	R-P-K-P-Q-Q-**F**-F-**G**-**L**-**M**-NH$_2$
Neurokinin A	H-K-T-D-S-**F**-V-**G**-**L**-**M**-NH$_2$
Neuropeptide K	D-A-D-S-S-I-E-K-Q-V-A-L-L-K-A-L-Y-G-H-G-Q-I-S-H-K-R-H-K-T-D-S-**F**-V-**G**-**L**-**M**-NH$_2$
Neuropeptide γ	D-A- G-H-G-Q-I-S-H-K-R-H-K-T-D-S-**F**-V-**G**-**L**-**M**-NH$_2$
Neurokinin B	D-M-H-D-**F**-V-**G**-**L**-**M**-NH$_2$
Chromosome 14 tachykinin-like peptide 1 (C14TKL-1)	R-H-R-T-P-M-**F**-Y-**G**-**L**-**M**-NH$_2$
Mouse/rat hemokinin 1	R-S-R-T-R-Q-**F**-Y-**G**-**L**-**M**-NH$_2$
Human hemokinin 1	T-G-K-A-S-Q-**F**-F-**G**-**L**-**M**-NH$_2$
Human endokinin A/B*	-G-K-A-S-Q-**F**-F-**G**-**L**-**M**-NH$_2$
Human endokinin C	K-K-A-Y-Q-L-E-H-T-**F**-Q-**G**-**L**-L-NH$_2$
Human endokinin D	V-G-A-Y-Q-L-E-H-T-**F**-Q-**G**-**L**-L-NH$_2$

* Shown is the C-terminal decapeptidic fragment common to Endokinin A (47 amino acids) and Endokinin B (41 amino acids), which are elongated forms of human Hemokinin 1 (11 amino acids).

instead of F-X-G-L-M-NH$_2$ (Fig. 17.1). While SP, NKA and NKB are conserved across mammalian species, the amino acid sequence of hemokinin 1 shows considerable variation between humans and rodents.

Most of the biological actions of tachykinins, particularly in the gastrointestinal tract, are mediated by three tachykinin receptors,[5,6,8] currently termed NK$_1$, NK$_2$ and NK$_3$ receptors and encoded by three genes, TACR1, TACR2 and TACR3 (Table 17.2). The membrane topology of these receptors is typical of metabotropic receptors with seven transmembrane domains. Although SP, NKA and NKB are agonists with preferential affinity for NK$_1$, NK$_2$ and NK$_3$ receptors, respectively (Table 17.2), they are full agonists at all three tachykinin receptors.[9] Human hemokinin 1 and C14TKL-1 are preferential NK$_1$ receptor agonists, while the receptor selectivity of endokinins A, B, C and D has not yet been reported.[8] By modification of the amino acid sequence of endogenous tachykinins, selective agonists for all three tachykinin receptors have been obtained, and this advance has been complemented by the design of potent and receptor-selective non-peptide antagonists for NK$_1$, NK$_2$ and NK$_3$ receptors (Table 17.2).

The amino acid sequence of the tachykinin receptors varies slightly across mammalian species,[3] which has little impact on the affinity of endogenous tachykinins and receptor-selective agonists but is the reason for remarkable species differences in the potency of non-peptide tachykinin receptor antagonists.[6] Being coupled to G-proteins, the tachykinin receptors utilize the phospholipase C/phosphoinositide system as major transduction pathway,[4–6] although other signaling mechanisms, such as the adenylate cyclase pathway, may also play a role.

Expression of tachykinins and tachykinin receptors in the gut

Since TAC1 mRNA prevails in the gut, SP and NKA are the predominant tachykinins in this organ system, whereas NKB has proved difficult to detect in the bowel[10,11] and the precise localization of TAC4 gene products in the gastrointestinal tract has not yet been determined. Although some SP is contained in enterochromaffin and immune cells of the gastrointestinal mucosa, the major source of tachykinins in the gut is the enteric nervous system.[10,11] In the guinea-pig intestine, SP is typically present in intrinsic primary afferent neurons (IPANs) of the myenteric and submucous plexus and, within the myenteric plexus, in ascending interneurons as well as in excitatory motoneurons to the longitudinal and circular muscle (Fig. 17.2).[12–14] Characteristically, most enteric neurons containing SP co-express choline acetyltransferase, which means that tachykinins are cotransmitters of cholinergic neurons. These tachykininergic enteric neurons can be further subgrouped by their content of calbindin/calretinin, neurofilament protein triplet and dynorphin/enkephalin-like immunoreactivity (Fig. 17.2). Primary afferent neurons that originate from dorsal root ganglia and reach the gut via sympathetic and sacral parasympa-

Chromosomal location	Gene	mRNAs	Peptides
Chromosome 7	TAC1 (PPT-A)	α-TAC1	Substance P
		β-TAC1	Substance P, neurokinin A, neuropeptide K
		γ-TAC1	Substance P, neurokinin A, neuropeptide γ
		δ-TAC1	Substance P
Chromosome 12	TAC3 (PPT-B)	α-TAC3	Neurokinin B
		β-TAC3	Neurokinin B
Chromosome 14			Chromosome 14 tachykinin-like peptide 1
Chromosome 17	TAC4 (PPT-C)	α-TAC4	Hemokinin 1, endokinin A, endokinin C
		β-TAC4	Hemokinin 1, endokinin B, endokinin D
		γ-TAC4	Hemokinin 1, endokinin B
		δ-TAC4	Hemokinin 1, endokinin B

Table 17.1 Human tachykinin genes and gene products

Table 17.2 Human tachykinin receptors, receptor agonists and receptor antagonists

Chromosomal location	Gene	Receptor	Endogenous agonist potency order	Selective agonists	Selective antagonists
Chromosome 2	TACR1	NK$_1$	SP = hHK1 = NKA > NKB	[Sar^9,Met(O$_2$)^{11}]-Substance P	Aprepitant (MK-869) Ezlopitant (CJ-11,974) Nolpitantium (SR-140,333) Vofovitant (GR-205,171)
Chromosome 10	TACR2	NK$_2$	NKA > NKB > SP = hHK1	(β-Ala^8)-Neurokinin A	Nepadutant (MEN-11420) Saredutant (SR-48,968)
	TACR3	NK$_3$	NKB > NKA > SP = hHK1	Senktide	Osanetant (SR-142,801) Talnetant (SB-223,412)

thetic nerves also contribute to the tachykinin content of the gut.[10,11] The peripheral fibers of these extrinsic sensory neurons project primarily to submucosal arterioles, but also supply the mucosa and enteric nerve plexuses (Fig. 17.2).

The distribution of tachykinin NK$_1$, NK$_2$ and NK$_3$ receptors to gastrointestinal neurons and effector cells (Fig 17.3) enables tachykinins to modify gastrointestinal motility, secretory activity, vascular diameter and permeability, immune function, gut sensitivity and nociception.[10,11,15–18] NK$_1$ receptors are found on longitudinal and circular muscle cells, interstitial cells of Cajal (ICCs), IPANs, excitatory and inhibitory mo-

toneurons, secretomotor neurons, epithelial cells and granulocytes of the rodent gut. In the human gastrointestinal tract, NK$_1$ receptors have also been localized to the muscularis mucosae, the media of submucosal blood vessels (Fig 17.3) and some immune cells. NK$_2$ receptors are typically expressed by the longitudinal muscle, circular muscle and muscularis mucosae and, in addition, are present on epithelial cells and enteric nerve endings (Fig 17.3). NK$_3$ receptors are largely confined to enteric neurons; in the rodent intestine IPANs, ascending and descending interneurons, excitatory and inhibitory motoneurons as well as secretomotor neurons are NK$_3$-positive (Fig. 17.3).

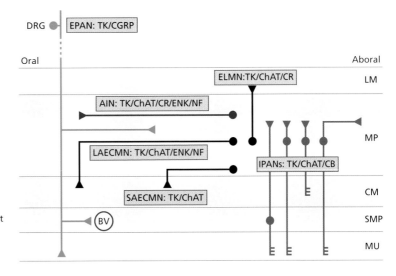

Fig. 17.2 Chemical coding and projections of the most important classes of tachykinin (TK)-immunoreactive neurons in the mammalian gut. AIN, ascending interneuron; BV, blood vessel; CB, calbindin; CGRP, calcitonin gene-related peptide; ChAT, choline acetyltransferase; CM, circular muscle; CR, calretinin; DRG, dorsal root ganglion; ELMN, excitatory longitudinal muscle motoneuron; ENK, enkephalin; EPAN, extrinsic primary afferent neuron; IPANs, intrinsic primary afferent neurons; LAECMN, long ascending excitatory circular muscle motor neuron; LM, longitudinal muscle; MP, myenteric plexus; MU, mucosa; NF, neurofilament protein; SAECMN, short ascending excitatory circular muscle motor neuron; SMP, submucous plexus.

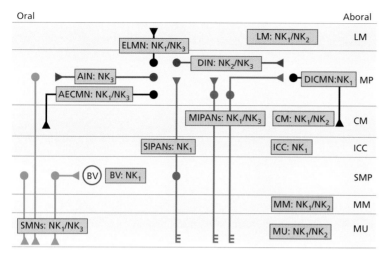

Fig. 17.3 Cellular expression of tachykinin NK_1, NK_2 and NK_3 receptors in the mammalian gut. Filled circles depict neuronal somata, filled triangles nerve endings. AECMN, ascending excitatory circular muscle motor neuron; AIN, ascending interneuron; BV, blood vessel; CM, circular muscle; DICMN, descending inhibitory circular muscle motor neuron; DIN, descending interneuron; ELMN, excitatory longitudinal muscle motor neuron; ICC, interstitial cell of Cajal; LM, longitudinal muscle; MIPANs, myenteric intrinsic primary afferent neurons; MM, muscularis mucosae; MP, myenteric plexus; MU, mucosa; SIPANs, submucosal intrinsic primary afferent neurons; SMN, secretomotor neuron; SMP, submucous plexus.

Physiological functions of tachykinins in the gut

Transmitter function

SP and NKA are cotransmitters of intrinsic enteric and extrinsic afferent neurons, which is consistent with their vesicular localization and calcium-dependent release upon nerve stimulation.[10,11,15,16] Within the enteric nervous system, tachykinins mediate slow postsynaptic excitation, a process that is relevant to the communication among IPANs (mediated primarily by NK_3 receptors), between IPANs and ascending as well as descending interneurons (mediated by NK_3 receptors), between ascending interneurons and excitatory motoneurons (mediated by NK_3 receptors) and between IPANs and inhibitory motoneurons (mediated by NK_1 receptors).[11,17–20] Furthermore, tachykinins participate in excitatory neuromuscular transmission (mediated by NK_2 and, to some extent, NK_1 receptors), although in this role they are subordinate to the principal transmitter acetylcholine.[11,16,21] Since NK_1, NK_2 and NK_3 receptors are present on SP-expressing neurons, it appears likely that presynaptic tachykinin autoreceptors exert feedback control of the transmission process.[11,22]

Motor regulation

Tachykinins can both stimulate and inhibit gastroin-testinal motility, the net response depending on the type and site of tachykinin receptors that are activated (see the text box: Motor actions and implications of tachykinins in the intestine). Facilitation of gastrointestinal motor activity is typically brought about by activation of NK_1 receptors on IPANs, ICCs and muscle cells, NK_2 receptors on muscle cells, and NK_3 receptors on IPANs, cholinergic interneurons and cholinergic motoneurons.[10,11,16,17,21] The stimulation of NK_1 receptors on ICCs enforces motility by prolonging the duration of the slow waves generated by these cells.[23] Tachykinin-induced muscle contraction in the human gut *in vitro* is prominently mediated by muscular NK_2 receptors,[11] and in the circular muscle of the isolated human sigmoid it appears as if tachykinins acting via NK_2 receptors are the main excitatory neurotransmitters released by nerve stimulation.[24] NK_2 receptors also make an important contribution to the effects of SP and NKA in stimulating motility in the human small intestine *in vivo* and in replacing the regular pattern of interdigestive motor activity by a pattern of irregular activity.[25,26] In contrast, the contractile response to NK_3 receptor stimulation is predominantly mediated by cholinergic neurons.[11]

NK_1 and NK_3 receptors on inhibitory motor pathways within the enteric nervous system enable tachykinins to depress motor activity (see the text box: Motor actions and implications of tachykinins in the intestine) via release of nitric oxide and adenosine triphosphate.[11,18,19,27] Accordingly, peristalsis in the guinea-pig small intestine is first stimulated, and then inhibited, by SP.[28] While NK_2 and NK_3 receptors are responsible for the stimulant response, NK_1 receptors mediate the inhibitory effect of SP through activation of nitrergic neurons.[29]

Despite the high pharmacological potency of tachykinins in modifying gastrointestinal motility, NK_1, NK_2 and NK_3 tachykinin receptor antagonists have little effect on gastrointestinal motor performance under physiological conditions, both *in vitro* and *in vivo*.[28,30] NK_1 receptor antagonists cause minor stimulation of peristaltic motility in the guinea-pig isolated small intestine[28] and enhance the velocity of propulsion in the rabbit isolated distal colon,[31] which is consistent with their ability to cause mild diarrhea in humans.[32,33] NK_2 receptor antagonists, on the contrary, do not alter small intestinal motility in humans[26] but lead to a minute inhibition of peristalsis in the guinea-pig small bowel.[28] Only when the overwhelming cholinergic component in the neural activation of smooth muscle has been compromised does blockade of tachykinin receptors impair peristalsis in the guinea-pig small intestine.[34,35] SP and NKA thus function as a backup system in the cholinergic activation of gastrointestinal muscle during peristalsis, a role that in the guinea-pig small intestine

is brought about by NK_1 and NK_2 receptors,[35] but in the human intestine is primarily mediated by NK_2 receptors.[36–38] However, when all three tachykinin receptors are blocked simultaneously, peristalsis in the guinea-pig distal colon is significantly depressed even without concomitant blockade of cholinergic transmission.[39]

From these findings it would appear that tachykinins regulate motility primarily in the colon, a hypothesis that has not yet been systematically tested. Furthermore, multi- or pan-tachykinin receptor antagonists may be more efficacious than monoreceptor antagonists in modifying gastrointestinal motor activity and, eventually, gastrointestinal motor disorders (see the text box: Motor actions and implications of tachykinins in the intestine).

Secretory regulation

Tachykinins modify endocrine and exocrine secretory processes in the gastrointestinal tract, including the stomach and pancreas.[11,14,15] Electrolyte and fluid output in the rodent intestine can be stimulated through activation of tachykinin NK_1 and NK_3 receptors on cholinergic and non-cholinergic secretomotor neurons in the submucous plexus as well as NK_1 and NK_2 receptors on epithelial cells. Mucosal ion transport in the isolated human colon is enhanced by both NK_1 and NK_2 receptor activation and subsequent stimulation of enteric neurons.[40–42]

Motor actions and implications of tachykinins in the intestine

Stimulation of motor activity is mainly via
- NK_1 receptors on ICCs and muscle cells;
- NK_2 receptors on muscle cells;
- NK_3 receptors on IPANs.

Inhibition of motor activity is mainly via
- NK_1 receptors on inhibitory motoneurons;
- NK_3 receptors on inhibitory motor pathways.

Effects of tachykinin receptor antagonists on gastrointestinal motility
- Minor effects of selective NK_1, NK_2 or NK_3 receptor antagonists on normal peristalsis.
- Inhibition of colonic peristalsis by NK_1, NK_2 and

NK_3 receptor antagonist combinations.
- Inhibition of atropine-compromised peristalsis by NK_1 or NK_2 receptor antagonists.

Pathophysiological implications in gastrointestinal motor control
- Tachykinins are cotransmitters and backup messengers of cholinergic enteric neurons.
- Gastrointestinal motor control by tachykinins is more important in the colon than in the small intestine.
- Multi- or pan-tachykinin receptor antagonists are more efficacious in gastrointestinal motor disorders than monotachykinin receptor antagonists.

The neurogenic actions of tachykinins in eliciting electrolyte and fluid secretion in the intestine are consistent with a role of SP and NKA as transmitters of enteric secretory reflexes. The implication of tachykinins in these reflexes may be threefold. Firstly, tachykinins released from IPANs or interneurons can activate cholinergic and non-cholinergic secretomotor neurons.[43–45] Secondly, SP can be released from axon collaterals of IPANs close to the epithelial effector cells and elicit chloride secretion via a mechanism resembling an axon reflex.[46] Thirdly, tachykinins released from extrinsic sensory nerve endings in response to capsaicin, *Clostridium difficile* toxin A or distension can stimulate enteric secretomotor neurons through activation of NK_1 and NK_3 receptors.[41,45,47]

Proinflammatory function

Tachykinins, particularly SP, are vasoactive peptides and may induce vasodilatation or vasoconstriction in the digestive tract, the type of action depending on the vascular bed and species under study.[11,15] The tachykinin-evoked vasodilatation in the intestine of cat, dog and guinea-pig is mediated by NK_1 receptors. Both SP and NKA enhance blood flow in the proximal small intestine of humans,[48] probably through activation of NK_1 receptors which have been localized to the media of submucosal blood vessels, at least in the human colon. Conversely, blood flow in the rat gastric mucosa is diminished by tachykinins by the constriction of collecting venules, a mechanism which may depend on the release of proteases from mast cells.[49]

Another effect of SP, acting via endothelial NK_1 receptors, is to increase venular permeability in the intestine and thereby to facilitate the extravasation of plasma proteins and leukocytes.[11,50] In addition, tachykinins can influence the activity of various immune cells in the gut.[51] Thus, NK_1 and NK_2 receptors have been localized to monocytes/macrophages, granulocytes, lymphoid cells and eosinophils, and stimulation of tachykinin receptors can lead to the recruitment and activation of granulocytes as well as mast cells in the gastrointestinal tract.[11,15]

Tachykinins and tachykinin receptors in gastrointestinal disease

Pathological changes in tachykinin expression

Many studies show that gastrointestinal infection, inflammation and mucosal injury are associated with time-related changes in the expression and release of tachykinins in the gut. However, the alterations in SP and NKA expression are variable, given that the intestinal tachykinin levels in patients with inflammatory bowel disease (IBD) have been reported to be either decreased, increased (see the text box: Pathological alterations of tachykinin (*TAC1* mRNA, SP, NKA) expression in the gastrointestinal tract) or unchanged.[11] Importantly, whole-mount analysis of the myenteric plexus has revealed that the chemical coding of enteric neurons in ulcerative colitis is shifted inasmuch as the ratio of SP-positive versus SP-negative cholinergic neurons is significantly increased.[52] Animal studies have shown that experimental infection and inflammation also causes changes in the gastrointestinal tachykinin levels (see the text box: Pathological alterations of tachykinin (*TAC1* mRNA, SP, NKA) expression in the gastrointestinal tract), which mirror those seen in IBD to a variable degree.[11]

Pathological changes in tachykinin receptor expression

Perturbations of tachykinin receptor expression in gastrointestinal disease are of particular relevance to disease mechanisms and may provide important therapeutic clues. Importantly, IBD is accompanied by increased expression of NK_1 and NK_2 receptors in the inflamed and non-inflamed regions of the human ileum and colon (see the text box: Pathological alterations of tachykinin receptor expression in the gastrointestinal tract).[53–55] The upregulation and ectopic occurrence of SP binding sites in pseudomembranous colitis due to *Clostridium difficile* infection[56] is reproduced by treatment of rats with *Clostridium difficile* toxin A.[57] Several other studies have shown that the expression of tachykinin receptors is either up- or downregulated under conditions of experimentally induced infection or inflammation (see the text box: Pathological alterations of tachykinin receptor expression in the gastrointestinal tract).[11]

Pathological alterations of tachykinin (*TAC1* mRNA, SP, NKA) expression in the gastrointestinal tract

Gastrointestinal disease

Increase in tachykinin expression
- Non-ulcer dyspepsia (stomach)
- Pancreatitis (pancreas)
- Pouchitis (ileum)
- Ulcerative colitis (colon)
- Irradiation (colon).

Decrease in tachykinin expression
- Gastro-esophageal reflux (stomach)
- Crohn's disease (colon)
- Ulcerative colitis (colon)
- Chronic obstipation (colon)

Experimental models of gastrointestinal disease

Increase in tachykinin expression
- *Helicobacter pylori* infection (mouse stomach)
- *Trichinella spiralis* infection (rat and mouse small intestine)

- *Schistosoma japonicum* infection (pig colon)
- Treatment with *Clostridium difficile* toxin A (rat small intestine)
- Inflammation caused by dextran sulfate (rat colon)

Decrease in tachykinin expression
- Treatment with *Escherichia coli* endotoxin (rat small intestine)
- *Schistosoma mansoni* infection (mouse small intestine)
- *Trichinella spiralis* infection (ferret and guinea-pig small intestine)
- *Trypanosoma cruzi* infection (mouse colon)
- Inflammation caused by trinitrobenzene sulfonic acid (guinea-pig small intestine, rat and rabbit colon)
- Inflammation caused by zymosan (rat colon)
- Immune complex-induced inflammation (rabbit colon)

Pathological alterations of tachykinin receptor expression in the gastrointestinal tract

Gastrointestinal disease

Upregulation of tachykinin receptors
- Crohn's disease (NK_1 receptors on lymphoid cells, epithelial cells, endothelial cells and enteric neurons, NK_2 receptors on eosinophils)
- Ulcerative colitis (NK_1 receptors on lymphoid cells and endothelial cells, NK_2 receptors on eosinophils)
- Pseudomembranous colitis due to *Clostridium difficile* infection (SP binding sites on small blood vessels and lymphoid aggregates)

Downregulation of tachykinin receptors
- Ulcerative colitis (downregulation of NK_1 receptors on epithelial cells)

Experimental models of gastrointestinal disease

Upregulation of tachykinin receptors
- Infection with *Cryptosporidium parvum* (NK_1 receptors in mouse intestine)
- Infection with *Salmonella dublin* (NK_1 receptors on macrophages in rat intestine)
- Treatment with *Clostridium difficile* toxin A (NK_1 receptors on epithelial cells in rat intestine)

Downregulation of tachykinin receptors
- Infection with *Nippostrongylus brasiliensis* (NK_1 receptors on myenteric neurons and NK_2 receptors on muscle cells in rat intestine)
- Inflammation caused by trinitrobenzene sulfonic acid (NK_1 and NK_2 receptors on vasculature, muscle and nerve of rat and rabbit colon)

Therapeutic potential of tachykinin receptor antagonists in gastrointestinal disease

Although the alterations in the expression of tachykinins and tachykinin receptors following gastrointestinal infection, inflammation and other injury are variable, they attest to the dynamic regulation of the gastrointestinal tachykinin system in health and disease and prompt the hypothesis that various gastrointestinal disorders involve an imbalanced function of SP and NKA.[11] If so, tachykinin receptor antagonists may provide therapeutic benefit in diseases in which the tachykinin system is upregulated. There is indeed preclinical evidence that tachykinin receptor antagonists should be useful in the treatment of gastrointestinal motor disorders, diarrhea, IBD, functional bowel disorders such as irritable bowel syndrome (IBS), abdominal hyperalgesia as well as nausea and vomiting.[11] While the antiemetic efficacy of the NK_1 receptor antagonist aprepitant has been proved,[7,32,58] clinical studies substantiating a therapeutic effect of tachykinin receptor antagonists in other conditions of gastrointestinal disease have not yet been published.

Motor disturbances

There is good reason to think that tachykinins are involved in pathological disturbances of gastrointestinal motility, because the motor effects of tachykinins are changed in certain gastrointestinal diseases and tachykinin receptor antagonists are beneficial in experimental models of gastrointestinal dysmotility. For instance, the efficacy of NK_2 receptor agonists in contracting the colonic circular muscle *in vitro* is attenuated in IBD.[36,59] Similarly, the responsiveness of the colonic musculature to tachykinin receptor agonists is depressed by trinitrobenzene sulfonic acid-induced colitis in the rat and rabbit, whereas in ricin-evoked ileitis of the rabbit tachykinin-mediated neurogenic contractions are amplified.[11] The ability of NK_2 receptor agonists to stimulate colonic circular muscle activity is increased in some patients with chronic idiopathic constipation,[59] while NK_2 receptor-mediated transmission to the colonic circular muscle is deficient in children with slow-transit constipation.[60]

Tachykinin receptor antagonists are able to correct many forms of experimentally disturbed motility in the gut (see the text box: Effects of tachykinin receptor antagonists in experimental models of gastrointestinal motor disturbances). Specifically, NK_1 receptor antagonists inhibit stress-induced defecation and correct the hypomotility and muscular hyporesponsiveness caused by anaphylaxis, inflammation and pain.[11] Postoperative and peritonitis-induced ileus is ameliorated by both NK_1 and NK_2 receptor antagonists, while the giant colonic contractions associated with inflammatory diarrhea are effectively suppressed by NK_2 receptor antagonists (see the text box: Effects of

---

Effects of tachykinin receptor antagonists in experimental models of gastrointestinal motor disturbances

Beneficial effects of NK_1 receptor antagonists on:
- Acid-induced relaxation of ferret lower esophageal sphincter
- Inhibition of rat gastric motility after peritoneal irritation
- Inhibition of rat gastrointestinal transit after abdominal surgery
- Disruption of migrating motor complex in rat intestine after ovalbumin anaphylaxis
- Hyporesponsiveness of rat colon muscle after trinitrobenzene sulfonic acid-induced inflammation

- Inhibition of rat colon motility by noxious rectal distension
- Increased defecation in rat and Mongolian gerbil after restraint stress

Beneficial effects of NK_2 receptor antagonists on:
- Inhibition of rat gastrointestinal transit after abdominal surgery
- Giant contractions of rat colon in castor oil-induced inflammatory diarrhea
- High-amplitude motility in rat colon after acetic acid irritation.

tachykinin receptor antagonists in experimental models of gastrointestinal motor disturbances). Although the usefulness of NK_3 receptor antagonists remains to be explored, it appears that NK_1 receptor antagonists are particularly useful in alleviating gastrointestinal motor inhibition, whereas NK_2 receptor antagonists are beneficial in attenuating pathological hypermotility without causing constipation.[11]

Apart from acting on mast cells, enteric neurons and muscle cells, tachykinin receptor antagonists may correct gastrointestinal dysmotility by inhibiting the function of extrinsic afferents which can contribute to gastrointestinal motor dysregulation in two ways.[11] Firstly, they participate in autonomic intestino-intestinal reflexes in which SP and NKA, released from the central endings of sensory neurons in the spinal cord or brainstem, mediate transmission to the efferent reflex arc. Secondly, tachykinins released from sensory nerve endings in the gut can disturb gastrointestinal motility, an instance that may be reflected by the ability of NK_1

receptor antagonists to ameliorate dysmotility caused by esophageal acidification, anaphylaxis and inflammation (see the text box: Effects of tachykinin receptor antagonists in experimental models of gastrointestinal motor disturbances).

Hypersecretion and inflammation

There is considerable evidence that the tachykinin system contributes to gastrointestinal mucosal pathologies associated with infection, inflammation and functional bowel disorders.[11] Thus, the secretory response to SP is blunted in mucosal tissues isolated from patients with Crohn's disease or ulcerative colitis,[41] and tachykinin receptor antagonists display beneficial effects in various models of experimental gastrointestinal infection, inflammation, injury and diarrhea (see the text box: Effects of tachykinin receptor antagonists in experimental models of gastrointestinal hypersecretion and inflammation). Tachykinins play a particular role in the inflammation (granulocyte, mast cell and macrophage

---

Effects of tachykinin receptor antagonists in experimental models of gastrointestinal hypersecretion and inflammation

Beneficial effects of NK_1 receptor antagonists
- Cerulein-induced acute pancreatitis in mouse
- Choline deficiency-induced necrotizing pancreatitis in mouse
- Ischemia–reperfusion-induced inflammation and hemorrhage in rat duodenum
- Milk protein allergy-induced hypermastocytosis and hypersecretion in rat jejunum
- Anti-IgE-induced mast cell degranulation in isolated human colon
- *Cholera* toxin-induced hypersecretion in rat jejunum
- *Clostridium difficile* toxin A-induced inflammation and hypersecretion in rat and mouse small intestine
- *Trichinella spiralis*-induced inflammation in mouse small intestine
- *Cryptosporidium parvum*-induced colitis in mouse
- Dinitrobenzene sulfonic acid-induced mast cell degranulation, plasma protein leakage and damage in mouse small intestine and colon
- Trinitrobenzene sulfonic acid-induced granulocyte

infiltration and damage in rat and mouse colon
- Dextran sulfate-induced colitis in rat
- Acetic acid-induced rectocolitis in guinea-pig

Beneficial effects of NK_2 receptor antagonists
- *Cholera* toxin-induced hypersecretion in rat jejunum
- *Clostridium difficile* toxin A/B-induced diarrhea in mouse
- *Escherichia coli* toxin STa-induced diarrhea in mouse
- Trinitrobenzene sulfonic acid-induced granulocyte infiltration and damage in guinea-pig ileum and rat colon
- Acetic acid-induced rectocolitis in guinea-pig
- Castor oil-induced diarrhea in rat

Beneficial effects of NK_3 receptor antagonists
- Trinitrobenzene sulfonic acid-induced granulocyte infiltration and damage in guinea-pig ileum

activation) and hypersecretion evoked by *Clostridium difficile* toxin A, which involves activation of capsaicin-sensitive extrinsic afferent neurons, release of SP and activation of NK_1 receptors on enteric neurons.[47,56,57,61] Many types of gastrointestinal hypersecretion and inflammation depend on multiple tachykinin receptors (see the text box: Effects of tachykinin receptor antagonists in experimental models of gastrointestinal hypersecretion and inflammation), which is exemplified by the observations that the intestinal hypersecretion evoked by *Cholera* toxin, the diarrhea caused by castor oil and the trinitrobenzene sulfonic acid-induced rectocolitis in the rat are inhibited by both NK_1 and NK_2 receptor antagonists.[62–64]

Of clinical relevance is the question of whether tachykinins play a role in the initiation and/or maintenance of gastrointestinal hypersecretion and inflammation. Experimental data indicate that SP and NKA participate primarily in the initial stage of trinitrobenzene sulfonic acid- and acetic acid-induced colitis.[65] If so, tachykinin receptor antagonists may be more beneficial in the initiation or reactivation of inflammation than in the suppression of an ongoing inflammatory process. This view is in keeping with the proinflammatory activity of tachykinins, which comprises vasodilatation, enhancement of venular permeability and modulation of immune cell activity.[11] The effect of SP in increasing vascular permeability in the gastrointestinal tract is amplified in the inflamed tissue because inflammation leads to downregulation of neutral endopeptidase, which in normal tissue maintains low levels of SP in the extracellular fluid and thus limits its proinflammatory effects.[50,66]

Preclinical studies suggest that various immune cells in the gut are under the influence of SP and NKA.[41,51,67] Of particular relevance to gastrointestinal inflammation and hypersecretion is a bidirectional interplay between mast cells and tachykininergic neurons acting via NK_1 receptors. Other tachykinin-responsive immune cells in the gut include lymphocytes and granulocytes. In addition, it needs to be borne in mind that immune cells are not only targets of tachykinin actions, but under pathological conditions can themselves be induced to synthesize and release tachykinins. This is true for macrophages in the mucosa of the rat ileum exposed to *Clostridium difficile* toxin A[68] and for eosinophils from the mucosa of IBD patients.[69]

Hyperalgesia and pain

Since most of the spinal afferents supplying the rodent gastrointestinal tract express SP, tachykinin receptor antagonists have been explored for their therapeutic potential in abdominal nociception and IBS.[11,70] A double-blind pilot study has shown that the NK_1 receptor antagonist CJ-11,974 reduces IBS symptoms and attenuates the emotional response to rectosigmoid distension.[71] This outcome is consistent with a number of preclinical studies which attest to a beneficial effect of tachykinin receptor antagonists in abdominal pain and hyperalgesia (see the text box: Effects of tachykinin receptor antagonists in experimental models of gastrointestinal hyperalgesia and pain).[11] In addition, genetic deletion of NK_1 receptors abolishes pseudoaffective pain responses to intracolonic capsaicin and prevents the development of mechanical hyperalgesia in response to inflammation.[72]

Experimental studies with selective receptor antagonists show that all three tachykinin receptors play a role in gastrointestinal nociception and inflammation-induced hyperalgesia.[73] In addressing the question of which tachykinin receptors should be targeted in the treatment of gastrointestinal pain, two issues need to be considered. Firstly, there are species differences, given that the pain responses to colorectal distension in the rat are preferentially inhibited by NK_2 and NK_3 receptor antagonists, whereas in the rabbit NK_1 receptor antagonists are clearly active (see the text box: Effects of tachykinin receptor antagonists in experimental models of gastrointestinal hyperalgesia and pain).[74–76] Secondly, it appears that the analgesic efficacy of multi- and pan-tachykinin receptor antagonists is superior to that of mono-receptor antagonists. Thus, the inflammation-induced hypersensitivity to noxious colorectal distension in rats is not affected by intrathecal treatment with an NK_1 or NK_2 receptor antagonist alone but inhibited by their combined administration.[73] Similarly, the afferent signaling of a noxious acid stimulus from the stomach to the rat brainstem is attenuated only by simultaneous administration of an NK_1, an NK_2 and a ionotropic NMDA-type glutamate receptor antagonist.[77]

Conceptually, tachykinin receptor antagonists may target multiple relays in the pathways of gastrointestinal nociception from the periphery to the brain (Fig. 17.4). Apart from blocking tachykininergic transmission

Effects of tachykinin receptor antagonists in experimental models of gastrointestinal hyperalgesia and pain

Beneficial effects of NK$_1$ receptor antagonists
- Cardiovascular pain response to peritoneal irritation and jejunal distension in rat
- Inflammation-induced hypersensitivity to noxious colonic distension in rabbit

Beneficial effects of NK$_2$ receptor antagonists
- Cardiovascular pain response to peritoneal irritation and jejunal distension in rat
- Visceromotor pain response to gastric and colorectal distension in rat
- Enhanced c-Fos expression in spinal cord after trinitrobenzene sulfonic acid-induced irritation of

rat colon
- Inflammation- and stress-induced hypersensitivity to noxious rectal distension in rat
- Enhanced firing of lumbosacral afferents after distension of inflamed rat colon
- *Nippostrongylus brasiliensis*-evoked hypersensitivity to noxious jejunal distension in rat

Beneficial effects of NK$_3$ receptor antagonists
- Visceromotor pain response to colorectal distension in rat
- Inflammation-induced hypersensitivity to noxious colorectal distension in rat

from primary afferents, NK$_1$, NK$_2$ and NK$_3$ receptor antagonists may be indirectly antihyperalgesic owing to their beneficial activities on disordered gut function.[11] By correcting hyper- or hypomotility, hypersecretion

and inflammation, they are likely to reduce the sensory gain of extrinsic afferents in the gastrointestinal tract. In IBS therapy, the effects of brain-penetrant NK$_1$ receptor antagonists at the level of the gut and afferent

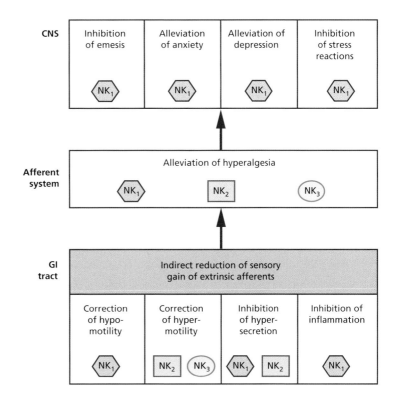

Fig. 17.4 Summary of the possible effects of tachykinin NK$_1$, NK$_2$ and NK$_3$ receptor antagonists in the treatment of gastrointestinal (GI) disease at the level of gut, primary afferent neurons and central nervous system (CNS).

system may combine favorably with their inhibitory actions on emesis, anxiety, depression and stress reactions in the brain (Fig. 17.4).[7,11,32,58,78,79]

Nausea and vomiting

In preclinical studies, NK_1 receptor antagonists inhibit vomiting caused by a variety of factors, including the anticancer agent cisplatin, irradiation, copper sulfate, morphine, apomorphine and motion.[7,78] This broad-spectrum profile of activity against peripherally and centrally acting emetogenic stimuli and the requirement for brain penetration demonstrate that NK_1 receptor antagonists interrupt the emetic reflex at a central site of action within the brainstem, close to the nucleus of the solitary tract and the Bötzinger complex.[7] The experimental observation that NK_1 receptor antagonists block both the acute and delayed phase of cisplatin-induced emesis has been reproduced in clinical trials. In particular, the NK_1 receptor antagonist aprepitant enhances the antiemetic efficacy of $5\text{-}HT_3$ receptor antagonists and dexamethasone in humans and, in this combination, provides significant control over the delayed phase of chemotherapy-induced nausea and emesis.[32,58] As a consequence, aprepitant was licensed in 2003, making this compound the first NK_1 receptor antagonist in clinical use. Trials to assess the activity of NK_1 receptor antagonists in motion sickness and postoperative vomiting are under way.

Acknowledgments

The artistry of Evelin Painsipp in preparing the figures is greatly appreciated. Work in the author's laboratory is supported by the Austrian Research Funds, the Jubilee Funds of the Austrian National Bank, the Austrian Federal Ministry of Education, Science and Culture and the Zukunftsfonds Steiermark.

References

1   Pernow B. Substance P. *Pharmacol Rev* 1983; **35**: 85–141.

2   Chang MM, Leeman SE. Isolation of a sialogogic peptide from bovine hypothalamic tissue and its characterization as substance P. *J Biol Chem* 1970; **245**: 4784–90.

3   Severini C, Improta G, Falconieri-Erspamer G, Salvadori S, Erspamer V. The tachykinin peptide family. *Pharmacol Rev* 2002; **54**: 285–322.

4   Maggio JE. Tachykinins. *Annu Rev Neurosci* 1988; **11**: 13–28

5   Nakanishi S. Mammalian tachykinin receptors. *Annu Rev Neurosci* 1991; **14**: 123–36.

6   Maggi CA. The mammalian tachykinin receptors. *Gen Pharmacol* 1995; **26**: 911–44.

7   Andrews PLR, Rudd JA. The role of tachykinins and the tachykinin NK_1 receptor in nausea and emesis. In: Holzer P, ed. *Tachykinins. Handbook of Experimental Pharmacology, Vol. 164.* Berlin: Springer, 2004: 359–440.

8   Patacchini R, Lecci A, Holzer P, Maggi CA. Newly discovered tachykinins raise new questions about their peripheral roles and the tachykinin nomenclature. *Trends Pharmacol Sci* 2004; **25**: 1–3.

9   Maggi CA, Schwartz TW. The dual nature of the tachykinin NK_1 receptor. *Trends Pharmacol Sci* 1997; **18**: 351–4.

10 Holzer P, Holzer-Petsche U. Tachykinins in the gut. Part I. Expression, release and motor function. *Pharmacol Ther* 1997; **73**: 173–217.

11 Holzer P. Role of tachykinins in the gastrointestinal tract. In: Holzer P, ed. *Tachykinins. Handbook of Experimental Pharmacology, Vol. 164.* Berlin: Springer, 2004: 511–58

12 Furness JB. Types of neurons in the enteric nervous system. *J Auton Nerv Syst* 2000; **81**: 87–96.

13 Brookes SJH. Classes of enteric nerve cells in the guinea-pig small intestine. *Anat Rec* 2001; **262**: 58–70.

14 Schemann M, Reiche D, Michel K. Enteric pathways in the stomach. *Anat Rec* 2001; **262**: 47–57.

15 Holzer P, Holzer-Petsche U. Tachykinins in the gut. Part II. Roles in neural excitation, secretion and inflammation. *Pharmacol Ther* 1997; **73**: 219–63.

16 Maggi CA. Principles of tachykininergic co-transmission in the peripheral and enteric nervous system. *Regul Pept* 2000; **93**: 53–64.

17 Furness JB, Sanger GJ. Intrinsic nerve circuits of the gastrointestinal tract: identification of drug targets. *Curr Opin Pharmacol* 2002; **2**: 612–22.

18 Alex G, Clerc N, Kunze WA, Furness JB. Responses of myenteric S neurones to low frequency stimulation of their synaptic inputs. *Neuroscience* 2002; **110**: 361–73.

19 Thornton PD, Bornstein JC. Slow excitatory synaptic potentials evoked by distension in myenteric descending interneurones of guinea-pig ileum. *J Physiol (Lond)* 2002; **539**: 589–602.

20 Tonini M, De Ponti F, Frigo G, Crema F. Pharmacology of the enteric nervous system. In: Brookes S, Costa M, eds. *Innervation of the Gastrointestinal Tract.* London: Taylor & Francis, 2002: 213–94.

21 Lecci A, Santicioli P, Maggi CA. Pharmacology of transmission to gastrointestinal muscle. *Curr Opin Pharmacol* 2002; **2**: 630–41.

22 Patacchini R, Maggi CA, Holzer P. Tachykinin autoreceptors in the gut. *Trends Pharmacol Sci* 2002; **21**: 166.

23 Huizinga JD, Thuneberg L, Vanderwinden JM, Rumessen JJ. Interstitial cells of Cajal as targets for pharmacological intervention in gastrointestinal motor disorders. *Trends Pharmacol Sci* 1997; **18**: 393–403.

24 Cao W, Pricolo VE, Zhang L, Behar J, Biancani P, Kirber MT. G_q-linked NK_2 receptors mediate neurally induced contraction of human sigmoid circular smooth muscle. *Gastroenterology* 2000; **119**: 51–61.

25 Lördal M, Theodorsson E, Hellström PM. Tachykinins influence interdigestive rhythm and contractile strength of human small intestine. *Dig Dis Sci* 1997; **42**: 1940–9.

26 Lördal M, Navalesi G, Theodorsson E, Maggi CA, Hellström PM. A novel tachykinin NK_2 receptor antagonist prevents motility-stimulating effects of neurokinin A in small intestine. *Br J Pharmacol* 2001; **134**: 215–23.

27 Lecci A, De Giorgio R, Barthó L *et al.* Tachykinin NK_1 receptor-mediated inhibitory responses in the guinea-pig small intestine. *Neuropeptides* 1999; **33**: 91–7.

28 Holzer P, Schluet W, Maggi CA. Substance P stimulates and inhibits intestinal peristalsis via distinct receptors. *J Pharmacol Exp Ther* 1995; **274**: 322–8.

29 Holzer P. Involvement of nitric oxide in the substance P-induced inhibition of intestinal peristalsis. *Neuroreport* 1997; **8**: 2857–60.

30 Crema F, Moro E, Nardelli G, de Ponti F, Frigo G, Crema A. Role of tachykininergic and cholinergic pathways in modulating canine gastric tone and compliance *in vivo*. *Pharmacol Res* 2002; **45**: 341–7.

31 Onori L, Aggio A, Taddei G *et al.* Peristalsis regulation by tachykinin NK_1 receptors in the rabbit isolated distal colon. *Am J Physiol* 2003; **285**: G325–31.

32 Campos D, Pereira JR, Reinhardt RR *et al.* Prevention of cisplatin-induced emesis by the oral neurokinin-1 antagonist, MK-869, in combination with granisetron and dexamethasone or with dexamethasone alone. *J Clin Oncol* 2001; **19**: 1759–67.

33 Goldstein DJ, Wang O, Gitter BD, Iyengar S. Dose-response study of the analgesic effect of lanepitant in patients with painful diabetic neuropathy. *Clin Neuropharmacol* 2001; **24**: 16–22.

34 Holzer P, Maggi CA. Synergistic role of muscarinic acetylcholine and tachykinin NK-2 receptors in intestinal peristalsis. *Naunyn Schmiedeberg's Arch Pharmacol* 1994; **349**: 194–201.

35 Holzer P, Lippe IT, Heinemann A, Barthó L. Tachykinin NK_1 and NK_2 receptor-mediated control of peristaltic propulsion in the guinea-pig small intestine *in vitro*. *Neuropharmacology* 1998; **37**: 131–8.

36 Al-Saffar A, Hellström PM. Contractile responses to natural tachykinins and selective tachykinin analogs in normal and inflamed ileal and colonic muscle. *Scand J Gastroenterol* 2002; **36**: 485–93.

37 Krysiak PS, Preiksaitis HG. Tachykinins contribute to nerve-mediated contractions in the human esophagus. *Gastroenterology* 2001; **120**: 39–48.

38 Mitolo-Chieppa D, Mansi G, Nacci C *et al.* Idiopathic chronic constipation: tachykinins as cotransmitters in colonic contraction. *Eur J Clin Invest* 2001; **31**: 349–55.

39 Tonini M, Spelta V, De Ponti F *et al.* Tachykinin-dependent and -independent components of peristalsis in the guinea pig isolated distal colon. *Gastroenterology* 2001; **120**: 938–45.

40 Riegler M, Castagliuolo I, So PT *et al.* Effects of substance P on human colonic mucosa in vitro. *Am J Physiol* 1999; **276**: G1473–83.

41 Moriarty D, Goldhill J, Selve N, O'Donoghue DP, Baird AW. Human colonic anti-secretory activity of the potent NK_1 antagonist, SR140333: assessment of potential antidiarrhoeal activity in food allergy and inflammatory bowel disease. *Br J Pharmacol* 2001; **133**: 1346–54.

42 Tough IR, Lewis CA, Fozard J, Cox HM. Dual and selective antagonism of neurokinin NK_1 and NK_2 receptor-mediated responses in human colon mucosa. *Naunyn-Schmiedeberg's Arch Pharmacol* 2003; **367**: 104–8.

43 Cooke HJ, Sidhu M, Wang YZ. Activation of 5-HT$_{1P}$ receptors on submucosal afferents subsequently triggers VIP neurons and chloride secretion in the guinea-pig colon. *J Auton Nerv Syst* 1997; **66**: 105–10.

44 Frieling T, Dobreva G, Weber E *et al.* Different tachykinin receptors mediate chloride secretion in the distal colon through activation of submucosal neurones. *Naunyn Schmiedeberg's Arch Pharmacol* 1999; **359**: 71–9.

45 Weber E, Neunlist M, Schemann M, Frieling T. Neural components of distension-evoked secretory responses in the guinea-pig distal colon. *J Physiol (Lond)* 2001; **536**: 741–51.

46 Cooke HJ, Sidhu M, Fox P, Wang YZ, Zimmermann EM. Substance P as a mediator of colonic secretory reflexes. *Am J Physiol* 1997; **272**: G238–45.

47 Pothoulakis C, Castagliuolo I, LaMont JT *et al.* CP-96,345, a substance P antagonist, inhibits rat intestinal responses to *Clostridium difficile* toxin A but not cholera toxin. *Proc Natl Acad Sci USA* 1994; **91**: 947–51.

48 Schmidt PT, Lördal M, Gazelius B, Hellström PM. Tachykinins potently stimulate human small bowel blood flow: a laser Doppler flowmetry study in humans. *Gut* 2003; **52**: 53–6.

49 Rydning A, Lyng O, Aase S, Grönbech JE. Substance P may attenuate gastric hyperemia by a mast cell-dependent mechanism in the damaged gastric mucosa. *Am J Physiol* 1999; **277**: G1064–73.

50 Sturiale S, Barbara G, Qiu B *et al*. Neutral endopeptidase (EC 3.4.24.11) terminates colitis by degrading substance P. *Proc Natl Acad Sci USA* 1999; **96**: 11653–8.

51 Maggi CA. The effects of tachykinins on inflammatory and immune cells. *Regul Pept* 1997; **70**: 75–90.

52 Neunlist M, Aubert P, Toquet C *et al*. Changes in chemical coding of myenteric neurones in ulcerative colitis. *Gut* 2003; **52**: 84–90.

53 Mantyh CR, Vigna SR, Bollinger RR, Mantyh PW, Maggio JE, Pappas TN. Differential expression of substance P receptors in patients with Crohn's disease and ulcerative colitis. *Gastroenterology* 1995; **109**: 850–60.

54 Goode T, O'Connell J, Anton P *et al*. Neurokinin-1 receptor expression in inflammatory bowel disease: molecular quantitation and localisation. *Gut* 2000; **47**: 387–96.

55 Renzi D, Pellegrini B, Tonelli F, Surrenti C, Calabro A. Substance P (neurokinin-1) and neurokinin A (neurokinin-2) receptor gene and protein expression in the healthy and inflamed human intestine. *Am J Pathol* 2000; **157**: 1511–22.

56 Mantyh CR, Maggio JE, Mantyh PW, Vigna SR, Pappas TN. Increased substance P receptor expression by blood vessels and lymphoid aggregates in *Clostridium difficile*-induced pseudomembranous colitis. *Dig Dis Sci* 1996; **41**: 614–20.

57 Pothoulakis C, Castagliuolo I, Leeman SE *et al*. Substance P receptor expression in intestinal epithelium in *Clostridium difficile* toxin A enteritis in rats. *Am J Physiol* 1998; **275**: G68–75.

58 de Wit R, Herrstedt J, Rapoport B *et al*. Addition of the oral NK$_1$ antagonist aprepitant to standard antiemetics provides protection against nausea and vomiting during multiple cycles of cisplatin-based chemotherapy. *J Clin Oncol* 2003; **21**: 4105–11.

59 Menzies JR, McKee R, Corbett AD. Differential alterations in tachykinin NK$_2$ receptors in isolated colonic circular smooth muscle in inflammatory bowel disease and idiopathic chronic constipation. *Regul Pept* 2001; **99**: 151–6.

60 Stanton MP, Hengel PT, Southwell BR *et al*. Cholinergic transmission to colonic circular muscle of children with slow-transit constipation is unimpaired, but transmission via NK$_2$ receptors is lacking. *Neurogastroenterol Motil* 2003; **15**: 669–78.

61 Castagliuolo I, Riegler M, Pasha A *et al*. Neurokinin-1 (NK-1) receptor is required in *Clostridium difficile*-induced enteritis. *J Clin Invest* 1998; **101**: 1547–50.

62 Croci T, Landi M, Emonds-Alt X, Le Fur G, Maffrand JP, Manara L. Role of tachykinins in castor oil diarrhoea in rats. *Br J Pharmacol* 1997; **121**: 375–80.

63 Mazelin L, Theodorou V, More J, Emonds-Alt X, Fioramonti J, Bueno L. Comparative effects of nonpeptide tachykinin receptor antagonists on experimental gut inflammation in rats and guinea-pigs. *Life Sci* 1998; **63**: 293–304.

64 Turvill JL, Connor P, Farthing MJ. Neurokinin 1 and 2 receptors mediate cholera toxin secretion in rat jejunum. *Gastroenterology* 2000; **119**: 1037–44.

65 Cutrufo C, Evangelista S, Cirillo R *et al*. Protective effect of the tachykinin NK$_2$ receptor antagonist nepadutant in acute rectocolitis induced by diluted acetic acid in guinea-pigs. *Neuropeptides* 2000; **34**: 355–9.

66 Kirkwood KS, Bunnett NW, Maa J *et al*. Deletion of neutral endopeptidase exacerbates intestinal inflammation induced by *Clostridium difficile* toxin A. *Am J Physiol* 2001; **281**: G544–51.

67 Wershil BK, Castagliuolo I, Pothoulakis C. Direct evidence of mast cell involvement in *Clostridium difficile* toxin A-induced enteritis in mice. *Gastroenterology* 1998; **114**: 956–64.

68 Castagliuolo I, Keates AC, Qiu BS *et al*. Increased substance P responses in dorsal root ganglia and intestinal macrophages during *Clostridium difficile* toxin A enteritis in rats. *Proc Natl Acad Sci USA* 1997; **94**: 4788–93.

69 Metwali A, Blum AM, Ferraris L, Klein JS, Fiocchi C, Weinstock JV. Eosinophils within the healthy or inflamed human intestine produce substance P and vasoactive intestinal peptide. *J Neuroimmunol* 1994; **52**: 69–78.

70 Lecci A, Valenti C, Maggi CA. Tachykinin receptor antagonists in irritable bowel syndrome. *Curr Opin Investig Drugs* 2002; **3**: 589–601.

71 Lee O-Y, Munakata J, Naliboff BD, Chang L, Mayer EA. A double blind parallel group pilot study of the effects of CJ-11,974 and placebo on perceptual and emotional responses to rectosigmoid distension in IBS patients. *Gastroenterology* 2000; **118**: A846.

72 Laird JM, Olivar T, Roza C, De Felipe C, Hunt SP, Cervero F. Deficits in visceral pain and hyperalgesia of mice with a disruption of the tachykinin NK$_1$ receptor gene. *Neuroscience* 2000; **98**: 345–52.

73 Kamp EH, Beck DR, Gebhart GF. Combinations of neurokinin receptor antagonists reduce visceral hyperalgesia. *J Pharmacol Exp Ther* 2001; **299**: 105–13.

74 Julia V, Morteau O, Bueno L. Involvement of neurokinin 1 and 2 receptors in viscerosensitive response to rectal distension in rats. *Gastroenterology* 1994; **107**: 94–102.

75 Julia V, Su X, Bueno L, Gebhart GF. Role of neurokinin 3 receptors on responses to colorectal distension in the rat: electrophysiological and behavioral studies. *Gastroenterology* 1999; **116**: 1124–31.

76 Okano S, Ikeura Y, Inatomi N. Effects of tachykinin NK$_1$ receptor antagonists on the viscerosensory response caused by colorectal distension in rabbits. *J Pharmacol Exp Ther* 2002; **300**: 925–31.

77 Jocic M, Schuligoi R, Schöninkle E, Pabst MA, Holzer P. Cooperation of NMDA and tachykinin NK$_1$ and NK$_2$ receptors

in the medullary transmission of vagal afferent input from the acid-threatened rat stomach. *Pain* 2001; **89**: 147–57.

78   Rupniak NMJ, Kramer MS. Discovery of the anti-depressant and anti-emetic efficacy of substance P receptor (NK_1) antagonists. *Trends Pharmacol Sci* 1999; **20**: 485–90.

79   Kramer MS, Winokur A, Kelsey J *et al.* Demonstration of the efficacy and safety of a novel substance P (NK_1) receptor antagonist in major depression. *Neuropsychopharmacology* 2004; **29**: 385–92.

CHAPTER 18

Serotonin Receptor Modulators

Fabrizio De Ponti

Serotonin (5-HT) and its receptors

It has been known for more than 60 years that there is a significant amount of serotonin (5-hydroxytryptamine or 5-HT) in the gut,[1] distributed mainly in enterochromaffin cells and, to a lesser extent, in enteric neurons.[2] 5-HT can be released in response to increased intraluminal pressure or to vagal stimulation.[3–5] 5-HT is also localized in descending interneurons, which project to other myenteric ganglia and/or submucous ganglia. Release of 5-HT from enteric neurons can be demonstrated in response to depolarizing stimuli (for a detailed review, see Tonini and De Ponti, 1995).[2]

Modulation of intestinal functions by 5-HT receptors

5-HT has a bewildering range of effects in the intestine, largely due to the presence of multiple receptor subtypes, which appear to be present on several classes of myenteric neurons and on smooth muscle cells (Table 18.1). The issue is further complicated by the recent report that genes for 5-HT receptors display marked population and molecular genetic complexity.[6]

Genetic complexity may also affect the transporter protein responsible for the 5-HT reuptake process (serotonin transporter or SERT). Apart from changes in the expression or pharmacological profile of SERT associated with dysfunctions of central serotonergic transmission (e.g. depression and migraine), it is noteworthy that, in guinea-pigs with experimental colitis, a concomitant increment of 5-HT availability and a decrease in mRNA SERT expression were detected in the inflamed colonic mucosa.[7] Clinical evidence suggests that similar alterations might also occur in patients with either irritable bowel syndrome (IBS) or inflammatory bowel disease.[8] Moreover, SERT polymorphisms may be responsible for pharmacogenetic differences, as suggested by the colonic transit response to alosetron in patients with diarrhea-predominant IBS.[9]

5-HT receptors that are known to affect gut motor function are those belonging to the 5-HT_1, 5HT_2, 5-HT_3, 5-HT_4, and 5-HT_7 subtypes.[2,10–13] In addition, the presence of 5-HT_{1P} receptors is reported in enteric neurons,[14] but it should be noted that they are not included in the official International Union of Pharmacology (IUPHAR) classification of 5-HT receptors and are still considered 'orphan' receptors.[15]

Serotonin in the gut

1 In the gut, 5-HT is distributed mainly (>90%) in enterochromaffin cells and, to a lesser extent, in enteric neurons.

2 5-HT released from EC cells may affect several subtypes of enteric neurons (intrinsic and extrinsic sensory neurons as well as motor and secretomotor neurons) and final effector cells (smooth muscle cells and enterocytes).

3 Several 5-HT receptor subtypes are now identified.

4 Therefore, manipulation of 5-HT levels or 5-HT receptor subtypes represents a rational target for therapeutic intervention.

Table18.1 Synopsis of major 5-HT receptor subtypes in the gut

	$5\text{-}HT_{1A}$	$5\text{-}HT_{1B/D}$	$5\text{-}HT_{2A}$	$5\text{-}HT_{2B}$	$5\text{-}HT_3$	$5\text{-}HT_4$	$5\text{-}HT_7$
Distribution in the gut	Enteric neurons	Enteric neurons (?), circular smooth muscle (?)	Smooth muscle	Longitudinal smooth muscle	Enteric neurons	Enteric neurons, smooth muscle	Smooth muscle
Functional response	Reduced transmitter release	Facilitation of peristalsis, contraction	Contraction	Contraction	Enhanced transmitter release	Enhanced transmitter release, relaxation	Relaxation
Agonists	8-OH-DPAT Buspirone	Sumatriptan Rizatriptan, naratriptan	α-Me-5-HT	α-Me-5-HT BW723C86	2-Me-5-HT CPBG	Tegaserod Prucalopride	5-CT 8-OH-DPAT
Antagonists	WAY100635	GR127935 ($5\text{-}HT1_{B/D}$ antagonist) SB216641 ($5\text{-}HT_{1B}$-selective) BRL15572 ($5\text{-}HT_{1D}$-selective)	Ketanserin, MDL100907	SB200646 SB204741	Ondansetron Alosetron Cilansetron	GR113808 GR125487 Piboserod	Methiotepin Metergoline SB258719 SB269970 SB656104
Effectors	$G_{i/o}$	$G_{i/o}$	$G_{q/11}$	$G_{q/11}$	Ligand-gated ion channel	G_s	G_s

Neuronal 5-HT receptors may enhance or inhibit transmitter release and include the $5\text{-}HT_{1A}$ (inhibitory)[16], the $5\text{-}HT_3$ and the $5\text{-}HT_4$ subtype (both excitatory). Smooth muscle 5-HT receptors may contract or relax the effector cells and belong to the $5\text{-}HT_{2A}$ (mediating contraction), $5\text{-}HT_4$ or $5\text{-}HT_7$ subtypes (both mediating relaxation). In the human small bowel, $5\text{-}HT_{2A}$ receptors mediating contraction and $5\text{-}HT_4$-receptors mediating relaxation coexist on smooth muscle cells.[17]

In the last 15 years, the increased availability of selective 5-HT receptor agonists and antagonists has given impetus to a large number of investigations aimed at developing therapeutic agents for functional gut disorders. However, selectivity for a given 5-HT receptor subtype is usually a relative concept and it should be acknowledged that the trend towards labeling a drug as a 'selective' ligand for a given 5-HT receptor subtype often leads us to overlook the fact that a single molecule may be endowed with multiple pharmacological actions at therapeutic doses, some of which may contribute to the desired effects, whereas others may be the source of side-effects. Table 18.2 illustrates the complex pharmacological profile of some serotonergic agents used in gut disorders. Conversely, although selectivity for a given receptor subtype is desirable to reduce side-effects, it is also true that single-receptor modulating drugs are less likely to achieve a substantial therapeutic gain because of the multifactorial pathophysiology of functional gut disorders. Indeed, designing clinical trials of new therapeutic agents for functional syndromes presents a considerable challenge.[18] Currently available agents for the treatment of functional disorders were

$5\text{-}HT_3$ receptors

$5\text{-}HT_3$ receptors are a key therapeutic target because they have the potential to control
- motility ($5\text{-}HT_3$ receptor stimulation may exert a prokinetic effect)
- fluid secretion ($5\text{-}HT_3$ receptor stimulation may increase intraluminal fluids)
- visceral sensitivity ($5\text{-}HT_3$ receptor stimulation may activate visceral afferents)

Table 18.2 Multiple pharmacological properties of some 5-HT receptor ligands

Compound	Proposed indications in gastroenterology	Main pharmacological property	Additional pharmacological properties
Cisapride	Gastro-esophageal reflux, prokinetic agent in several gut motor disorders	5-HT$_4$ receptor agonist	5-HT$_3$ receptor antagonist (this action may impair the prokinetic effect) HERG K$^+$ channel blocker (this action may theoretically favor the prokinetic effect and certainly has a pro-arrhythmic effect that led to withdrawal from the market)
Mosapride	Gastro-esophageal reflux, prokinetic agent in gut motor disorders	5-HT$_4$ receptor agonist	Its metabolite is a potent 5-HT$_3$ receptor antagonist
Buspirone	Functional dyspepsia (patients with impaired gastric accommodation)	5-HT$_{1A}$ receptor agonist	Dopamine D$_2$ receptor antagonist Its metabolite 1-(2-pyrimidinyl)piperazine is an α_2-adrenoceptor antagonist
Sumatriptan	Functional dyspepsia (patients with impaired gastric accommodation)	5-HT$_{1B/D}$ receptor agonist	5-HT$_{1F}$ receptor agonist Low-affinity 5-HT$_7$ receptor agonist Some authors consider this compound as a 5-HT$_{1P}$ receptor agonist (see text)

developed in the past three decades, focusing mainly on the underlying motor disorder (e.g. delayed gastric emptying), which indeed affects a significant proportion of patients. More recently, visceral hypersensitivity (altered peripheral sensation or central processing of peripheral sensory signals) has become a major target for drug development.

These difficulties in clearly defining a drug target explain why the exponential growth of compounds of potential interest for the treatment of functional gut disorders[19] has not yet filled the gap between basic and clinical research. Indeed, only a few 5-HT receptor ligands have received marketing authorization for the treatment of gut disorders.

5-HT$_3$ and 5-HT$_4$ receptors are the most extensively studied in the gut and will be dealt with in detail in the next two sections. Other 5-HT receptor subtypes are not yet established targets for therapeutic intervention: they will be covered later (see Emerging serotonergic agents for functional disorders).

5-HT$_3$ receptors

5-HT$_3$ receptors are located at several peripheral and central sites and have the potential to control motility, intestinal secretion and visceral sensitivity (Figs 18.1 and 18.2; Table 18.3).

From a functional standpoint, *in vitro* studies in the isolated ileum have repeatedly shown that 5-HT$_3$ receptor antagonists do not affect peristalsis when ap-

---

5-HT$_4$ receptors

5-HT$_4$ receptors are another key therapeutic target. Their stimulation has the potential to
• exert a prokinetic effect
• favor fluid secretion
The effect on visceral perception is still unclear.

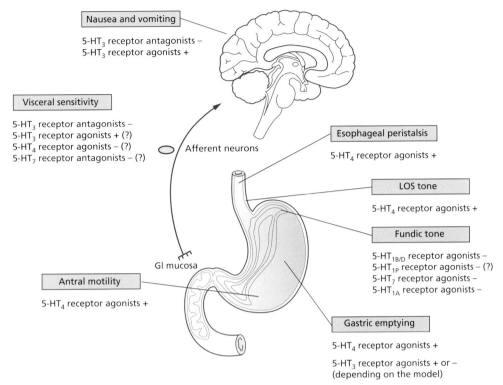

Fig. 18.1 Therapeutic targets in patients with functional disorders of the upper gut and effects of serotonin (5-HT) receptor ligands. Stimulation is indicated by + and inhibition by –; ? indicates that there is debate in the literature or that the effect is not conclusively proved. LOS, lower esophageal sphincter; GI, gastrointestinal.

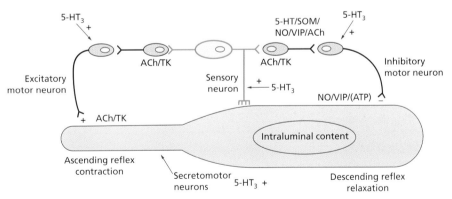

Fig. 18.2 Modulation of intestinal motility by 5-HT₃ receptors. Distension by intraluminal contents stimulates sensory neurons (intrinsic primary afferent neurons), which trigger an ascending excitatory reflex (leading to contraction) and a descending inhibitory reflex (leading to relaxation). Transmitters released by interneurons in the ascending reflex include acetylcholine (ACh) and Substance P (a tachykinin), whereas descending interneurons belonging to different subpopulations may use serotonin (5-HT), somatostatin (SOM), vasoactive intestinal polypeptide (VIP), nitric oxide (NO), ACh and other mediators as transmitters. Excitatory motor neurons release ACh and tachykinins (TK) at the neuromuscular junction, whereas inhibitory motor neurons may release NO, VIP or ATP depending on the gut level and on the animal species. + indicates stimulation; – indicates inhibition; ? indicates circumstantial evidence.

Table 18.3 Potential mechanisms by which 5-HT receptor ligands may influence gut function

	Examples	Motility	Absorption/secretion	Visceral sensitivity
5-HT$_3$ receptor antagonists	Alosetron Cilansetron	Reduced transmitter release from excitatory and inhibitory neurons: hence, inhibition of peristalsis and enhanced compliance	Increased absorption/reduced secretion through an action on secretomotor neurons: hence, inhibition of diarrhea	Reduced visceral sensitivity through an action on intrinsic or extrinsic primary afferent neurons Antiemetic effect
5-HT$_3$ receptor agonists	MKC-733	Enhanced transmitter release from enteric neurons, hence accelerated gut transit (the reported delay in gastric emptying in humans may be a consequence of nausea)	Increased secretion, hence diarrhea	Stimulation of vagal afferents with possible occurrence of nausea
5-HT$_4$ receptor agonists	Tegaserod Prucalopride	Enhanced transmitter release (acetylcholine, tachykinins, etc.) from excitatory, inhibitory and sensory neurons, hence prokinesia Direct relaxation of smooth muscle cells (increased compliance with indirect effect on visceral sensitivity)	Increased secretion, hence loose stools and diarrhea	Reduced visceral sensitivity through an action on afferent pathways (circumstantial evidence)
5-HT$_4$ receptor antagonists	Piboserod	Reduced transmitter release, hence delay in transit	Decreased secretion	?
5-HT$_{1B/D}$ receptor agonists	Sumatriptan Naratriptan Rizatriptan	Gastric relaxation, increased gastric accommodation, possibly via facilitation of nitrergic inhibitory pathways	–	Reduced sensitivity to gastric distension secondary to increased accommodation
5-HT$_{1A}$ receptor agonists	Buspirone Flesinoxan	Gastric relaxation, increased gastric accommodation (independent of nitrergic pathways?)	–	Reduced sensitivity to distension through a central site of action
5-HT$_7$ receptor antagonists	SB269970 SB656104	Inhibition of smooth muscle relaxation, hence decreased compliance	–	Reduced visceral sensitivity through a direct effect on visceral afferents?

plied to the serosal side.[2] Conversely, they exert an inhibitory effect when applied intraluminally, suggesting blockade of 5-HT$_3$ receptors on intrinsic sensory neurons.[20,21] Both neurogenic contraction and relaxation (Fig. 18.2) can be induced *in vitro* by 5-HT$_3$-receptor activation in experimental animals.[22,23]

In vivo, more complex interactions seem to occur because of the multiple peripheral and central sites of action.[2,19] In rodents, the observation that 5-HT- and re-straint stress-induced increase in fecal pellet output were antagonized by the 5-HT$_3$ receptor antagonists ondansetron, granisetron or YM 114 and by FK 1052 (a mixed 5-HT$_3$/5-HT$_4$ receptor antagonist) was suggestive for a role for 5-HT$_3$ receptors in modulating colonic transit.[24,25] Autoradiographic studies indeed detected high densities of $[^{125}I](S)$-iodozacopride (a 5-HT$_3$ receptor ligand) in the myenteric plexus of the human colon.[26,27]

In humans, ondansetron has no effect on small bowel transit in healthy volunteers,[28] or in patients with diarrhea-predominant IBS.[29] However, ondansetron slows colonic transit[30,31] and inhibits the colonic motor response to a meal[32] in healthy subjects. In a double-blind, placebo-controlled study on 50 IBS patients, ondansetron reduced bowel frequency and improved stool consistency in the diarrhea-predominant subgroup (28 patients).[33]

Further evidence in favor of a role for 5-HT$_3$ receptors in humans was provided by Prior and Read,[34] who found a dose-dependent reduction in postprandial colonic motility with granisetron, and by von der Ohe and colleagues,[35] who reported reduction of the postprandial colonic hypertonic response in carcinoid diarrhea with ondansetron.

5-HT$_4$ receptors

5-HT$_4$ receptors mediate a number of responses in the gut (Figs 18.1 and 18.3; Table 18.3).[19] Prokinesia may result from increased release of acetylcholine (and tachykinins) from excitatory neurons and may operate in human small bowel and stomach,[36,37] but early studies failed to identify this pathway in the human colonic circular muscle.[38] Besides these actions, 5-HT$_4$ receptors also affect secretory processes at the mucosal level.[39]

It should be noted that, in contrast with what is observed in one of the most widely used experimental models (the guinea-pig colon, where neuronal 5-HT$_4$ receptors mediate contractile responses that are mainly cholinergic in nature),[40,41] human colonic circular muscle strips are endowed with 5-HT$_4$ receptors located on smooth muscle cells, where they mediate relaxation.[26,42,43] A recent report[44] suggests the presence of 5-HT$_4$ receptors on cholinergic neurons supplying the longitudinal muscle in the human colon. All these findings should be considered in the light of some clinical studies reporting a colonic prokinetic effect of cisapride, while in others cisapride was found to have no effect on stool frequency or transit time (for a review, see De Ponti and Malagelada).[19] These conflicting results are not unexpected if one considers that the net *in vivo* response to 5-HT$_4$ receptor stimulation is the result of a number of actions at different levels, that cisapride is a mixed 5-HT$_4$ receptor agonist/5-HT$_3$ receptor antagonist, and that the underlying pathophysiology may strongly influence the clinical effect.

There are animal[45] and human[46] data suggesting that 5-HT released by mucosal stimulation initiates a peristaltic reflex by activating 5-HT$_4$ receptors on sensory neurons containing calcitonin gene-related peptide (CGRP). These effects are mimicked by mu-

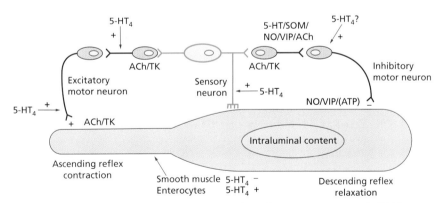

Fig. 18.3 Modulation of intestinal motility by 5-HT$_4$ receptors. Distension by intraluminal contents stimulates sensory neurons (intrinsic primary afferent neurons), which trigger an ascending excitatory reflex (leading to contraction) and a descending inhibitory reflex (leading to relaxation). Transmitters released by interneurons in the ascending reflex include acetylcholine (ACh) and substance P (a tachykinin), whereas descending interneurons belonging to different subpopulations may use serotonin (5-HT), somatostatin (SOM), vasoactive intestinal polypeptide (VIP), nitric oxide (NO), ACh and other mediators as transmitters. Excitatory motor neurons release ACh and tachykinins (TK) at the neuromuscular junction, whereas inhibitory motor neurons may release NO, VIP or ATP depending on the gut level and on the animal species. + indicates stimulation; – indicates inhibition; ? indicates circumstantial evidence.

cosal application of selective 5-HT$_4$ receptor agonists (prucalopride and tegaserod).[47] However, experimental evidence for this mechanism in humans is so far limited to the small bowel.

Whether 5-HT$_4$ receptor agonists can affect visceral sensitivity is controversial. In healthy volunteers, cisapride significantly lowered thresholds for perception and for discomfort during gastric distension, but also significantly enhanced the size of the meal-induced fundus relaxation (i.e. improved gastric accommodation).[48] In another study,[49] eight healthy subjects were studied on two different days, each after 7 days' treatment either with placebo or cisapride. Intraduodenal infusion of lipids caused relaxation of gastric fundus, and this effect was unchanged by cisapride. Cisapride did not influence gastric sensitivity to distension or gastric compliance.

A study carried out in awake rats also suggests an effect of tegaserod on colorectal sensitivity not linked to alterations in compliance at the doses of 0.1 and 0.3 mg/kg i.p.: tegaserod was found to increase pain threshold to colorectal but not to gastric distension.[50]

In healthy subjects, tegaserod is reported to decrease sensitivity to rectal distension, as assessed by inhibition of the RIII reflex.[51]

5-HT$_3$ receptor modulators

5-HT$_3$ receptor antagonists

Among 5-HT$_3$ receptor antagonists, alosetron was initially approved by the US Food and Drug Administration (FDA) for the treatment of diarrhea-predominant IBS in women, but safety concerns (ischemic colitis affecting between 1 in 700 and 1 in 1000 patients receiving the drug) led to drug withdrawal only a few months after approval. Recently, alosetron was reintroduced into the market with restrictions on its use. It has an indication only for women with severe diarrhea-predominant IBS who have failed to respond to conventional therapy (see the FDA dedicated internet address: http://www.fda.gov/cder/drug/infopage/lotronex/lotronex.htm). The starting dose of alosetron is now 1 mg once daily, which, if well tolerated, after 4 weeks may be increased to 1 mg twice daily (i.e. the dose used in controlled trials) in case the control of symptoms is not adequate.

Other 5-HT$_3$ receptor antagonists are now under development. Apart from the well-known antiemetic effect, theoretically 5-HT$_3$ receptor antagonists may act on multiple therapeutic targets in functional gut disorders:[52–54] by modulating visceral sensitivity;[55] by increasing compliance (i.e. increasing the ability of the gut to adapt to distension);[56] by blocking excitatory 5-HT$_3$ receptors located on sensory, ascending and descending neuronal pathways involved in peristalsis; and by increasing jejunal fluid absorption.[52] For this reason, 5-HT$_3$-receptor antagonists may slow transit. A recent study,[57] which failed to observe a significant effect of alosetron on transit parameters, discusses important issues in the optimization of experimental design of trials designed to find mechanistic explanations for drug action in functional gut disorders.

Several animal models point to the role of 5-HT$_3$ receptors in modulating visceral sensitivity.[19] Granisetron and tropisetron (but not ondansetron) were found to inhibit the fall in blood pressure and intragastric pressure observed in rats after duodenal distension.[58] Whether the site of 5-HT receptors modulating afferent information is on peripheral afferent nerve fibers or outside the gut, however, is unclear. For instance, alosetron, administered either centrally or peripherally in dogs, seems to modulate the visceral nociceptive effect of rectal distension in dogs.[59]

In humans, reduced perception of colonic distension may also depend on increased compliance of the colon to distension.[56] In other studies, granisetron was found to reduce rectal sensitivity in patients with IBS,[34] whereas ondansetron had no effect.[60] Interestingly,

---

Constipation-predominant IBS (C-IBS)

1 The relative risk of being a responder in terms of global relief of gastrointestinal symptoms in C-IBS is significantly higher with tegaserod 12 and 4 mg compared with placebo, with a number needed to treat of 14 and 20, respectively.

2 Diarrhea is the most frequent side-effect.

however, ondansetron reduced nausea and gastric sensitivity to distension during intraduodenal lipid infusion in healthy subjects.[61]

As regards the possible use of 5-HT$_3$ receptor antagonists in functional dyspepsia, Talley and colleagues[62] performed a pilot, dose-ranging, placebo-controlled, multicenter, randomized trial with 320 functional dyspepsia patients, who received placebo ($n = 81$) or alosetron 0.5 mg b.d. ($n = 77$), 1.0 mg b.d. ($n = 79$) or 2.0 mg b.d. ($n = 83$) for 12 weeks, followed by 1 week of follow-up. The measure of primary efficacy was the 12-week average rate of adequate relief of upper abdominal pain or discomfort. Twelve-week average rates of adequate relief of pain or discomfort were 46, 55, 55 and 47% in the placebo and 0.5 mg, 1.0 mg and 2.0 mg in the alosetron groups, respectively. Alosetron 0.5 or 1.0 mg showed potential benefit over placebo for early satiety and postprandial fullness. Constipation was the most commonly reported adverse event. Thus, the therapeutic gain with alosetron appeared to be relatively modest in this population of dyspeptic patients.

Another trial carried out in 36 healthy volunteers[63] assessed the effects of placebo and alosetron 0.5 and 1 mg b.d. on fasting and postprandial gastric volumes (using single photon emission computed tomography) and symptoms based on a 100 mm visual analog scale, 30 minutes after the maximum volume had been ingested. Alosetron significantly reduced postprandial symptoms (1 mg alosetron reduced aggregate score by approximately 40% with respect to placebo) and nausea, and tended to reduce bloating. Effects on pain and fullness were not statistically significant. There was no significant effect of the 5-HT$_3$ antagonist on the volume of meal tolerated. Since 5-HT$_3$ receptors are unlikely to be involved in the control of gastric tone,[64] these observations are probably to be interpreted as effects on visceral afferents and are not due to increased postprandial gastric volume.

5-HT$_3$ receptor antagonists have also been tested in IBS. In a double-blind, placebo-controlled, parallel-group study,[65] a total of 462 patients with IBS (335 females) had a 12-week treatment period with the following doses of alosetron: 0.1, 0.5 and 2 mg b.i.d. In the total population and in the female subpopulation (but not in the males), alosetron 2 mg b.i.d. significantly increased the proportion of pain-free days and decreased the visual analog scale score for diarrhea. It also led to a significant hardening of stool and a reduction in stool frequency in the total population.

In another study,[66] 623 non-constipated females with IBS were randomized to receive alosetron 1 mg twice daily or mebeverine 135 mg three times daily for 12 weeks. The primary efficacy end-point was monthly responders for adequate relief of IBS-related abdominal pain and discomfort (defined as patients reporting adequate relief in at least 2 out of 4 weeks). There were significantly more responders in the alosetron group compared with mebeverine at months 2 and 3 ($P < 0.01$).

Camilleri and colleagues[67] studied 647 female IBS patients with diarrhea-predominant or alternating bowel patterns: 324 patients were assigned 1 mg alosetron and 323 placebo orally twice daily for 12 weeks. Once again, adequate relief of abdominal pain and discomfort was the primary end-point. The dropout rate was 24% in the alosetron group and 16% in the placebo group. The difference was mainly due to a greater occurrence of constipation in the alosetron group. Adequate relief for all 3 months of treatment was reported in a greater proportion of alosetron-treated patients (difference 12%). Alosetron also decreased urgency and stool frequency. Constipation occurred in 30% and 3% of patients in the alosetron and placebo groups, respectively.

A recent meta-analysis of the efficacy of alosetron in IBS concluded that the average number need to treat is approximately 7 and that one in four patients may develop constipation.[68]

Cilansetron, a new 5HT$_3$ receptor antagonist, underwent recently clinical trials.[70,71] It showed efficacy for relief of urgency and improvement of stool frequency and consistency in the treatment (6 months) of male and female patients suffering from IBS with diarrhea predominance.[71] At the dose of 2 mg t.i.d, Cilansetron was well tolerated with a low constipation rate.

5-HT$_3$ receptor agonists

Stimulation of 5-HT$_3$ receptors can exert a prokinetic effect, but it can also stimulate nausea and vomiting. Indeed, the 5-HT$_3$ receptor agonist MKC-733 can accelerate gastric emptying in animal models, but it was recently reported to delay gastric emptying in humans,[72] possibly as a consequence of the induction of nausea. In a recent study,[72] Coleman and colleagues determined the effect of oral MKC-733 (0.2, 1 and 4 mg) on upper gastrointestinal motility compared with placebo in three randomized, double-blind, crossover studies in healthy males. Antroduodenal manometry was recorded for 8 hours during fasting and 3 hours postprandially ($n = 12$). Gastric emptying and small intestinal transit were determined by gamma-scintigraphy ($n = 16$). Gastric emptying, accommodation and antral motility were determined by echoplanar magnetic resonance imaging ($n = 12$). MKC-733 (4 mg) increased the number of migrating motor complexes recorded in the antrum and duodenum, but had no effect on postprandial motility. MKC-733 delayed scintigraphically assessed liquid gastric emptying and accelerated small intestinal transit. Echoplanar magnetic resonance imaging confirmed the delayed gastric emptying and demonstrated a significant increase in cross-sectional area of the proximal stomach. Thus, MKC-733 delays liquid gastric emptying in association with relaxation of the proximal stomach, stimulates fasting antroduodenal migrating motor complex activity and accelerates small intestinal transit.

To date, no other studies are available in the literature on the gastrointestinal effects on 5-HT$_3$ receptor agonists in humans.

5-HT$_4$ receptor modulators

5-HT$_4$ receptor agonists

The most extensively studied 5-HT$_4$ receptor agonists are cisapride, tegaserod and prucalopride. However, the potential of cisapride to induce ventricular arrhythmias and prolongation of the QT interval through blockade of human ether-à-go-go related gene (HERG) K$^+$ channels[73] led to withdrawal of the compound, which is now available on a limited access basis. A large number of studies have been published on cisapride, but these will not be discussed here because cisapride is no longer used.

Among second-generation 5-HT$_4$ receptor agonists, tegaserod[74,75] and prucalopride[76,77] have already

undergone clinical trials, which have been targeted mainly to the treatment of lower gut disorders.[78] However, because of carcinogenicity in animals, it is unclear whether prucalopride will reach clinical practice.

Second-generation 5-HT$_4$ receptor agonists such as tegaserod and mosapride seem to be devoid of HERG K$^+$ channel-blocking properties,[73,79–81] and at least some of them (tegaserod,[82] prucalopride[77,83,84]) may be more active at the colonic level than cisapride. Interestingly, mosapride, whose main metabolite is a 5-HT$_3$ receptor antagonist,[85] displays little or no prokinetic activity in the colon,[86] similarly to what is observed with the mixed 5-HT$_4$ receptor agonist/5-HT$_3$ receptor antagonist cisapride. Mosapride is marketed in Japan and is targeted for the treatment of upper gut disorders, such as gastro-esophageal reflux disease.[87] It was found not different from placebo in the treatment of functional dyspepsia.[88]

In healthy subjects, Degen and colleagues[89] have shown that intravenous (0.6 mg) and oral (6 mg) tegaserod accelerate gastric emptying, and small bowel and colonic transit. Tack and colleagues[90] reported that tegaserod 6 mg b.i.d. enhances fasting gastric compliance and allows larger intragastric volumes, both before and after a meal. The absolute bioavailability of tegaserod is approximately 10% and food reduces tegaserod C$_{max}$ and the area under the plasma concentration curve. The terminal elimination half-life is approximately 11 hours.[75]

As regards the use of tegaserod in functional gut disorders, Prather and colleagues studied the effects of tegaserod on gastric, small bowel and colonic transit in 24 patients with constipation-predominant IBS, who were randomized to 1 week of tegaserod (2 mg twice daily) or placebo.[91] Interestingly, tegaserod accelerated orocecal transit, leaving gastric emptying unaltered, and also tended to accelerate colonic transit. No serious adverse events were reported.

Tegaserod results in global relief of IBS symptoms in females with symptoms of constipation-predominant

---

Diarrhea-predominant IBS

1 In patients with IBS, alosetron induces adequate relief of pain or global improvement of symptoms with an average number needed to treat of 7

2 one in four patients may develop constipation.

IBS.[92–94] The effective doses of tegaserod are 4–12 mg per day in two divided doses (2 or 6 mg twice daily). Relief was associated with significant improvement in a number of secondary end-points, such as pain-free days, frequency of bowel movements, and stool consistency. The drug was significantly effective, providing 8–21% advantage over placebo in female patients, particularly in those with documented constipation during the baseline run-in period. Tegaserod appears to be relatively safe, with no serious adverse effects reported in the clinical trials program and in the cohort treated in open evaluation for over 6 months.[95]

The other 5-HT$_4$ receptor agonist, prucalopride, is being investigated for a range of conditions including constipation-predominant IBS and slow-transit constipation. In a double-blind, crossover study in 24 healthy volunteers,[76] prucalopride 1 and 2 mg for 1 week significantly increased the number of stools and the percentage of loose/watery stools compared with placebo. These parameters returned to baseline within 1 week after stopping prucalopride. Prucalopride also significantly shortened mean colonic transit time and total gut transit time.

Administration of prucalopride 1 and 2 mg for 1 week in healthy volunteers significantly increased the number of stools and the percentage of loose/watery stools.[96] Prucalopride accelerated orocecal and whole-gut transit, while having no effect on gut sensitivity to distension and electrical stimulation.

In a randomized, double-blind study in 50 healthy volunteers, prucalopride 0.5–4 mg daily for 7 days significantly accelerated colonic transit at 4, 8, 24 and 48 hours and proximal colonic emptying, while having no significant effects on gastric emptying or small bowel transit.[83]

In a multicenter, randomized, double-blind study in 251 patients with chronic constipation, prucalopride 0.5–2 mg b.i.d. for 12 weeks significantly increased stool frequency and consistency throughout the study period, with a dose-dependent increase in the number of responding patients.[97]

Diarrhea is the most common side-effect reported with tegaserod and prucalopride and occurs in approximately 10% of the subjects.[95]

5-HT$_4$ receptor antagonists

Because of the different locations of 5-HT$_4$ receptors in the gut, it is difficult to predict the net effect of a selective antagonist *in vivo*. 5-HT$_4$ receptor antagonists do not seem to affect normal bowel motility in animals[98] or humans,[99] although they may antagonize both the ability of 5-HT to sensitize the peristaltic reflex and 5-hydroxytryptophan-induced defecation/diarrhea, at least in animals.[98,100,101]

Preliminary clinical data on the possible role of selective 5-HT$_4$ receptor antagonists in the treatment of functional gastrointestinal disorders are now available. Piboserod (SB207266A) is one of the best characterized 5-HT$_4$ receptor antagonists so far. It displays subnanomolar affinity (pK$_B$ 9.98) in the human intestine[98] and, at single oral doses of 0.5–5 mg in healthy male volunteers, significantly and dose-dependently antagonized the effects of cisapride in a pharmacodynamic model of 5-HT$_4$ receptor activation (increase in plasma aldosterone levels).[102] Dynamic modeling in this study predicted that a dose of approximately 1 mg piboserod would block 90% of the cisapride-induced aldosterone response.

Piboserod prolongs orocecal transit time in patients with diarrhea-predominant IBS,[103] hence the proposed indication in this subset of patients. The ability of piboserod to affect visceral sensitivity is unclear. At variance with 5-HT$_3$ receptors, limited data are available to support a role for 5-HT$_4$ receptors in controlling visceral sensitivity.[104] Although oral piboserod (20 mg daily for 10 days) tended to increase the distension volume required to induce the sensation of discomfort in diarrhea-predominant IBS patients, this effect did not reach statistical significance.[103] Interestingly, in a rat model of intestinal hyperalgesia,[105] piboserod *per se* had no effect but potentiated the effects of submaximal doses of granisetron, suggesting that 5-HT$_4$ receptors may cooperate with 5-HT$_3$ receptors in inhibiting intestinal hyperalgesia. This observation poses a rationale for the development of dual antagonists (5-HT$_3$/5-HT$_4$ receptor antagonists).[25]

Emerging serotonergic agents for functional disorders

5-HT$_1$ receptor agonists

In the past decade, several studies have documented the effects of the 5-HT$_{1B/D}$ receptor agonist sumatriptan on gastric motility and sensitivity in the same dose range used in migraine.[106–108] Houghton and colleagues[109] were the first to show that intravenous administration of sumatriptan in healthy subjects delayed gastric emptying of a nutrient liquid meal. Subsequently, Coulie et al.[107] showed that sumatriptan in humans caused a notable delay in gastric emptying of both liquids and solids. Of course, this effect is not desirable in dyspeptic patients in whom gastric emptying is already delayed. However, the same authors[108] reported that, in healthy volunteers, sumatriptan caused significant relaxation of the gastric fundus and enabled accommodation of considerably larger volumes before thresholds for perception or discomfort were reached during isovolumetric distension. The fact that perception thresholds were altered by sumatriptan in response to isovolumetric, not isobaric, distension suggests that the effect of sumatriptan was determined by the change in gastric tone rather than by an effect on visceral sensitivity. These observations provide a rationale for testing sumatriptan as a means for relieving symptoms in dyspeptic patients with defective postprandial gastric accommodation. In dyspeptic patients, the injection of subcutaneous sumatriptan was shown to restore gastric accommodation, improving the symptoms of early satiety.[110]

Malatesta et al.[111] evaluated the effect of sumatriptan and of the anticholinergic agent hyoscine on gastric accommodation after liquid ingestion in normal subjects and dyspeptic patients. This study showed that, both in dyspeptic patients and in normal controls, gastric size measured after water distension was modified by sumatriptan, with a reduction in transverse and an increase in longitudinal size. Gastric distension with 500 ml of water induced the onset of nausea, bloating, heartburn and, to lesser extent, epigastric pain. As expected, the symptom score was higher in dyspeptics than in controls. In this study, sumatriptan showed a beneficial effect only on the nausea induced by gastric distension both in dyspeptics and in controls, without affecting the other symptoms.

Because distension of the proximal stomach is a potent stimulus for the occurrence of transient lower esophageal sphincter relaxations (TLESRs, a major mechanism of reflux in patients with gastro-esophageal reflux disease), the effect of sumatriptan on the frequency of postprandial TLOSRs and gastro-esophageal reflux was also studied in healthy subjects.[112]

Esophageal manometry and pH monitoring were performed in 13 healthy volunteers for 30 minutes before and 90 minutes after a semiliquid meal. Sumatriptan 6 mg subcutaneously or placebo were administered on separate days 30 minutes after the meal. Sumatriptan significantly increased postprandial lower esophageal sphincter (LES) pressure, but did not reduce reflux events. On the contrary, reflux was more frequent after sumatriptan than after placebo. TLESRs were more frequent after sumatriptan, particularly in the second 30-minute period after drug administration. The authors concluded that sumatriptan prevents the natural decay in rate of TLESRs that occurs after a meal and favors the occurrence of gastro-esophageal reflux in spite of the increase in LES pressure. The sustained postprandial high rate of transient LES relaxations after sumatriptan may be a consequence of a prolonged fundic relaxation and retention of the meal in the proximal stomach.

The use of animal models has provided more insight into the possible mechanism mediating the gastric motor effects of sumatriptan. Coulie and colleagues,[106] using an in vivo cat model, suggested that sumatriptan-induced fundic relaxation occurs through the activation of a nitrergic pathway. However, they did not provide evidence on the 5-HT receptor subtype involved in this response. In guinea-pigs, it was demonstrated that 5-HT-induced gastric relaxations are mediated through activation of a $5-HT_1$-like receptor.[113] Some authors also considered $5-HT_{1P}$ receptors, since their presence is reported in enteric neurons,[14] and suggested that sumatriptan might act via this receptor subtype.[108] However, $5-HT_{1P}$ receptors are not included in the official International Union of Pharmacology (IUPHAR) classification of serotonin receptors,[15] and none of the authors reporting the gastric motor effects of sumatriptan in vivo has ever tested the effect of $5-HT_{1P}$ receptor antagonists because of the lack of selective agents suitable for in vivo use. The fact that the effect of sumatriptan was fully reversed by GR127935 (dual $5-HT_{1B/D}$ receptor antagonist) and SB216641 (selective $5-HT_{1B}$ receptor antagonist) supports the involvement of $5-HT_{1B}$ receptors (Fig. 18.4).[114,115] The involvement of $5-HT_7$ receptors in the response to sumatriptan is unlikely, because the affinity value of sumatriptan for this receptor subtype is low.

Gastric relaxation and enhanced accommodation to a distending stimulus seem to be a class effect of trip-

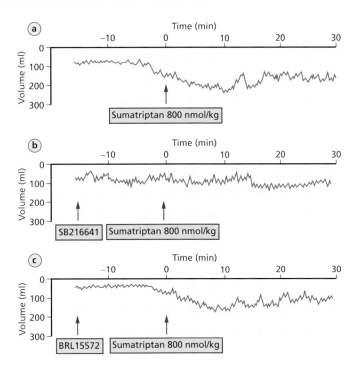

Fig. 18.4 Representative tracings of intragastric volume in the canine proximal stomach, measured by a barostat at a distending pressure of 2 mmHg before and after intravenous administration of sumatriptan 800 nmol/kg alone (a) or combined with the selective 5-HT$_{1B}$ receptor antagonist SB216641 (559 nmol/kg) (b) or the selective 5-HT$_{1D}$ receptor antagonist BRL15572 (676 nmol/kg) (c). Note that sumatriptan causes an immediate volume increase reflecting fundic relaxation. Note that SB216641, but not BRL15572, totally prevents sumatriptan-induced relaxation. Reproduced with permission from reference 115.

tans, since they occur not only with sumatriptan but also with second-generation triptans (rizatriptan and naratriptan), at least in a canine model (Fig. 18.5).[115]

Whether the site of action of sumatriptan is central or peripheral remains to be determined. The fact that the compound penetrates poorly the blood–brain barrier and can relax the guinea-pig isolated stomach[116] would argue against a central site of action, although evidence for the presence of 5-HT$_{1B/D}$ receptors in the gut is still lacking.

Rouzade and colleagues studied 5-HT$_{1A}$ receptors by using flesinoxan (a 5-HT$_{1A}$ receptor agonist). They suggested that activation of these receptors in the central nervous system can increase gastric tone and decrease gastric sensitivity to distension in rats.[117] However, Xue and colleagues[118] have recently reported a peripheral inhibitory effect exerted by the 5-HT$_{1A}$ receptor agonist buspirone on murine fundic tone. Likewise, flesinoxan induced gastric relaxation in conscious dogs via 5-HT$_{1A}$ receptors (as indicated by blockade with the selective 5-HT$_{1A}$ receptor antagonist WAY-100635), a response mediated through a non-nitrergic vagal pathway.[119] Interestingly, a preliminary account of a crossover study of buspirone in patients with functional dyspepsia

showed a reduction in symptoms and enhanced gastric accommodation to a meal.[120]

In conclusion, in dyspeptic patients with impaired fundic relaxation to a meal or altered gastric sensitivity to distension, prokinetics (such as motilin receptor agonists) are contraindicated (because of the possible further impairment of fundic relaxation), whereas a gastric-relaxing drug could decrease early satiety, a cardinal symptom of dyspepsia. Long-term studies with different classes of orally active fundus-relaxing drugs seem warranted to confirm their therapeutic potential.

5-HT$_7$ receptor ligands

The pharmacological profile of the 5-HT$_7$ receptor is similar to that of the 5-HT$_{1A}$ receptor subtype. Indeed, 8-OH-DPAT [8-hydroxy-2-(di-n-propylaminotetralin)], a compound previously considered a selective 5-HT$_{1A}$ receptor agonist, is now known to be a partial agonist at the 5-HT$_7$ receptor.[121]

5-HT$_7$ receptors mediate relaxation in human colonic smooth muscle[13] and in the guinea-pig ileum.[122] Janssen and colleagues also proposed that the 5-HT$_7$ receptors may modulate relaxation of the proximal stomach in conscious dogs by a mechanism not involv-

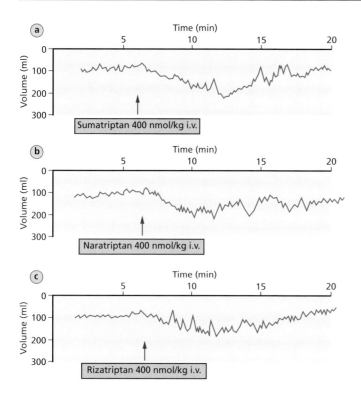

Fig. 18.5 Representative tracings of intragastric volume in the canine proximal stomach, measured by a barostat at a distending pressure of 2 mmHg before and after intravenous administration of sumatriptan (a), naratriptan (b) and rizatriptan (c), all at the dose of 400 nmol/kg. Reproduced with permission from reference 115.

ing nitric oxide.[123,124] 5-HT$_7$ receptors are also involved in the inhibitory effect of 5-HT on peristalsis.[125]

One intriguing finding is that 5-HT$_7$ receptors are expressed by rat primary afferent nociceptors which terminate in the superficial layers of the spinal cord dorsal horn, and that the 5-HT$_7$ receptor subtype is involved in nociceptor activation by 5-HT.[126]

To the best of our knowledge, no selective 5-HT$_7$ receptor ligands are yet available for clinical use, but selective antagonists suitable for *in vivo* administration are being developed and are expected soon.

5-HT reuptake inhibitors (antidepressants)

Although, strictly speaking, antidepressants are not 5-HT receptor ligands, they are briefly discussed in this section because, by prolonging the availability of physiologically released 5-HT, they may modulate gut sensorimotor function.

Antidepressants (both tricyclic compounds and selective 5-HT reuptake inhibitors) are indeed included in management algorithms for functional gastrointestinal syndromes, but their role is still debated because only a few controlled studies are available. Antidepressants are recommended for severe or refractory symptoms of pain, and most of the studies on the use of antidepressants in functional syndromes were carried out in patients with the irritable bowel syndrome.[127]

Because of their complex pharmacological properties (both central and peripheral), antidepressants may exert useful actions at more than one site along the brain–gut axis. Two studies showed that imipramine can prolong orocecal and whole-gut transit times in diarrhea-predominant IBS subjects and controls, while paroxetine reduced orocecal transit times with no effect on whole-gut transit times.[128,129] Although, as the authors acknowledge, demonstration of altered transit by antidepressants does not imply therapeutic usefulness, the above studies have shown that antidepressants can alter motor function independently of mood effects, since the antidepressants were taken only for 4–5 days. As regards the modulation of afferent information from the gut by antidepressants, a report[130] suggests that this is a possible mechanism of action. In healthy volunteers, imipramine can increase pain and perception thresholds to esophageal balloon disten-

---

Antidepressants and IBS

The mechanism of action of antidepressants on colonic sensorimotor function is unclear. They may exert both central and peripheral actions.

Antidepressants have a different side-effect profile:

- tricyclic compounds tend to induce constipation because of their anticholinergic properties;
- selective 5-HT reuptake inhibitors tend to be prokinetic.

---

sion. Thus, antidepressants seem to have analgesic and neuromodulatory properties independent of their psychotropic effects, and these effects may occur sooner and at lower doses than is the case when these drugs are used for the treatment of depression.[131,132]

Several authors have investigated the effects of 5-HT reuptake inhibitors, such as paroxetine,[133,134] sertraline[135] and venlafaxine[134] on gastric sensorimotor function. In particular, Tack and colleagues[133] reported that pretreatment with oral paroxetine (20 mg daily for 7 days) had no influence on fasting gastric tone, fasting gastric compliance or the perception of gastric distensions in healthy volunteers studied with a barostat. The authors suggested an effect of paroxetine on gastric accommodation to a meal because of a significant difference in the postprandial fundic relaxation between paroxetine and placebo. However, it should be noticed that the difference was small and that, in another study,[134] paroxetine did not have any effect on fasting or postprandial gastric volume, measured using single photon emission computed tomography (SPECT) imaging of the stomach.

Mertz and colleagues[136] tried to determine how amitryptiline affects digestive symptoms and perceptual responses to gastric distension. Patients were randomized to 4 weeks of amitryptiline 50 mg taken at bedtime, versus placebo. Seven out of seven patients reported significantly less severe gastrointestinal symptoms after 4 weeks on amitryptiline compared with placebo. Five of seven patients had evidence for altered perception of gastric balloon distension during placebo treatment. However, the subjective symptom improvement on amitryptiline was not associated with normalization of the perceptual responses to gastric distension. The authors concluded that the beneficial effect of low-dose amitryptiline was not related to changes in the perception of gastric distension and that increased tolerance to aversive visceral sensations might play a role in the

therapeutic effect, but the results need to be confirmed in sufficiently powered studies.

Although recent studies on the effects of antidepressants on colonic sensorimotor function only partly match initial expectations,[137,138] it is probably too early to dismiss the hypothesis of a beneficial effect in IBS.

Conclusions

I have provided an overview of several investigational agents targeting 5-HT receptors for the treatment of functional gut disorders. On the basis of currently available information, 5-HT$_3$ receptor antagonists have a strong rationale for the treatment of female patients with diarrhea-predominant IBS, who may also benefit from the reduction of visceral sensitivity. However, the safety issues of alosetron limit its use to severe cases of IBS. Ongoing studies will determine whether IBS and other functional gut disorders are responsive to other 5-HT$_3$ receptor antagonists. Because accelerated delivery of colonic contents into the rectum with reduced compliance is not specific for IBS (it may occur in inflammatory conditions or radiation-induced colonic damage), 5-HT$_3$ receptor antagonists may turn out to be useful even in some organic conditions with altered bowel habits and lower abdominal pain.

Selective 5-HT$_4$ receptor agonists and antagonists have the potential to become new classes of drugs with colonic prokinetic or antiprokinetic effect, respectively. However, their role in functional disorders still needs to be fully characterized, especially as regards the control of visceral sensitivity. Among 5-HT$_4$ receptor agonists, tegaserod is already marketed in several parts of the world (though not yet in the European Union) for constipation-predominant IBS in women.

The 5-HT$_1$ receptor agonist sumatriptan, in spite of its interesting profile with respect to gastric sensorimotor function in dyspeptic patients, is an unlikely contender for the everyday management of functional dyspepsia, because of several uncertainties about possible undesired effects: its promotion of TLOSRs associated with a delay in gastric emptying, its possible enhancement of esophageal visceral sensitivity (induction of chest pain), and its vasoconstrictive effect on coronary arteries. More basic work is needed to define the exact mechanism of action of sumatriptan in dyspeptic patients and to clarify whether $5\text{-HT}_{1B/D}$ receptor agonists deserve further clinical development.

5-HT_7 receptor ligands may offer interesting opportunities for drug development, but in the present state of knowledge a deeper insight into the function of 5-HT_7 receptors along the brain–gut axis is a prerequisite for targeted drug development in this area.

Conflict of interest statement

The author has declared no conflicts of interest.

References

1 Vialli M, Erspamer V. Ricerche sul secreto delle cellule enterocromaffini. IX. Intorno alla natura chimica della sostanza specifica. *Boll Soc Med Chir Pavia* 1937; **51**: 1111–30.

2 Tonini M, De Ponti F. Serotonin modulation of gastrointestinal motility. In: Gaginella TS, Galligan JJ, eds. *Serotonin and Gastrointestinal Function*. Boca Raton: CRC Press, 1995: 53–84.

3 Bülbring E, Lin RCY. The effect of intraluminal application of 5-hydroxytryptamine and 5-hydroxytryptophan on peristalsis: the local production of 5-HT and its release in relation to intraluminal pressure and propulsive activity. *J Physiol (Lond)* 1958; **140**: 381–98.

4 Bülbring E, Crema A. The release of 5-hydroxytryptamine in relation to pressure exerted on the intestinal mucosa. *J Physiol (Lond)* 1959; **146**: 18–28.

5 Bülbring E, Gershon MD. 5-hydroxytryptamine participation in the vagal inhibitory innervation of the stomach. *J Physiol (Lond)* 1967; **192**: 23–46.

6 Glatt CE, Tampilic M, Christie C, DeYoung J, Freimer NB. Re-screening serotonin receptors for genetic variants identifies population and molecular genetic complexity. *Am J Med Genet* 2004; **124B**: 92–100.

7 Linden DR, Chen JX, Gershon MD, Sharkey KA, Mawe GM. Serotonin availability is increased in mucosa of guinea pigs with TNBS-induced colitis. *Am J Physiol* 2003; **285**: G207–16.

8 Coates MD, Mahoney CR, Linden DR *et al.* Molecular defects in mucosal serotonin content and decreased serotonin reuptake transporter in ulcerative colitis and IBS. *Gastroenterology* 2004; **126**: 1657–64.

9 Camilleri M, Atanasova E, Carlson PJ *et al.* Serotonin-transporter polymorphism pharmacogenetics in diarrhea-predominant irritable bowel syndrome. *Gastroenterology* 2002; **123**: 425–32.

10 Briejer MR, Akkermans LM, Schuurkes JA. Gastrointestinal prokinetic benzamides: the pharmacology underlying stimulation of motility. *Pharmacol Rev* 1995; **47**: 631–51.

11 Read NW, Gwee KA. The importance of 5-hydroxytryptamine receptors in the gut. *Pharmacol Ther* 1994; **62**: 159–73.

12 Galligan JJ. Electrophysiological studies of 5-hydroxytryptamine receptors on enteric neurons. In: Gaginella TS, Galligan JJ, eds. *Serotonin and Gastrointestinal Function*. Boca Raton: CRC Press, 1995: 109–26.

13 Prins NH, Briejer MR, Van Bergen PJ, Akkermans LM, Schuurkes JA. Evidence for 5-HT7 receptors mediating relaxation of human colonic circular smooth muscle. *Br J Pharmacol* 1999; **128**: 849–52.

14 Mawe GM, Branchek TA, Gershon MD. Peripheral neural serotonin receptors: identification and characterization with specific antagonists and agonists. *Proc Natl Acad Sci USA* 1986; **83**: 9799–803.

15 Hoyer D, Clarke DE, Fozard JR *et al.* International Union of Pharmacology classification of receptors for 5-hydroxytryptamine (serotonin). *Pharmacol Rev* 1994; **46**: 157–203.

16 Dietrich C, Kilbinger H. 5-HT1A receptor-mediated inhibition of acetylcholine release from guinea pig myenteric plexus: potential mechanisms. *Neuropharmacology* 1996; **35**: 483–8.

17 Kuemmerle JF, Murthy KS, Grider JR, Martin DC, Makhlouf GM. Coexpression of 5-HT2A and 5-HT4 receptors coupled to distinct signaling pathways in human intestinal muscle cells. *Gastroenterology* 1995; **109**: 1791–800.

18 Malagelada JR. Review article: clinical pharmacology models of irritable bowel syndrome. *Aliment Pharmacol Ther* 1999; **13** (Suppl. 2): 57–64.

19 De Ponti F, Malagelada JR. Functional gut disorders: from motility to sensitivity disorders. A review of current and investigational drugs for their management. *Pharmacol Ther* 1998; **80**: 49–88.

20 Tuladhar BR, Kaisar M, Naylor RJ. Evidence for a 5-HT3 receptor involvement in the facilitation of peristalsis on mucosal application of 5-HT in the guinea pig isolated ileum. *Br J Pharmacol* 1997; **122**: 1174–8.

21 Jin JG, Foxx-Orenstein AE, Grider JR. Propulsion in guinea pig colon induced by 5-hydroxytryptamine (HT) via 5-HT4 and 5-HT3 receptors. *J Pharmacol Exp Ther* 1999; **288**:

93–7.

22 Miyata K, Kamato T, Nishida A *et al*. Pharmacologic profile of (R)-5-[(1-methyl-3-indolyl)carbonyl]-4,5,6,7-tetrahydro-1H-benzimidazole hydrochloride (YM060), a potent and selective 5-hydroxytryptamine3 receptor antagonist, and its enantiomer in the isolated tissue. *J Pharmacol Exp Ther* 1991; **259**: 15–21.

23 Messori E, Candura SM, Coccini T, Balestra B, Tonini M. 5-HT3 receptor involvement in descending reflex relaxation in the rabbit isolated distal colon. *Eur J Pharmacol* 1995; **286**: 205–8.

24 Miyata K, Kamato T, Nishida A *et al*. Role of serotonin 3 receptor in stress-induced defecation. *J Pharmacol Exp Ther* 1992; **261**: 297–303.

25 Kadowaki M, Nagakura Y, Tomoi M, Mori J, Kohsaka M. Effect of FK1052, a potent 5-hydroxytryptamine 3 and 5-hydroxytryptamine 4 receptor dual antagonist, on colonic function in vivo. *J Pharmacol Exp Ther* 1993; **266**: 74–80.

26 Sakurai-Yamashita Y, Yamashita K, Yoshimura M, Taniyama K. Differential localization of 5-hydroxytryptamine 3 and 5-hydroxytryptamine 4 receptors in the human rectum. *Life Sci* 2000; **66**: 31–4.

27 Sakurai-Yamashita Y, Yamashita K *et al*. Differential distribution of 5-hydroxytryptamine 3 receptor in the colon between human and guinea pig. *Chin J Physiol* 1999; **42**: 195–8.

28 Talley NJ, Phillips SF, Haddad A *et al*. Effect of selective 5HT3 antagonist (GR 38032F) on small intestinal transit and release of gastrointestinal peptides. *Dig Dis Sci* 1989; **34**: 1511–15.

29 Steadman CJ, Talley NJ, Phillips SF, Zinsmeister AR. Selective 5-hydroxytryptamine type 3 receptor antagonism with ondansetron as treatment for diarrhea-predominant irritable bowel syndrome: a pilot study. *Mayo Clin Proc* 1992; **67**: 732–8.

30 Talley NJ, Phillips SF, Haddad A *et al*. GR 38032F (ondansetron), a selective 5-HT3 receptor antagonist, slows colonic transit in healthy man. *Dig Dis Sci* 1990; **35**: 477–80.

31 Gore S, Gilmore IT, Haigh CG, Brownless SM, Stockdale H, Morris AI. Colonic transit in man is slowed by ondansetron (GR38032F), a selective 5-hydroxytryptamine receptor (type 3) antagonist. *Alim Pharmacol Ther* 1990; **4**: 139–44.

32 von der Ohe M, Hanson RB, Camilleri M. Serotonergic mediation of postprandial colonic tonic and phasic responses in humans. *Gut* 1994; **35**: 536–41.

33 Maxton DG, Morris J, Whorwell PJ. Selective 5-hydroxytryptamine antagonism: a role in irritable bowel syndrome and functional dyspepsia? *Alim Pharmacol Ther* 1996; **10**: 595–9.

34 Prior A, Read NW. Reduction of rectal sensitivity and post-prandial motility by granisetron, a 5 HT3-receptor

antagonist, in patients with irritable bowel syndrome. *Alim Pharmacol Ther* 1993; **7**: 175–80.

35 von der Ohe MR, Camilleri M, Kvols LK. A 5-HT3 antagonist corrects the postprandial colonic hypertonic response in carcinoid diarrhea. *Gastroenterology* 1994; **106**: 1184–9.

36 Schuurkes JAJ, Meulemans AL, Obertop H, Akkermans LMA. 5-HT4 receptors on the human stomach [abstract]. *J Gastrointest Motil* 1991; **3**: 199.

37 Sakurai-Yamashita Y, Takada K, Takemura K *et al*. Ability of mosapride to bind to 5-HT4 receptor in the human stomach. *Jpn J Pharmacol* 1999; **79**: 493–6.

38 Burleigh DE, Trout SJ. Evidence against an acetylcholine releasing action of cisapride in the human colon. *Br J Clin Pharmacol* 1985; **20**: 475–8.

39 Borman RA, Burleigh DE. Evidence for the involvement of a 5-HT4 receptor in the secretory response of human small intestine to 5-HT. *Br J Pharmacol* 1993; **110**: 927–8.

40 Briejer MR, Akkermans LM, Meulemans AL, Lefebvre RA, Schuurkes JA. Cisapride and a structural analogue, R 76,186, are 5-hydroxytryptamine 4 (5-HT4) receptor agonists on the guinea-pig colon ascendens. *Naunyn Schmiedebergs Arch Pharmacol* 1993; **347**: 464–70.

41 Wardle KA, Sanger GJ. The guinea-pig distal colon – a sensitive preparation for the investigation of 5-HT4 receptor-mediated contractions. *Br J Pharmacol* 1993; **110**: 1593–9.

42 Tam FS, Hillier K, Bunce KT, Grossman C. Differences in response to 5-HT4 receptor agonists and antagonists of the 5-HT4-like receptor in human colon circular smooth muscle. *Br J Pharmacol* 1995; **115**: 172–6.

43 McLean PG, Coupar IM. Stimulation of cyclic AMP formation in the circular smooth muscle of human colon by activation of 5-HT4-like receptors. *Br J Pharmacol* 1996; **117**: 238–9.

44 Prins NH, Akkermans LMA, Lefebvre RA, Cheyns P, Schuurkes JAJ. Cholinergic 5-HT4 receptor stimulation enhances canine and human colon longitudinal muscle contractility [abstract]. *Neurogastroenterol Motil* 2000; **12**: 267.

45 Grider JR, Kuemmerle JF, Jin JG. 5-HT released by mucosal stimuli initiate peristalsis by activating 5-HT4/5-HT1p receptors on sensory CGRP neurons. *Am J Physiol* 1996; **270**: 778–82.

46 Foxx-Orenstein AE, Kuemmerle JF, Grider JR. Distinct 5-HT receptors mediate the peristaltic reflex induced by mucosal stimuli in human and guinea-pig intestine. *Gastroenterology* 1996; **111**: 1281–90.

47 Grider JR, Foxx-Orenstein AE, Jin JG. 5-Hydroxytryptamine 4 receptor agonists initiate the peristaltic reflex in human, rat, and guinea pig intestine. *Gastroenterology* 1998; **115**: 370–80.

48 Tack J, Broeckaert D, Coulie B, Janssens J. The influence

of cisapride on gastric tone and the perception of gastric distension. *Aliment Pharmacol Ther* 1998; **12**: 761–6.

49 Manes G, Dominguez-Munoz JE, Leodolter A, Malfertheiner P. Effect of cisapride on gastric sensitivity to distension, gastric compliance and duodeno-gastric reflexes in healthy humans. *Dig Liver Dis* 2001; **33**: 407–13.

50 Coelho AM, Rovira P, Fioramonti J, Buéno L. Antinociceptive properties of HTF 919 (tegaserod), a 5-HT4 receptor partial agonist, on colorectal distension in rats [abstract]. *Gastroenterology* 2000; **118** (Suppl. 2): A835.

51 Coffin B, Farmachidi JP, Rueegg P, Bastie A, Bouhassira D. Tegaserod, a 5-HT4 receptor partial agonist, decreases sensitivity to rectal distension in healthy subjects. *Aliment Pharmacol Ther* 2003; **17**: 577–85.

52 Gunput MD. Review article: clinical pharmacology of alosetron. *Aliment Pharmacol Ther* 1999; **13** (Suppl. 2): 70–6.

53 Humphrey PP, Bountra C, Clayton N, Kozlowski K. Review article: the therapeutic potential of 5-HT3 receptor antagonists in the treatment of irritable bowel syndrome. *Aliment Pharmacol Ther* 1999; **13** (Suppl. 2): 31–8.

54 Balfour JA, Goa KL, Perry CM. Alosetron [see Guest Commentaries]. *Drugs* 2000; **59**: 511–18.

55 Kozlowski CM, Green A, Grundy D, Boissonade FM, Bountra C. The 5-HT3 receptor antagonist alosetron inhibits the colorectal distention induced depressor response and spinal c-fos expression in the anaesthetised rat. *Gut* 2000; **46**: 474–80.

56 Delvaux M, Louvel D, Mamet JP, Campos-Oriola R, Frexinos J. Effect of alosetron on responses to colonic distension in patients with irritable bowel syndrome. *Aliment Pharmacol Ther* 1998; **12**: 849–55.

57 Thumshirn M, Coulie B, Camilleri M, Zinsmeister AR, Burton DD, Van Dyke C. Effects of alosetron on gastrointestinal transit time and rectal sensation in patients with irritable bowel syndrome. *Aliment Pharmacol Ther* 2000; **14**: 869–78.

58 Moss HE, Sanger GJ. The effects of granisetron, ICS 205–930 and ondansetron on the visceral pain reflex induced by duodenal distension. *Br J Pharmacol* 1990; **100**: 497–501.

59 Miura M, Lawson DC, Clary EM, Mangel AW, Pappas TN. Central modulation of rectal distension-induced blood pressure changes by alosetron, a 5-HT3 receptor antagonist. *Dig Dis Sci* 1999; **44**: 20–4.

60 Goldberg PA, Kamm MA, Setti-Carraro P, van der Sijp JR, Roth C. Modification of visceral sensitivity and pain in irritable bowel syndrome by 5-HT3 antagonism (ondansetron). *Digestion* 1996; **57**: 478–83.

61 Feinle C, Read NW. Ondansetron reduces nausea induced by gastroduodenal stimulation without changing gastric motility. *Am J Physiol* 1996; **261**: G591–7.

62 Talley NJ, Van Zanten SV, Saez LR *et al.* A dose-ranging, placebo-controlled, randomized trial of alosetron in patients with functional dyspepsia. *Aliment Pharmacol Ther* 2001; **15**: 525–37.

63 Kuo B, Camilleri M, Burton D, Viramontes B *et al.* Effects of 5-HT3 antagonism on postprandial gastric volume and symptoms in humans. *Aliment Pharmacol Ther* 2002; **16**: 225–33.

64 Zerbib F, Bruley des Varannes S, Oriola RC, McDonald J, Isal JP, Galmiche JP. Alosetron does not affect the visceral perception of gastric distension in healthy subjects. *Aliment Pharmacol Ther* 1994; **8**: 403–7.

65 Bardhan KD, Bodemar G, Geldof H *et al.* A double-blind, randomized, placebo-controlled dose-ranging study to evaluate the efficacy of alosetron in the treatment of irritable bowel syndrome. *Aliment Pharmacol Ther* 2000; **14**: 23–34.

66 Jones RH, Holtmann G, Rodrigo L *et al.* Alosetron relieves pain and improves bowel function compared with mebeverine in female nonconstipated irritable bowel syndrome patients. *Aliment Pharmacol Ther* 1999; **13**: 1419–27.

67 Camilleri M, Northcutt AR, Kong S, Dukes GE, McSorley D, Mangel AW. Efficacy and safety of alosetron in women with irritable bowel syndrome: a randomised, placebo-controlled trial. *Lancet* 2000; **355**: 1035–40.

68 Cremonini F, Delgado-Aros S, Camilleri M. Efficacy of alosetron in irritable bowel syndrome: a meta-analysis of randomized controlled trials. *Neurogastroenterol Motil* 2003; **15**: 79–86.

69 Stacher G. Cilansetron. Solvay. *Curr Opin Investig Drugs* 2001; **2**: 1432–6.

70 Stacher G, Weber U, Stacher-Janotta G *et al.* Effects of the 5-HT3 antagonist cilansetron vs placebo on phasic sigmoid colonic motility in healthy man: a double-blind crossover trial. *Br J Clin Pharmacol* 2000; **49**: 429–36.

71 Clouse R.E., Caras S., Cataldi F., et al. Cilansetron is efficacious for relief of urgency in patients with irritable bowel syndrome with diarrhea predominance (IBS-D). JPGN 2004; **39** (Suppl. 3): S777.

72 Coleman NS, Marciani L, Blackshaw E *et al.* Effect of a novel 5-HT3 receptor agonist MKC-733 on upper gastrointestinal motility in humans. *Aliment Pharmacol Ther* 2003; **18**: 1039–48.

73 Tonini M, De Ponti F, Di Nucci A, Crema F. Review article: cardiac adverse effects of gastrointestinal prokinetics. *Alim Pharmacol Ther* 1999; **13**: 1585–91.

74 Camilleri M. Review article: tegaserod. *Aliment Pharmacol Ther* 2001; **15**: 277–89.

75 Wagstaff AJ, Frampton JE, Croom KF. Tegaserod: a review of its use in the management of irritable bowel syndrome with constipation in women. *Drugs* 2003; **63**: 1101–20.

76 Poen AC, Felt-Bersma RJ, Van Dongen PA, Meuwissen

SG. Effect of prucalopride, a new enterokinetic agent, on gastrointestinal transit and anorectal function in healthy volunteers. *Aliment Pharmacol Ther* 1999; **13**: 1493–7.

77 Camilleri M, McKinzie S, Burton D, Thomforde GM, Zinsmeister A, Bouras EP. Prucalopride accelerates small bowel and colonic transit in patients with chronic functional constipation (FC) or constipation-predominant irritable bowel syndrome (C-IBS) [abstract]. *Gastroenterology* 2000; **118** (Suppl. 2): A845.

78 De Ponti F, Tonini M. Irritable bowel syndrome: new agents targeting serotonin receptor subtypes. *Drugs* 2001; **61**: 317–32.

79 Carlsson L, Amos GJ, Andersson B, Drews L, Duker G, Wadstedt G. Electrophysiological characterization of the prokinetic agents cisapride and mosapride *in vivo* and *in vitro*: implications for proarrhythmic potential? *J Pharmacol Exp Ther* 1997; **282**: 220–7.

80 Drici MD, Ebert SN, Wang WX *et al.* Comparison of tegaserod (HTF 919) and its main human metabolite with cisapride and erythromycin on cardiac repolarization in the isolated rabbit heart. *J Cardiovasc Pharmacol* 1999; **34**: 82–8.

81 Whorwell PJ, Krumholz S, Muller-Lissner S, Schmitt C, Dunger-Baldauf C, Rueegg PC. Tegaserod has a favorable safety and tolerability profile in patients with constipation predominant and alternating forms of irritable bowel syndrome (IBS) [abstract]. *Gastroenterology* 2000; **118** (Suppl. 2): A1204.

82 Nguyen A, Camilleri M, Kost LJ *et al.* SDZ HTF 919 stimulates canine colonic motility and transit *in vivo*. *J Pharmacol Exp Ther* 1997; **280**: 1270–6.

83 Bouras EP, Camilleri M, Burton DD, McKinzie S. Selective stimulation of colonic transit by the benzofuran 5HT4 agonist, prucalopride, in healthy humans. *Gut* 1999; **44**: 682–6.

84 Emmanuel AV, Nicholls T, Roy AJ, Antonelli K, Kamm MA. Prucalopride (PRU) improves colonic transit and stool frequency in patients (pts) with slow and normal transit constipation [abstract]. *Gastroenterology* 2000; **118** (Suppl. 2): A846.

85 Yoshida N, Omoya H, Kato S, Ito T. Pharmacological effects of the new gastroprokinetic agent mosapride citrate and its metabolites in experimental animals [abstract]. *Arzneimittelforschung* 1993; **43**: 1078–83.

86 Mine Y, Yoshikawa T, Oku S, Nagai R, Yoshida N, Hosoki K. Comparison of effect of mosapride citrate and existing 5-HT4 receptor agonists on gastrointestinal motility *in vivo* and *in vitro*. *J Pharmacol Exp Ther* 1997; **283**: 1000–8.

87 Ruth M, Hamelin B, Röhss K, Lundell L. The effect of mosapride, a novel prokinetic, on acid reflux variables in patients with gastro-oesophageal reflux disease. *Alim Phar-*

macol Ther 1998; **12**: 35–40.

88 Hallerback BI, Bommelaer G, Bredberg E *et al.* Dose finding study of mosapride in functional dyspepsia: a placebo-controlled, randomized study. *Aliment Pharmacol Ther* 2002; **16**: 959–67.

89 Degen L, Matzinger D, Merz M. Tegaserod (HTF919), a 5-HT4 receptor partial agonist, accelerates gastrointestinal transit. *Gastroenterology* 2000; **118**: A845.

90 Tack J, Vos R, Janssens J, Salter J, Jauffret S, Vandeplassche G. Influence of tegaserod on proximal gastric tone and on the perception of gastric distension. *Aliment Pharmacol Ther* 2003; **18**: 1031–7.

91 Prather CM, Camilleri M, Zinsmeister AR, McKinzie S, Thomforde G. Tegaserod accelerates orocecal transit in patients with constipation-predominant irritable bowel syndrome. *Gastroenterology* 2000; **118**: 463–8.

92 Muller-Lissner SA, Fumagalli I, Bardhan KD *et al.* Tegaserod, a 5-HT(4) receptor partial agonist, relieves symptoms in irritable bowel syndrome patients with abdominal pain, bloating and constipation. *Aliment Pharmacol Ther* 2001; **15**: 1655–66.

93 Novick J, Miner P, Krause R *et al.* A randomized, double-blind, placebo-controlled trial of tegaserod in female patients suffering from irritable bowel syndrome with constipation. *Aliment Pharmacol Ther* 2002; **16**: 1877–88.

94 Kellow J, Lee OY, Chang FY *et al.* An Asia-Pacific, double blind, placebo controlled, randomised study to evaluate the efficacy, safety, and tolerability of tegaserod in patients with irritable bowel syndrome. *Gut* 2003; **52**: 671–6.

95 Tougas G, Snape WJ Jr, Otten MH *et al.* Long-term safety of tegaserod in patients with constipation-predominant irritable bowel syndrome. *Aliment Pharmacol Ther* 2002; **16**: 1701–8.

96 Emmanuel AV, Kamm MA, Roy AJ, Antonelli K. Effect of a novel prokinetic drug, R093877, on gastrointestinal transit in healthy volunteers. *Gut* 1998; **42**: 511–16.

97 Otten M, Schneider H, Wurzer H *et al.* A double-blind, placebo controlled evaluation of safety and efficacy of 12-week, twice-daily treatment with prucaloprid in patients with chronic constipation. *Gastroenterology* 1999; **116**: 1055.

98 Sanger GJ, Banner SE, Smith MI, Wardle KA. SB-207266: 5-HT4 receptor antagonism in human isolated gut and prevention of 5-HT-evoked sensitization of peristalsis and increased defaecation in animal models. *Neurogastroenterol Motil* 1998; **10**: 271–9.

99 Bharucha AE, Camilleri M, Ferber I, Zinsmeister AR. Effects of a serotonin (5-HT4) receptor antagonist on gastrointestinal (GI) transit, colonic motor and sensory function in health. *Gastroenterology* 1999; **116**: A958.

100 Sanger GJ. 5-Hydroxytryptamine and functional bowel

disorders. *Neurogastroenterol Motil* 1996; **8**: 319–31.

101 Sanger GJ, Yoshida M, Yahyah M, Kitazumi K. Increased defecation during stress or after 5-hydroxytryptophan: selective inhibition by the 5-HT4 receptor antagonist, SB-207266. *Br J Pharmacol* 2000; **130**: 706–12.

102 Cooper SM, Haydock SF, Tompson DJ, Higgins RG, Fitzpatrick KL. A pharmacodynamic model of 5-HT4 receptor activation in man: antagonism by the 5-HT4 receptor antagonist SB-207266. *Gastroenterology* 1999; **116**: A598.

103 Houghton LA, Jackson NA, Whorwell PJ, Cooper SM. 5-HT4 receptor antagonism in irritable bowel syndrome: effect of SB-207266-A on rectal sensitivity and small bowel transit. *Aliment Pharmacol Ther* 1999; **13**: 1437–44.

104 Sanger GJ. Hypersensitivity and hyperreactivity in the irritable bowel syndrome: an opportunity for drug discovery. *Dig Dis* 1999; **17**: 90–9.

105 Smith MI, Banner SE, Sanger GJ. 5-HT4 receptor antagonism potentiates inhibition of intestinal allodynia by 5-HT3 receptor antagonism in conscious rats. *Neurosci Lett* 1999; **271**: 61–4.

106 Coulie B, Tack J, Sifrim D, Andrioli A, Janssens J. Role of nitric oxide in fasting gastric fundus tone and in 5-HT1 receptor-mediated relaxation of gastric fundus. *Am J Physiol* 1999; **276**: G373–7.

107 Coulie B, Tack J, Maes B, Geypens B, De Roo M, Janssens J. Sumatriptan, a selective 5-HT1 receptor agonist, induces a lag phase for gastric emptying of liquids in humans. *Am J Physiol* 1997; **272**: G902–8.

108 Tack J, Coulie B, Wilmer A, Andrioli A, Janssens J. Influence of sumatriptan on gastric fundus tone and on the perception of gastric distension in man. *Gut* 2000; **46**: 468–73.

109 Houghton LA, Fowler P, Keene ON, Read NW. Effect of sumatriptan, a new selective 5HT1-like agonist, on liquid gastric emptying in man. *Aliment Pharmacol Ther* 1992; **6**: 685–91.

110 Tack J, Piessevaux H, Coulie B, Caenepeel P, Janssens J. Role of impaired gastric accommodation to a meal in functional dyspepsia. *Gastroenterology* 1998; **115**: 1346–52.

111 Malatesta MG, Fascetti E, Ciccaglione AF *et al.* 5-HT1-receptor agonist sumatriptan modifies gastric size after 500 ml of water in dyspeptic patients and normal subjects. *Dig Dis Sci* 2002; **47**: 2591–5.

112 Sifrim D, Holloway RH, Tack J *et al.* Effect of sumatriptan, a 5HT1 agonist, on the frequency of transient lower esophageal sphincter relaxations and gastroesophageal reflux in healthy subjects. *Am J Gastroenterol* 1999; **94**: 3158–64.

113 Meulemans AL, Helsen LF, Schuurkes JA. The role of nitric oxide (NO) in 5-HT-induced relaxations of the guinea-pig stomach. *Naunyn Schmiedebergs Arch Pharmacol* 1993; **348**: 424–30.

114 De Ponti F, Crema F, Moro E, Nardelli G, Frigo G, Crema A. Role of 5-HT1B/D receptors in canine gastric accommodation: effect of sumatriptan and 5-HT1B/D receptor antagonists. *Am J Physiol* 2003; **285**: G96–104.

115 Moro E, Crema F, De Ponti F, Frigo G. Triptans and gastric accommodation: pharmacological and therapeutic aspects. *Dig Liver Dis* 2004; **36**: 85–92.

116 Meulemans AL, Elsen LF, de Ridder WJA, Schuurkes JAJ. Effects of sumatriptan on the guinea-pig isolated stomach. *Neurogastroenterol Motil* 1996; **8**: A183.

117 Rouzade ML, Fioramonti J, Bueno L. Decrease in gastric sensitivity to distension by 5-HT1A receptor agonists in rats. *Dig Dis Sci* 1998; **43**: 2048–54.

118 Xue L, Locker GRI, Schuurkes JAJ, Meulemans A, Coulie B, Szurszewski JH. Serotonergic modulation of murine fundic tone. *Gastroenterology* 2003; **124**: A580.

119 Janssen P, Prins NH, Moreaux B, Meulemans AL, Lefebvre RA. *In vivo* characterization of 5-HT1A receptor-mediated gastric relaxation in conscious dogs. *Br J Pharmacol* 2003; **140**: 913–20.

120 Tack J, Piessevaux H, Coulie B, Fischler B, DeGucht VA. Placebo controlled trial of buspirone, a fundus relaxing drug, in functional dyspepsia: effect on symptoms and gastric sensory and motor function. *Gastroenterology* 1999; **116**: G1423.

121 Vanhoenacker P, Haegeman G, Leysen JE. 5-HT7 receptors: current knowledge and future prospects. *Trends Pharmacol Sci* 2000; **21**: 70–7.

122 Carter D, Champney M, Hwang B, Eglen RM. Characterization of a postjunctional 5-HT receptor mediating relaxation of guinea-pig isolated ileum. *Eur J Pharmacol* 1995; **280**: 243–50.

123 Janssen P, Prins NH, Meulemans AL, Lefebvre RA. 5-HT7 receptors mediate canine stomach relaxation, an *in vivo* study. *Neurogastroenterol Motil* 2002; **14**: 571.

124 Janssen P, Prins NH, Meulemans AL, Lefebvre RA. Pharmacological characterization of the 5-HT receptors mediating contraction and relaxation of canine isolated proximal stomach smooth muscle. *Br J Pharmacol* 2002; **136**: 321–9.

125 Tuladhar BR, Ge L, Naylor RJ. 5-HT7 receptors mediate the inhibitory effect of 5-HT on peristalsis in the isolated guinea-pig ileum. *Br J Pharmacol* 2003; **138**: 1210–14.

126 Meuser T, Pietruck C, Gabriel A, Xie GX, Lim KJ, Pierce PP. 5-HT7 receptors are involved in mediating 5-HT-induced activation of rat primary afferent neurons. *Life Sci* 2002; **71**: 2279–89.

127 Jackson JL, O'Malley PG, Tomkins G, Balden E, Santoro J, Kroenke K. Treatment of functional gastrointestinal disorders with antidepressant medications: a meta-analysis. *Am J Med* 2000; **108**: 65–72.

128 Gorard DA, Libby GW, Farthing MJ. Influence of antidepressants on whole gut and orocaecal transit times in

health and irritable bowel syndrome. *Aliment Pharmacol Ther* 1994; **8**: 159–66.

129 Gorard DA, Libby GW, Farthing MJ. Effect of a tricyclic antidepressant on small intestinal motility in health and diarrhea predominant irritable bowel syndrome. *Dig Dis Sci* 1995; **40**: 86–95.

130 Peghini PL, Katz PO, Castell DO. Imipramine decreases oesophageal pain perception in human male volunteers. *Gut* 1998; **42**: 807–13.

131 Drossman DA, Whitehead WE, Camilleri M. Irritable bowel syndrome: a technical review for practice guideline development. *Gastroenterology* 1997; **112**: 2120–37.

132 Onghena P, Van Houdenhove B. Antidepressant-induced analgesia in chronic non-malignant pain: a meta-analysis of 39 placebo-controlled studies. *Pain* 1992; **49**: 205–19.

133 Tack J, Broekaert D, Coulie B, Fischler B, Janssens J. Influence of the selective serotonin re-uptake inhibitor, paroxetine, on gastric sensorimotor function in humans. *Aliment Pharmacol Ther* 2003; **17**: 603–8.

134 Chial HJ, Camilleri M, Burton D, Thomforde G, Olden KW, Stephens D. Selective effects of serotonergic psychoactive agents on gastrointestinal functions in health. *Am J Physiol* 2003; **284**: G130–7.

135 Ladabaum U, Glidden D. Effect of the selective serotonin reuptake inhibitor sertraline on gastric sensitivity and compliance in healthy humans. *Neurogastroenterol Motil* 2002; **14**: 395–402.

136 Mertz H, Fass R, Kodner A, Yan-Go F, Fullerton S, Mayer EA. Effect of amitriptyline on symptoms, sleep, and visceral perception in patients with functional dyspepsia. *Am J Gastroenterol* 1998; **93**: 160–5.

137 Kuiken SD, Tytgat GNJ, Boeckxstaens GEE. The selective serotonin reuptake inhibitor fluoxetine does not change rectal sensitivity and symptoms in patients with irritable bowel syndrome: a double blind, randomized, placebo-controlled study. *Clin Gastroenterol Hepatol* 2003; **1**: 219–28.

138 Chial HJ, Camilleri M, Ferber I *et al*. Effects of venlafaxine, buspirone, and placebo on colonic sensorimotor functions in healthy humans. *Clin Gastroenterol Hepatol* 2003; **1**: 211–18.

CHAPTER 19

Emerging Transmitters

Lionel Bueno

Many transmitters involved in the physiological functioning of the gastrointestinal tract have been identified during the last 20 years. The hypothesis that their release and/or the distribution of their receptors may be altered in both inflammatory and functional bowel disorders has recently emerged. In addition to serotonin (5-HT), several other neurotransmitters, such as tachykinins, corticotropin releasing factor (CRF), nerve growth factor (NGF), proteases and glutamate, may participate in alterations in enteric nervous system functioning and brain–gut communications or sensory signaling of the gut.

Peripheral versus central CRF in initiating enteric nervous system mediated gastrointestinal disorders

Corticotropin releasing factor is the primary mediator of the hypothalamic–pituitary–adrenal endocrine limb of the stress response. In the late 1980s, CRF was identified as an important factor involved at central nervous system level in the effects of stress on gastrointestinal[1] and colonic[2] motility. More recently, it has been shown that CRF participates in stress-induced alterations of gut sensitivity[3] and immune reaction.[4–6]

Centrally mediated effects

In several animal species, most of the gastrointestinal motor effects of stress are suppressed by central administration of a non-selective CRF antagonist, such as α-helical CRF_{9-41} or CRF antibodies. For example, slowing of gastric emptying induced by acoustic stress is blocked by i.c.v. administration of both α-helical CRF_{9-41} and CRF antibodies.[1,2] However, CRF does not appear to be the only peptide involved at brain level in the genesis of stress-induced slowing of gastric emptying, and thyrotropin-releasing hormone plays

---

Three emerging transmitters

Corticotropin releasing factor
Many effects of stress on digestive functions are linked to the central and peripheral release of this neuromediator. Blockade of its receptor to prevent its deleterious effects on visceral sensitivity is a relevant target and selective antagonists are now available.

Nerve growth factor
This growth factor plays an important role in long-term effects of stress and inflammation on the sensory system and the mucosal barrier in relation to mast cells. Further research is needed to confirm its

major role in the genesis of functional bowel disorders such as irritable bowel syndrome, but antagonists for its receptors are not presently available.

Proteinase-activated receptor 2
This is a very promising target as it is widely distributed in the gastrointestinal tract. At colonic level, it can be cleaved directly and subsequently activated by luminal serine proteases (trypsin, bacterial proteases), triggering alterations of the mucosal barrier and subsequently hypersensitivity to distension similar to that observed in irritable bowel syndrome.

---

an important role in cold-stress-induced alterations of gastrointestinal motility.[7]

CRF also plays an important role in stress-induced colonic motor and transit stimulation. In a model of emotional stress, fear of receiving electric footshocks increases colonic motility through the central release of CRF.[8] Defecation induced by passive avoidance stress was also shown to be mediated through the hypothalamic release of CRF (see Chapter 8). These effects are not mediated through the stimulation of the hypothalamic–pituitary–adrenal axis, since CRF-induced motor effects of stress persisted after hypophysectomy or adrenalectomy.[8]

CRF is also involved at brain level in the modulation of visceral pain. Indeed, the hypersensitivity of the gastrointestinal tract initiated by restraint stress is blunted by i.c.v. administration of α-helical CRF_{9-41} and mimicked by central administration of CRF.[3] This effect of central CRF is linked to the peripheral activation of mast cells within the gastrointestinal tract, which sensitizes mechanoreceptors in the gut or favors mast cell degranulation in response to a baric stimulus such as distension.[10] CRF may also be involved in mast cell degranulation induced by restraint stress, but the mechanism involved remains unclear.[11]

In contrast, brain CRF is not involved in the deleterious effect of stress on gut inflammatory responses, and the release of CRF by the brain has an anti-inflammatory influence.[4] However, colitis induces hypothalamic CRF expression and blunts the CRF gene response to stress in rats.[12] Several important findings have suggested that, in addition to its role at brain level in the control of gastrointestinal function, CRF also plays a role at peripheral level.

Peripherally mediated effects

Although the origin of peripherally circulating CRF and its distribution, or that of its related peptides, in various tissues is still debated, numerous recent studies suggest that CRF may act peripherally to modulate several gastrointestinal functions, including motility, permeability and inflammatory response (see Chapter 8). Moreover, urocortin gene expression has been found in peripheral tissues, particularly in the colonic enteric nervous system, and CRF is expressed in peripheral inflamed tissues of rodents[13] and humans.[14] Peripheral administration of CRF or analogs such as urocortin

and sauvagine alters colonic motility and induces fecal output in rats.[15]

A local proinflammatory role of CRF has been demonstrated in acute models of gut inflammation[16] and the peripheral origin is supported by the observations that CRF stimulates *in vitro* the secretion of cytokines[17] and the proliferation of immunocytes.[13] Peripheral CRF is secreted by both T and B cells stimulated by lipopolysaccharide or concanavalin A,[18] and recent evidence indicates that both CRF1 and CRF2 receptors are present in the lamina propria mononuclear cells of the human colonic mucosa[19] and that CRF2 receptors are overexpressed in inflamed tissues. In a model of *Clostridium difficile* toxin A-induced ileal inflammation, CRF1 receptor antagonist was found to be anti-inflammatory.[16] CRF has also been proposed to be directly responsible for the enhancement of colonic epithelial permeability induced by stress. This peripheral site of action is supported by the increase in macromolar permeability induced by CRF in Ussing chambers.[20] The mechanism by which stress or CRF increases gut paracellular permeability is not completely elucidated, but it has been suggested recently that it involves CD4[+] lymphocytes, interferon γ (IFNγ) and the contraction of the epithelial cell cytoskeleton through the activation of myosin light chain kinase.[6]

No studies have yet shown that the involvement of CRF in stress-induced visceral pain is of peripheral origin. However, acute restraint stress-induced rectal hypersensitivity to rectal distension is linked to increased colonic paracellular permeability, and this increase in colonic paracellular permeability may be of peripheral origin.[20]

Types of receptors involved in the gastrointestinal effects of CRF and related peptides

Recently, two genes encoding G-protein-coupled CRF receptors – putative targets for CRF-related peptides – have been cloned.[21] CRF1 receptors are expressed widely in the brain and gastrointestinal tract, while three different CRF2 receptor splice variants have been described, also distributed within the brain and the gut, though not always in the same structures. Additionally, CRF2 receptors are also localized on vagal afferents.[22] The discovery of endogenous selective CRF2 receptor agonists – the type 2 urocortins (Ucn 2 and Ucn 3) – has improved our knowledge about the type of receptor involved in the effects of stress and/or CRF (see Chapter 8).

Nerve growth factor: its role in modulating motility, viscerosensitivity and inflammation

One of the family of neurotrophins, NGF has a key role in the survival and establishment of the phenotype of responsive primary afferent neurons during development.[23] NGF is produced by a range of cell types from smooth muscle cells to neurons, including macrophages, mast cells and epithelial cells. Recent studies have revealed that these trophic factors also play a critical role throughout life by regulating neurotransmitter and neuropeptide synthesis, and by influencing neuronal morphology and synaptic functions.[24] Responsiveness to NGF is conferred by the high-affinity trkA receptor but also, to a lesser extent, by a less specific low-affinity p75 receptor.[25]

NGF and motility

Very few data are available concerning the influence of NGF on gut motility. Diarrhea is a side-effect in patients treated with brain-derived neurotrophic factor (BDNF) and neurotrophin 3 (NT-3), and in patients with severe constipation, treatment with subcutaneously injected recombinant BDNF or NT-3 increased stool frequency. The rapid onset of action has suggested a direct effect on neurotransmission at the level of the enteric nervous system.[26]

NGF and visceral pain

Injected locally or systematically, NGF has hyperalgesic effects by acting: (1) at the peripheral terminals of primary sensory neurons either indirectly, via mast cell degranulation,[27] or directly, by a tyrosine kinase-mediated change in transduction/receptor sensitivity, or (2) in dorsal root ganglion cell bodies following its retrograde transport.[28] More recently, it was shown that NGF-induced hyperalgesia in some conditions may require the presence of the normal sympathetic postganglionic terminals[29] or may be dependent on circulating neutrophils.[30] Similar observations have been made concerning visceral pain. Indeed, the pronociceptive role of NGF has been identified in the urinary bladder in a model of turpentine-induced cystitis associated with an increase in NGF expression.[31] Administration of exogenous NGF into the lumen of urinary bladder produces a rapid and sustained bladder hyper-reflexia, and pretreatment with a soluble receptor (a molecule consisting of two trkA receptors) attenuates viscerovisceral hyper-reflexia.[32]

In rats, intraperitoneal injection of NGF dose-dependently decreases the threshold of pain in response to colonic distension. Moreover, in a model of hypersensitivity to colonic distension triggered by experimental colitis in rats, it was shown that antibodies against NGF restore a normal threshold of abdominal response to colonic distension.[33] In this model, it has also been suggested that other growth factors, such as BDNF, may also participate in trinitrobenzene sulfonic acid-(TNBS) induced lowering of the threshold to colonic distension.

Neonatal stress resulting from maternal deprivation initiates long-term alterations in gut permeability and gut hypersensitivity to distension, and these two effects have been linked.[34] Maternal deprivation is associated with central overexpression of NGF.[35] Recently, it has been shown that these long-term effects of NGF on colonic sensitivity and permeability are suppressed by neonatal treatment with NGF antibodies. These long-term alterations are mimicked by NGF administration during the neonatal period. All these data support an important role of NGF in the long-term development of gut hypersensitivity.[36]

NGF and gut inflammatory reactions

NGF has a pivotal role in modulating sensory neuropeptide release, which plays a role in gut inflammatory reactions. NGF expression in the gut mucosa is increased in various inflammatory conditions. Mucosal NGF upregulation was observed in TNBS colitis and in inflammatory bowel disease.[37] NGF has a protective effect on TNBS-induced colitis in rats, as pretreatment with anti-NGF causes a significant two- to threefold increase in the severity of the experimental inflammation, as assessed by a macroscopic damage score, a histological ulceration score, and myeloperoxidase activity in the tissues. The amount of calcitonin gene-related peptide, but not that of substance P, in the colon is significantly reduced by NGF immunoneutralization.[38]

The anti-inflammatory properties of NGF in experimental colitis have been attributed in part to its action on sensory nerves. However, immunoregulatory cells, such as T cells, express different neurotrophins and neurotrophin receptors, such as trk and p75. This suggests multidirectional communication between immune cells and neuronal structures as well as epithelial cells, in which NGF plays a major role. This is evidenced by the fact that NGF reduces apoptosis in CD4+ cells extracted from the inflamed colon of CD4+ cell-repopulated SCID mice.[39]

Proteinase-activated receptor 2: consequences of their activation for gastrointestinal functions

Proteinase-activated receptors (PARs) are G-protein-coupled receptors that are activated by the proteolytic cleavage of their N-terminal domain. The new N-terminal sequence that is exposed by proteolysis acts as a tethered ligand, which binds to and activates the receptor. PAR-2 is highly expressed in the gastrointestinal tract, where it is found in endothelial cells, colonic myocytes, enterocytes (on both basolateral and apical membranes), enteric neurons, terminals of mesenteric afferent nerves and immune cells. The discovery of this novel receptor family has highlighted a new role for proteinases as signaling molecules that can affect tissue functions via the PARs. In the gastrointestinal tract, PAR-2 may be activated by tryptase from mast cells but also by luminal proteases such as trypsin and possibly bacterial proteases.

Activation of PAR-2 and motility

From the pioneering work of Corvera and colleagues[40] showing that PAR-2 activating peptide (PAR2-AP) and trypsin inhibit *in vitro* colonic motility, much has been published concerning the site of action. Because this response was unaffected by indomethacin, l-NG-nitroarginine methyl ester, a bradykinin B_2 receptor antagonist and tetrodotoxin, and because PAR-2 is highly expressed by colonic myocytes, a direct action on smooth muscle has been postulated. However, enteric neurons express PAR-2[41] and local application of trypsin and tryptase evokes slowly activating excitatory responses reminiscent of slow synaptic excitation in enteric neurons.[42] This type of effect suggests that one component of the motor inhibition linked to PAR-2 activation corresponds to the selective activation of uniaxonal S-type neurons immunoreactive for nitric

oxide synthase, which are characteristic of inhibitory neurons projecting to the circular muscle layer.[43]

PAR-2 and visceral pain

Prolonged thermal and mechanical hyperalgesia is observed shortly after intraplantar administration of PAR-2 agonists, these effects being mediated through the central activation of neurokinin 1 (NK1) receptors and the release of prostaglandins.[44] In rats, intracolonic infusion of PAR-2 agonists (PAR2-activating peptide (SLIGRL), trypsin) initiates delayed hypersensitivity to colonic distension, occurring 6–24 hours after their administration. These effects are mediated locally, since they are not observed after systemic administration.[45] They are also inhibited by an NK1 receptor antagonist but not by indomethacin, suggesting that afferent nerves containing substance P are involved. Interestingly, this pronociceptive effect of local activation of PAR-2 is associated with increased colonic paracellular permeability. Blockade of such increased permeability to ^{51}Cr-EDTA prevents the occurrence of hypersensitivity to rectal distension, suggesting that activation of the local immune system by luminal toxins and antigens is responsible for the sensitization of primary afferent terminals to mechanical stimuli.

PAR-2 and the immune system of the gut

In vitro, the activation of PAR-2 at the mucosal site of the intestinal wall generates the release of prostanoids,[46] and in Ussing chambers the effects of PAR-2 on short-circuit current is suppressed by indomethacin.[47] In mice, it has been shown that intraluminal infusion of PAR2-AP and trypsin triggers an inflammatory reaction with neutrophilic attraction, increased cytokine expression (interleukin 1β, interleukin 2, IFNγ), increased paracellular permeability and bacterial translocation.[48] It has been recently evidenced that these effects partly involved afferent nerves and nitric oxide and in part depends upon the release of IFNγ from CD4+ cells.[49] However, low doses of intracolonic PAR2-AP directly activate receptors located on epithelial cells to promote cytoskeletal contraction by activating myosin light chain kinase, and subsequently the increase in paracellular permeability. In contrast to its local proinflammatory effects, systemic administration of SLIGRL has been shown to reduce inflammation in a model of TNBS colitis in mice.[50]

References

1 Bueno L, Gue M. Evidence for the involvement of corticotropin-releasing factor in the gastrointestinal disturbances induced by acoustic and cold stress in mice. *Brain Res* 1988: **441**: 1–4.

2 Williams CL, Peterson JM, Villar RG, Burks TF. Corticotropin-releasing factor directly mediates colonic responses to stress. *Am J Physiol* 1987; **253**: G582–6.

3 Gue M, Del Rio-Lacheze C, Eutamene H, Theodorou V, Fioramonti J, Bueno L. Stress-induced visceral hypersensitivity to rectal distension in rats: role of CRF and mast cells. *Neurogastroenterol Motil* 1997; **9**: 271–9.

4 Gue M, Bonbonne C, Fioramonti J et al. Stress-induced enhancement of colitis in rats: CRF and arginine vasopressin are not involved. *Am J Physiol* 1997; **272**: G84–91.

5 Soderholm JD, Yates DA, Gareau MG, Yang PC, MacQueen G, Perdue MH. Neonatal maternal separation predisposes adult rats to colonic barrier dysfunction in response to mild stress. *Am J Physiol Gastrointest Liver Physiol* 200; **283**: G1257–63.

6 Ferrier L, Mazelin L, Cenac N et al. Stress-induced disruption of colonic epithelial barrier: role of interferon-gamma and myosin light chain kinase in mice. *Gastroenterology* 2003; **125**: 795–804.

7 Diop L, Pascaud X, Junien JL, Bueno L. CRF triggers the CNS release of TRH in stress-induced changes in gastric emptying. *Am J Physiol* 1991; **260**: G39–44.

8 Gue M, Junien JL, Bueno L. Conditioned emotional response in rats enhances colonic motility through the central release of corticotropin-releasing factor. *Gastroenterology* 1991; **100**: 964–70.

9 Eutamene H, Theodorou V, Fioramonti J, Bueno L. Acute stress modulates the histamine content of mast cells in the gastrointestinal tract through interleukin-1 and corticotropin-releasing factor release in rats. *J Physiol* 2003; **553**: 959–66.

10 Bradesi S, Eutamene H, Garcia-Villar R, Fioramonti J, Bueno L. Stress-induced visceral hypersensitivity in female rats is estrogen-dependent and involves tachykinin NK1 receptors. *Pain* 2003; **102**: 227–34.

11 Castagliuolo I, Lamont JT, Qiu B et al. Stress causes mucin release from rat colon: role of corticotropin releasing factor and mast cells. *Am J Physiol* 1996; **271**: G884–92.

12 Kresse AE, Million M, Saperas E, Tache Y. Colitis induces CRF expression in hypothalamic magnocellular neurons and blunts CRF gene response to stress in rats. *Am J Physiol Gastrointest Liver Physiol* 2001; **281**: G1203–13.

13 Karalis K, Sano H, Redwine J, Listwak S, Wilder RL, Chrousos GP. Autocrine or paracrine inflammatory actions of corticotropin-releasing hormone in vivo. *Science* 1991; **254**: 421–3.

14 Crofford LJ, Sano H, Karalis K et al. Corticotropin-releasing hormone in synovial fluids and tissues of patients with rheumatoid arthritis and osteoarthritis. *J Immunol* 1993; **151**: 1587–96.

15 Maillot C, Million M, Wei JY, Gauthier A, Tache Y. Peripheral corticotropin-releasing factor and stress-stimulated colonic motor activity involve type 1 receptor in rats. *Gastroenterology* 2000; **119**: 1569–79.

16 Wlk M, Wang CC, Venihaki M et al. Corticotropin-releasing hormone antagonists possess anti-inflammatory effects in the mouse ileum. *Gastroenterology* 2002; **123**: 505–15.

17 Singh VK, Leu SJ. Enhancing effect of corticotropin-releasing neurohormone on the production of interleukin-1 and interleukin-2. *Neurosci Lett* 1990; **120**: 151–4.

18 Kravchenco IV, Furalev VA. Secretion of immunoreactive corticotropin releasing factor and adrenocorticotropic hormone by T- and B-lymphocytes in response to cellular stress factors. *Biochem Biophys Res Commun* 1994; **204**: 828–34.

19 Muramatsu Y, Fukushima K, Iino K et al. Urocortin and corticotropin-releasing factor receptor expression in the human colonic mucosa. *Peptides* 2000; **21**: 1799–809.

20 Saunders PR, Santos J, Hanssen NP, Yates D, Groot JA, Perdue MH. Physical and psychological stress in rats enhances colonic epithelial permeability via peripheral CRH. *Dig Dis Sci* 2002; **47**: 208–15.

21 Dautzenberg FM, Hauger RL. The CRF peptide family and their receptors: yet more partners discovered. *Trends Pharmacol Sci* 2002; **23**: 71–7.

22 Zorrilla EP, Tache Y, Koob GF. Nibbling at CRF receptor control of feeding and gastrocolonic motility. *Trends Pharmacol Sci* 2003; **24**: 421–7.

23 Barde YA. Trophic factors and neuronal survival. *Neuron* 1989; **2**: 1525–34.

24 von Boyen GB, Reinshagen M, Steinkamp M, Adler G, Kirsch J. Nervous plasticity and development: dependence on neurotrophic factors. *J Gastroenterol* 2002; **37**: 583–8.

25 Kaplan DR, Hempstead BL, Martin-Zanca D, Chao MV, Parada LF. The trk proto-oncogene product: a signal transducing receptor for nerve growth factor. *Science* 1991 **252**: 554–8.

26 Coulie B, Szarka LA, Camilleri M et al. Recombinant human neurotrophic factors accelerate colonic transit and relieve constipation in humans. *Gastroenterology* 2000; **119**: 41–50.

27 Tal M, Liberman R. Local injection of nerve growth factor (NGF) triggers degranulation of mast cells in rat paw. *Neurosci Lett* 1997; **221**: 129–32.

28 Zhou XF, Deng YS, Xian CJ, Zhong JH. Neurotrophins from dorsal root ganglia trigger allodynia after spinal nerve

injury in rats. *Eur J Neurosci* 2000; **12**: 100–5.

29   Andreev NYu, Dimitrieva N, Koltzenburg M, McMahon SB. Peripheral administration of nerve growth factor in the adult rat produces a thermal hyperalgesia that requires the presence of sympathetic post-ganglionic neurones. *Pain* 1995; **63**: 109–15.

30   Bennett DL, Koltzenburg M, Priestley JV, Shelton DL, McMahon SB. Endogenous nerve growth factor regulates the sensitivity of nociceptors in the adult rat. *Eur J Neurosci* 1998; **10**: 1282–91.

31   Oddiah D, Anand P, McMahon SB, Rattray M. Rapid increase of NGF, BDNF and NT-3 mRNAs in inflamed bladder. *Neuroreport* 1998; **9**: 1455–8.

32   Dmitrieva N, Shelton D, Rice AS, McMahon SB. The role of nerve growth factor in a model of visceral inflammation. *Neuroscience* 1997; **78**: 449–59.

33   Delafoy L, Raymond F, Doherty AM, Eschalier A, Diop L. Role of nerve growth factor in the trinitrobenzene sulfonic acid-induced colonic hypersensitivity. *Pain* 2003; **105**: 489–97.

34   Barreau F, Ferrier L, Fioramonti J, Bueno L. Neonatal maternal deprivation triggers long term alterations in colonic epithelial barrier and mucosal immunity in rats. *Gut* 2004; **53**: 501–6.

35   Cirulli F, Micera A, Alleva E, Aloe L. Early maternal separation increases NGF expression in the developing rat hippocampus. *Pharmacol Biochem Behav* 1998; **59**: 853–8.

36   Barreau F, Cartier C, Fioramonti J, Bueno L. Neonatal maternal deprivation triggers long term alterations in colonic epithelial barrier and mucosal immunity in rats. *Gut* 2004; **53**(4): 501–6.

37   Lommatzsch M, Braun A, Mannsfeldt A *et al.* Abundant production of brain-derived neurotrophic factor by adult visceral epithelia. Implications for paracrine and target-derived neurotrophic functions. *Am J Pathol* 1999; **155**: 1183–93.

38   Reinshagen M, Rohm H, Steinkamp M *et al.* Protective role of neurotrophins in experimental inflammation of the rat gut. *Gastroenterology* 2000; **119**: 368–76.

39   Reinshagen M, von Boyen G, Adler G, Steinkamp M. Role of neurotrophins in inflammation of the gut. *Curr Opin Investig Drugs* 2002; **3**: 565–8.

40   Corvera CU, Dery O, McConalogue K *et al.* Mast cell tryptase regulates rat colonic myocytes through proteinase-activated receptor 2. *J Clin Invest* 1997; **100**: 1383–93.

41   Corvera CU, Dery O, McConalogue K *et al.* Thrombin and mast cell tryptase regulate guinea-pig myenteric neurons through proteinase-activated receptors-1 and -2. *J Physiol* 1999; **517**: 741–56.

42   Gao C, Liu S, Hu HZ *et al.* Serine proteases excite myenteric neurons through protease-activated receptors in guinea pig small intestine. *Gastroenterology* 2002; **123**: 1554–64.

43   Brookes SJ. Classes of enteric nerve cells in the guinea-pig small intestine. *Anat Rec* 2001; **262**: 58–70.

44   Steinhoff M, Vergnolle N, Young SH *et al.* Agonists of proteinase-activated receptor 2 induce inflammation by a neurogenic mechanism. *Nat Med* 2000; **6**: 151–8.

45   Coelho AM, Vergnolle N, Guiard B, Fioramonti J, Bueno L. Proteinases and proteinase-activated receptor 2: a possible role to promote visceral hyperalgesia in rats. *Gastroenterology* 2002; **122**: 1035–47.

46   Kong W, McConalogue K, Khitin LM *et al.* Luminal trypsin may regulate enterocytes through proteinase-activated receptor 2. *Proc Natl Acad Sci USA* 1997; **94**: 8884–9.

47   Vergnolle N, Macnaughton WK, Al-Ani B, Saifeddine M, Wallace JL, Hollenberg MD. Proteinase-activated receptor 2 (PAR2)-activating peptides: identification of a receptor distinct from PAR2 that regulates intestinal transport. *Proc Natl Acad Sci USA* 1998; **95**: 7766–71.

48   Cenac N, Coelho AM, Nguyen C *et al.* Induction of intestinal inflammation in mouse by activation of proteinase-activated receptor-2. *Am J Pathol* 2002; **161**: 1903–15.

49   Cenac N, Garcia-Villar R, Ferrier L *et al.* Proteinase-activated receptor-2-induced colonic inflammation in mice: possible involvement of afferent neurons, nitric oxide, and paracellular permeability. *J Immunol* 2003; **170**: 4296–300.

50   Fiorucci S, Mencarelli A, Palazzetti B *et al.* Proteinase-activated receptor 2 is an anti-inflammatory signal for colonic lamina propria lymphocytes in a mouse model of colitis. *Proc Natl Acad Sci USA* 2001; **98**: 13936–41.

Index

Please note: page numbers in italic refer to figures and tables